Women's Health

Editor

MELISSA MCNEIL

MEDICAL CLINICS
OF NORTH AMERICA

www.medical.theclinics.com

Consulting Editor
JACK ENDE

March 2023 • Volume 107 • Number 2

ELSEVIER

1600 John F. Kennedy Boulevard • Suite 1800 • Philadelphia, Pennsylvania, 19103-2899

http://www.theclinics.com

MEDICAL CLINICS OF NORTH AMERICA Volume 107, Number 2
March 2023 ISSN 0025-7125, ISBN-13: 978-0-323-93927-0

Editor: Taylor Hayes
Developmental Editor: Diana Grace Ang

Medical Clinics of North America (ISSN 0025-7125) is published bimonthly by Elsevier Inc., 360 Park Avenue South, New York, NY 10010-1710. Months of publication are January, March, May, July, September, and November. Business and editorial offices: 1600 John F. Kennedy Boulevard, Suite 1800, Philadelphia, PA 19103-2899. Periodicals postage paid at New York, NY, and additional mailing offices. Subscription prices are USD $332.00 per year (US individuals), $786.00 per year (US institutions), $100.00 per year (US Students), $416.00 per year (Canadian individuals), $1023.00 per year (Canadian institutions), $200.00 per year for (foreign students), $100.00 per year for (Canadian students), $461.00 per year (foreign individuals), and $1023.00 per year (foreign institutions). To receive student/resident rate, orders must be accompanied by name of affiliated institution, date of term, and the signature of program/residency coordinator on institution letterhead. Orders will be billed at individual rate until proof of status is received. Foreign air speed delivery is included in all Clinics' subscription prices. All prices are subject to change without notice. **POSTMASTER:** Send address changes to *Medical Clinics of North America*, Elsevier Health Sciences Division, Subscription Customer Service, 3251 Riverport Lane, Maryland Heights, MO 63043. **Customer Service: Telephone: 1-800-654-2452** (U.S. and Canada); **1-314-447-8871** (outside U.S. and Canada). **Fax: 314-447-8029. E-mail: journalscustomerserviceusa@elsevier.com** (for print support); **journalsonlinesupport-usa@elsevier.com** (for online support).

Reprints. For copies of 100 or more of articles in this publication, please contact the Commercial Reprints Department, Elsevier Inc., 360 Park Avenue South, New York, NY 10010-1710. Tel.: 212-633-3874; Fax: 212-633-3820; E-mail: reprints@elsevier.com.

Medical Clinics of North America is also published in Spanish by McGraw-Hill Interamericana Editores S. A., P.O. Box 5-237, 06500 Mexico, D.F., Mexico.

Medical Clinics of North America is covered in *MEDLINE/PubMed (Index Medicus), Current Contents, ASCA, Excerpta Medica, Science Citation Index,* and *ISI/BIOMED.*

PROGRAM OBJECTIVE
The goal of the *Medical Clinics of North America* is to keep practicing physicians up to date with current clinical practice by providing timely articles reviewing the state of the art in patient care.

TARGET AUDIENCE
All practicing physicians and other healthcare professionals.

LEARNING OBJECTIVES
Upon completion of this activity, participants will be able to:
1. Review health conditions, diseases, and diagnoses common in women.
2. Explain signs and symptoms of menopause and potential side effects peri and post-menopause that can affect women.
3. Discuss advances in screening, alternative therapy, and treatment options in cancer care for women.

ACCREDITATION
The Elsevier Office of Continuing Medical Education (EOCME) is accredited by the Accreditation Council for Continuing Medical Education (ACCME) to provide continuing medical education for physicians.

The EOCME designates this journal-based CME activity for a maximum of 14 *AMA PRA Category 1 Credit*(s)™. Physicians should claim only the credit commensurate with the extent of their participation in the activity.

All other healthcare professionals requesting continuing education credit for this enduring material will be issued a certificate of participation.

DISCLOSURE OF CONFLICTS OF INTEREST
The EOCME assesses conflict of interest with its instructors, faculty, planners, and other individuals who are in a position to control the content of CME activities. All relevant conflicts of interest that are identified are thoroughly vetted by EOCME for fair balance, scientific objectivity, and patient care recommendations. EOCME is committed to providing its learners with CME activities that promote improvements or quality in healthcare and not a specific proprietary business or a commercial interest.

The planning committee, staff, authors, and editors listed below have identified no financial relationships or relationships to products or devices they or their spouse/life partner have with commercial interest related to the content of this CME activity:
Hannah Abumusa, MD; Deidra Beshear, MD; Rachel A. Bonnema, MD, MS; Andrea E. Carter, MD, MS; Rosemarie L. Conigliaro, MD; Shanice Cox, MS, BS; Deborah DiNardo, MD, MS; Kristen L. Eckstrand, MD, PhD; Jack Ende, MD; Morgan Faeder, MD, PhD; Amy H. Farkas, MD, MS; Katherine Gavinski, MD, MPH; Stefanie Gerstberger, MD, PhD; Deborah Gomez Kwolek, MD, FACP; Vidya Gopinath, MD; Rebecca Green, MD, MS; Sarah Jones, MD, MS; Lynette Jones, MSN, RN-BC; Agnes Koczo, MD; Jillian Kyle, MD; Elena Lebduska, MD, MS; Melissa McNeil, MD, MPH, MACP; Sarah Merriam, MD, MS; Elena Michaels, MD; Ryan Nasseri, MD; Rebeca Ortiz Worthington, MD, MS; Merlin Packiam; Jeanna M. Qiu, AB; Brianna Rossiter, MD, MS; Rachel S. Rubin, MD; Jennifer Rusiecki, MD, MS; Yahir Santiago-Lastra, MD Sneha Shrivastava, MD, MSEd; Swati Shroff, MD, MS; Brielle M. Spataro, MD, MS; Sarah Tait, MD; Sarah Tilstra, MD, MS; Eloho Ufomata, MD, MS.

UNAPPROVED/OFF-LABEL USE DISCLOSURE
The EOCME requires CME faculty to disclose to the participants;
1. When products or procedures being discussed are off-label, unlabelled, experimental, and/or investigational (not US Food and Drug Administration [FDA] approved); and
2. Any limitations on the information presented, such as data that are preliminary or that represent ongoing research, interim analyses, and/or unsupported opinions. Faculty may discuss information about pharmaceutical agents that is outside of FDA-approved labelling. This information is intended solely for CME and is not intended to promote off-label use of these medications. If you have any questions, contact the medical affairs department of the manufacturer for the most recent prescribing information.

TO ENROLL
To enroll in the *Medical Clinics of North America* Continuing Medical Education program, call customer service at 1-800-654-2452 or sign up online at http://www.theclinics.com/home/cme. The CME program is available to subscribers for an additional annual fee of USD 324.00.

METHOD OF PARTICIPATION

In order to claim credit, participants must complete the following;

1. Complete enrolment as indicated above.
2. Read the activity.
3. Complete the CME Test and Evaluation. Participants must achieve a score of 70% on the test. All CME Tests and Evaluations must be completed online.

CME INQUIRIES/SPECIAL NEEDS

For all CME inquiries or special needs, please contact elsevierCME@elsevier.com.

MEDICAL CLINICS OF NORTH AMERICA

Contributors

CONSULTING EDITOR

JACK ENDE, MD, MACP
The Schaeffer Professor of Medicine, Perelman School of Medicine, University of Pennsylvania, Philadelphia, Pennsylvania

EDITOR

MELISSA MCNEIL, MD, MPH, MACP
Professor of Medicine, Clinical Educator, The Warren Alpert School of Medicine of Brown University, Rhode Island Hospital, Senior Women's Health Consultant, Women's Health, VHA Central Office, Narragansett, Rhode Island

AUTHORS

HANNAH ABUMUSA, MD
Division of General Internal Medicine, University of Pittsburgh School of Medicine, UPMC VAPT, VA Pittsburgh Healthcare System, Pittsburgh, Pennsylvania

DEIDRA BESHEAR, MD
University of Kentucky, Lexington, Kentucky

RACHEL A. BONNEMA, MD, MS
Associate Professor, Internal Medicine, The University of Texas Southwestern Medical Center, Dallas, Texas

ANDREA E. CARTER, MD, MS
Assistant Professor of Medicine, Division of General Internal Medicine, Department of Medicine, University of Pittsburgh School of Medicine, Pittsburgh, Pennsylvania

ROSEMARIE L. CONIGLIARO, MD
Section Chief, Women's Health, Division of General Internal Medicine, Director, Katz Institute for Women's Health, Internal Medicine, Professor of Medicine, Donald and Barbara Zucker School of Medicine at Hofstra/Northwell, Lake Success, New York

SHANICE COX, MS, BS
Texas Christian University School of Medicine

DEBORAH DINARDO, MD, MS
Clinical Assistant Professor, VA Pittsburgh Healthcare System, University of Pittsburgh School of Medicine, Pittsburgh, Pennsylvania

KRISTEN L. ECKSTRAND, MD, PhD
Assistant Professor, Department of Psychiatry, University of Pittsburgh School of Medicine, Pittsburgh, Pennsylvania

MORGAN FAEDER, MD, PhD
Assistant Professor of Psychiatry and Neurology, University of Pittsburgh School of Medicine, UPMC Psychiatry CL, Pittsburgh, Pennsylvania

AMY H. FARKAS, MD, MS
Assistant Professor of Medicine, Division of General Internal Medicine, Medical College of Wisconsin, Milwaukee VA Medical Center, Milwaukee, Wisconsin

KATHERINE GAVINSKI, MD, MPH
Academic Clinician-Educator Scholars Fellow, University of Pittsburgh Medical Center, Pittsburgh, Pennsylvania

STEFANIE GERSTBERGER, MD, PhD
Department of Medicine, Massachusetts General Hospital, Boston, Massachusetts; Memorial Sloan Kettering Cancer Center, New York, New York

DEBORAH GOMEZ KWOLEK, MD, FACP
Lead, Women's Health and Sex and Gender Medicine Program, Department of Medicine, Massachusetts General Hospital, Assistant Professor of Medicine, Harvard Medical School, Boston, Massachusetts

VIDYA GOPINATH, MD
Assistant Professor of Medicine, Director of the Women's Health Track, The Warren Alpert Medical School of Brown University, Internal Medicine Residency Programs, Rhode Island Hospital, Providence, Rhode Island

REBECCA GREEN, MD, MS
Assistant Professor, Department of Medicine, University of Pittsburgh School of Medicine, UPMC General Internal Medicine Clinic, Pittsburgh, Pennsylvania

SARAH JONES, MD, MS
Assistant Professor of Medicine, Division of General Internal Medicine, University of Pittsburgh Medical Center, Pittsburgh, Pennsylvania

AGNES KOCZO, MD
T32 Postdoctoral Research Scholar, Clinical Instructor of Medicine, Division of Cardiology, University of Pittsburgh Medical Center, Pittsburgh, Pennsylvania

JILLIAN KYLE, MD, MS
Assistant Professor of Medicine, Division of General Internal Medicine, University of Pittsburgh, Pittsburgh, Pennsylvania

ELENA LEBDUSKA, MD, MS
University of Colorado, UC Heath Internal Medicine, Denver, Colorado

MELISSA MCNEIL, MD, MPH, MACP
Professor of Medicine, Clinical Educator, The Warren Alpert School of Medicine of Brown University, Rhode Island Hospital, Senior Women's Health Consultant, Women's Health, VHA Central Office, Narragansett, Rhode Island

SARAH MERRIAM, MD, MS
Clinical Assistant Professor of Medicine, Division of General Internal Medicine, Department of Medicine, University of Pittsburgh School of Medicine, Veterans Affairs Pittsburgh Healthcare System, Pittsburgh, Pennsylvania

ELENA MICHAELS, MD
Department of Medicine, University of Chicago, Chicago, Illinois

RYAN NASSERI, MD
UC San Diego Health, San Diego, California

JEANNA M. QIU, AB
Department of Medicine, Massachusetts General Hospital, Harvard Medical School, Boston, Massachusetts

BRIANNA ROSSITER, MD, MS
Division of General Internal Medicine, University of Pittsburgh School of Medicine, UPMC VAPT, VA Pittsburgh Healthcare System, Pittsburgh, Pennsylvania

RACHEL S. RUBIN, MD
Georgetown University, Washington, DC

JENNIFER RUSIECKI, MD, MS
Assistant Professor of Medicine, Department of Medicine, University of Chicago, Chicago, Illinois

YAHIR SANTIAGO-LASTRA, MD
UC San Diego Health, San Diego, California

SNEHA SHRIVASTAVA, MD, MSEd
Director, Women's Health Education, Division of General Internal Medicine, Northwell Health, Assistant Professor of Medicine, Donald and Barbara Zucker School of Medicine at Hofstra/Northwell, Glen Oaks, New York

SWATI SHROFF, MD, MS, FACP
Clinical Associate Professor of Medicine, Internal Medicine, Thomas Jefferson University, Jefferson Women's Primary Care, Philadelphia, Pennsylvania

BRIELLE M. SPATARO, MD, MS
University of Pittsburgh, Pittsburgh, Pennsylvania

SARAH TAIT, MD
Department of Medicine, Massachusetts General Hospital, Boston, Massachusetts

SARAH TILSTRA, MD, MS
Associate Professor, Department of Medicine, University of Pittsburgh School of Medicine, UPMC General Internal Medicine Clinic, Pittsburgh, Pennsylvania

ELOHO UFOMATA, MD, MS
Associate Professor, Department of Medicine, University of Pittsburgh School of Medicine, UPMC General Internal Medicine Clinic, Pittsburgh, Pennsylvania

REBECA ORTIZ WORTHINGTON, MD, MS
Assistant Professor of Medicine, Department of Medicine, University of Pittsburgh, Pittsburgh, Pennsylvania

Contents

Menopause, which is defined as the point in time 12 months after a woman's final menstrual period, is marked by a decrease in estrogen and accompanying symptoms including vasomotor and genitourinary symptoms. Hormone therapy is the most effective treatment of vasomotor symptoms and is first-line in women with moderate-to-severe vasomotor symptoms who are early in the menopausal transition and do not have a contraindication. Nonhormonal pharmacologic and nonpharmacologic treatments are also available for the treatment of menopause-related symptoms for women who prefer to avoid hormones or who have a contraindication to hormone therapy.

Osteoporosis is the most common bone disease in adults and confers significant morbidity and mortality in women. Universal screening is recommended for women above the age of 65 years; however, screening rates remain low. Bisphosphonates are the treatment of choice despite a decline in their use due to concerns about rare side effects. Treatment of osteoporosis dramatically decreases the likelihood of fragility fractures.

Polycystic ovarian syndrome (PCOS) is a complex, familial, polygenetic metabolic condition. The Rotterdam criteria are commonly used to diagnose PCOS. Lifestyle changes are the first-line treatment of PCOS. Treatment options for menstrual irregularities and hirsutism are based on the clinical goals and preferences of the patient. Along with treating the symptoms of PCOS, it is essential to screen and treat the comorbid conditions commonly associated with PCOS, including type 2 diabetes mellitus, obesity, nonalcoholic fatty liver disease, hyperlipidemia, obstructive sleep apnea, anxiety, depression, infertility, and vitamin D deficiency.

Abnormal uterine bleeding is a common problem in premenopausal women and refers to uterine bleeding that is abnormal in frequency, duration, volume, and/or regularity. Etiologies can be classified using the PALM-COIEN system. Patients should receive a comprehensive history and physical with special attention to menstrual, sexual, and family history. Physical examination needs to include a pelvic examination with speculum and bimanual components. All patients need to have a pregnancy test and CBC with platelets. Treatments vary by etiology. Medical treatments include levonorgestrel intrauterine devices, oral contraceptive pills, and tranexamic acid. Surgical treatment options include endometrial ablation and hysterectomy.

This article outlines the basics of all contraceptive options available in the United States, providing providers necessary information to best provide equitable contraceptive care for women. Long-acting reversible contraception should be considered in all women as there are few contraindications to use. Levonorgestrel intrauterine devices have been found to be safe for use for longer periods of time, in some cases up to eight years. Combination hormone contraceptives remain popular and offer benefits beyond contraception; importantly newer formulations exist providing patients with more contraceptive options. Education regarding emergency contraception should be provided to all patients.

Cervical cancer screening is an essential component of preventative health care. Although rates of cervical cancer have decreased over the last 50 years, survival has not changed dramatically, and there are significant discrepancies in disease detection by race. Multiple national organizations contribute to the recommendations for cervical cancer screening timing, testing modalities, and management. This article aims to summarize the current understanding of cervical cancer pathogenesis, options for cervical cancer screening, and the shift in guidelines toward risk-based clinical management.

This review provides an outline of a risk-based approach to breast cancer screening and prevention. All women should be assessed for breast cancer risk starting at age 18 with identification of modifiable and non-modifiable risk factors. Patients can then be stratified into average, moderate, and high-risk groups with personalized screening and prevention plans. Counseling on breast awareness and lifestyle changes is recommended for all women, regardless of risk category. High-risk individuals may benefit from additional screening modalities such as MRI and chemoprevention and should be managed closely by a multidisciplinary team.

Cardiovascular disease (CVD) is the leading cause of death for American women. CVD is preventable although risk reduction goals are not achieved for women compared with men. Considering a woman's cardiometabolic profile for prevention counseling and prescribing may help. Coronary artery calcium scores provide additional risk assessment and reproductive and menopause histories identify risk enhancers. Diagnosis of CVD is often delayed, and treatment is less optimal for women compared with men. Differences in presentation and underlying CVD etiology (Including spontaneous coronary artery dissection and microvascular disease) may partially account for these disparities. Improvements in CVD imaging to better diagnose these etiologies may benefit women's care.

deaths annually. Routine screening protocols do not detect these malignancies; thus, the recognition of risk factors and evaluation of worrisome symptoms are essential for early detection and improved prognoses. Treatment is managed by gynecologic oncologists, and often involves a combination of surgery, chemotherapy, and possible radiation treatments. Survivor care is managed by the primary-care clinician: expert attention to the mental, physical, and sexual health of each patient will ensure the best outcomes and quality of life.

Introduced in 2014, genitourinary syndrome of menopause (GSM) describes a variety of unpleasant genital, sexual and urinary symptoms that can either be isolated or coexisting and are not related to other medical conditions. GSM is a chronic and progressive condition that requires early recognition and appropriate management to preserve urogenital health. Despite the importance of early detection and treatment, the condition is consistently underdiagnosed and undertreated. Herein, we emphasize how to diagnose GSM in postmenopausal, hypoestrogenic, and hypoandrogenic women and summarize evidence-based treatments focusing on prescription treatments and adjunctive therapies.

Gender identity is a deeply felt internal sense of self, which may correspond (cisgender) or not correspond (transgender) with the person's assigned sex at birth. Transgender, nonbinary, and gender diverse people may choose to affirm their gender in any number of ways including medical gender affirmation. This is a primer on the medical care of transgender individuals which covers an introduction to understanding a common language, history of transgender medical care, creating a welcoming environment, hormone therapy, surgical therapies, fertility considerations, and cancer screening in transgender people.

IPV is a widespread and destructive public health problem that impacts women across the world and the lifespan. IPV encompasses a wide range of negative behaviors towards a person's romantic partner which include physical aggression, sexual violence, stalking, psychological torment, and coercive behaviors. Persons who experience IPV face a wide range of debilitating physical, mental health, and financial outcomes compared to those who have never experienced violence. Physicians play an important role in caring for patients who have experienced violence; knowledge of IPV's impact, consequences, treatment, and patient preferences around IPV discussions can lead to improved patient satisfaction and outcomes.

Foreword

Equity, Diversity, and Inclusion— and Women's Health

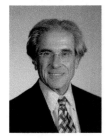

Jack Ende, MD, MACP
Consulting Editor

Like all professions, medicine is defined by its values. The values of medicine include many that are time-honored and central to our profession for as long as medicine has been accorded the status of being more than a trade or enterprise, but a profession. These values include altruism, or putting the interests of patients first; practicing within evidence-based guidelines and to the best of one's abilities; doing no harm, of course; being honest and truthful and avoiding conflicts of interests; treating colleagues with respect; trying always to improve the quality of care, and one's knowledge and skills; and just distribution of resources. There are others, of course, but this list, I believe, captures the traditional values of our profession.

But these are not traditional times. We live in a world, or at least in a country, that has come to appreciate other values that are no less important for, and germane to, medical practice as those listed above. I refer here to the values of equity, diversity, and inclusion. I was reminded of these values as I worked through the table of contents of this comprehensive review of Women's Health that comprises the March 2023 issue of *Medical Clinics of North America*, along with the insightful, on-target Preface by our guest editor, Dr Melissa McNeil.

Equity can be defined as the creation of opportunities for historically underrepresented populations. While the concept fits well in the domain of medical education and administrative leadership, and we all can be proud of the gains made in gender equity in medical school admissions and, to a lesser extent, but still emerging, in medical center leadership, so too does the concept of equity as a professional value pertains to medical practice and development of clinical guidelines. The article on Affirming Care of Transgender Patients exemplifies equity in medical practice.

Diversity refers to the multitude of identity factors that define who we are and what we believe in. These factors include race, age, sexual orientation, and, of

Med Clin N Am 107 (2023) xv–xvi
https://doi.org/10.1016/j.mcna.2022.11.001
0025-7125/23/© 2022 Published by Elsevier Inc.

course, gender. Just as we should strive to make our institutions more representative of who we are as a city, state, or nation, so too we should strive to make certain that our corpus of medical knowledge and systems of care address the needs of diverse populations. Women have been left out for too long in clinical trials, and the differences between men and women in terms of clinical presentations and outcomes have not received the attention they deserve. The article on Cardiovascular Disease Prevention, Diagnosis, and Treatment in Women addresses this straight on.

Finally, inclusion, which overlaps with equity and diversity, reminds us that systems of care should be allocated to all groups, women included, of course. That is why I am so proud of this entire remarkable issue. Its inclusion as a full issue of *Medical Clinics of North America* is a statement not just of the uniqueness of women's health but also of its importance.

I hope you find this issue clinically useful and, indeed, inspirational.

Jack Ende, MD, MACP
Perelman School of Medicine of the University of Pennsylvania
Philadelphia, PA 19104, USA

E-mail address:
jack.ende@pennmedicine.upenn.edu

Preface

Not a 70-Kilogram Man

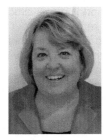

Melissa McNeil, MD, MPH, MACP
Editor

The explosion of information about gender-specific conditions in the last two decades highlights the need for providers with an interest and knowledge about conditions unique to women (eg, menopause), more common in women (eg, osteoporosis), or which present differently in women (eg, cardiovascular disease). One has only to look at the changing views regarding hormone therapy (HT) to understand the need for up-to-date practitioners. In 1995, HT was thought to be beneficial for both primary and secondary cardiac prevention, to be effective in reducing osteoporotic fractures, and to pose no increased risk for breast cancer or thromboembolic events. Beginning with the early release of the Women's Health Initiative results in 2001, these views have radically changed. We now would not use HT for either primary or secondary prevention of cardiac disease, and we appreciate increased risks of both breast cancer and thrombosis. The only "medical certainty" still standing is the belief that HT reduces osteoporotic fractures. However, the advent of new therapies, such as bisphosphonates and selective estrogen receptor modulators, has made even osteoporosis prevention a dubious indication for HT as a first-line treatment for osteoporosis.

A knowledge of the differences in disease presentation and treatment in women is crucial to any provider with a desire to provide comprehensive, evidence-based care for women. This issue of the *Medical Clinics of North America* focusing on Women's Health seeks to highlight those conditions that have gendered differences in diagnosis and treatment, including conditions wherein biologic sex and gender preference are different. For many years, women have either received fragmented care with "gendered conditions" being managed only by our gynecologist colleagues and with little appreciation of how these conditions impact the overall health of women. It is very hard to imagine, for example, how a primary provider of women could manage breast health, bone health, and heart health without understanding the impact of menopause and reproductive hormones on all of these conditions. There are new data that suggest that a woman's reproductive history impacts her subsequent risk

Med Clin N Am 107 (2023) xvii–xviii
https://doi.org/10.1016/j.mcna.2022.10.015
0025-7125/23/© 2023 Published by Elsevier Inc.

of cardiovascular disease. Preeclampsia, gestational hypertension, and gestational diabetes (just to name a few) all are risk factors for early cardiovascular disease in women and should be factored into risk assessment by providers. Increasingly, with cervical cancer screening becoming less frequent, women see gynecologists with less regularity, and thus, primary providers need to be aware of signs of symptoms of gynecologic malignancies, such as postmenopausal bleeding and abdominal bloating. A thorough understanding of all of these conditions and more is crucial to providing exceptional gender-specific care to the women we serve.

It is my hope that this issue of the *Medical Clinics of North America* will highlight these important gender-specific conditions, their diagnosis, and their treatment. The goal is to provide a roadmap to comprehensive care for women with specific recommendations and management strategies provided so that a provider, after reading this issue, will have the knowledge and skills necessary to view women as unique, complex, and endlessly interesting patients! The fragmentation of care for women has not served our patients well, and this is one attempt to end the "patchwork quilt" of care that women have so often experienced and to empower us as providers to see our women patients as more than just 70-kilogram men!

Melissa McNeil, MD, MPH, MACP
Warren Alpert School of Medicine of Brown University
Rhode Island Hospital
Women's Health, VHA Central Office
593 Eddy Street, Suite JB0105
Providence, RI 02903, USA

E-mail address:
mmcneil4@lifespan.org

Menopause

Andrea E. Carter, MD, MS[a], Sarah Merriam, MD, MS[b,*]

KEYWORDS

- Menopause • Vasomotor symptoms • Genitourinary syndrome of menopause
- Hormone therapy

KEY POINTS

- Menopause, which is defined as the point in time 12 months after a woman's final menstrual period, is marked by a decrease in estrogen and accompanying symptoms including vasomotor and genitourinary symptoms.
- Hormone therapy is the most effective treatment of vasomotor symptoms and is first-line in women with moderate-to-severe vasomotor symptoms who are early in the menopausal transition and do not have a contraindication.
- Nonhormonal pharmacologic and nonpharmacologic treatments are also available for the treatment of menopause-related symptoms for women who prefer to avoid hormones or who have a contraindication to hormone therapy.

BACKGROUND
Definition of Menopause

Menopause is defined as the point in time 12 months after a women's last menstrual period. Menopause reflects the loss of ovarian follicular function with resulting decreased estrogen concentration and increased follicle-stimulating hormone (FSH) concentration. Natural menopause occurs at median age of 51.[1] The period before menopause where women begin to experience changes in menstrual bleeding patterns and hormonal fluctuations is referred to as the menopausal transition, or perimenopause, and begins at a median age of 47 years.

Induced menopause refers to the cessation of mensuration after bilateral oophorectomy or other iatrogenic reason for ending ovarian function, such as chemotherapy or pelvic radiation. Premature menopause refers to menopause that occurs before age 40, generally from primary ovarian insufficiency. Primary ovarian insufficiency is associated with a variety of genetic conditions, autoimmune diseases, and medications and toxins.

[a] Division of General Internal Medicine, Department of Medicine, University of Pittsburgh School of Medicine, 200 Lothrop Street, MUH W923, Pittsburgh, PA 15213, USA; [b] Division of General Internal Medicine, Department of Medicine, University of Pittsburgh School of Medicine and Veterans Affairs Pittsburgh Healthcare System, University Drive C, Pittsburgh, PA 15240, USA
* Corresponding author.
E-mail address: sullivansb@upmc.edu

Med Clin N Am 107 (2023) 199–212
https://doi.org/10.1016/j.mcna.2022.10.003
0025-7125/23/© 2022 Elsevier Inc. All rights reserved.

Menopause and menopause-related symptoms can be experienced by all people born with a uterus and ovaries including cisgender women, transgender men, gender nonbinary people, and other people across the spectrum of gender diversity. We will use the term woman for the remainder of this article but we acknowledge that this term does not encapsulate the full spectrum of people who experience menopause.

Stages of Menopause

The Stages of Reproductive Aging Workshop (STRAW) staging system lays out system to characterize reproductive aging from the reproductive years through menopause.[2] STRAW divides the adult female life into 3 broad phases: reproductive, the menopausal transition, and postmenopause. The 3 phases are subdivided into 7 total stages centered on the final menstrual period (FMP) which is Stage 0. The early menopausal transition (Stage −2) is marked by the beginning of menstrual cycle irregularity, with persistent differences of over 7 days between consecutive cycles. The late menopausal transition (Stage −1) is marked by intervals of at least 60 days of amenorrhea between cycles.

Diagnosis of Menopause

In women aged older than 45 years, a diagnosis of the menopausal transition can be made if there is menstrual cycle irregularity with or without symptoms of menopause. Laboratory evaluation is not necessary.

In women aged younger than 45 years, other causes of menstrual cycle irregularity, such as pregnancy, hyperprolactinemia, and thyroid hormone abnormalities, should be ruled out first. In women with underlying menstrual cycle disorders, such as polycystic ovarian syndrome, the diagnosis of menopause can be more difficult and measuring FSH is helpful. An FSH level of greater than 25 IU/L indicates that the patient has likely entered the menopausal transition. Women taking combined oral contraceptives often do not develop irregular bleeding or menopause symptoms and may want reassurance that they are postmenopausal before stopping their medication. However, FSH measurement can be unreliable in these women because the hypothalamic-pituitary axis is suppressed by exogenous estrogen, so we suggest measuring the FSH level at least 2 to 4 weeks after stopping the contraceptive pill.

Clinical Manifestations of Menopause

The hallmark symptoms of the menopausal transition and early postmenopausal years are vasomotor symptoms (VMS), including hot flashes and night sweats. Women may experience several other symptoms including genitourinary symptoms, depression, and sleep disturbances. In the postmenopausal period, there is increased bone loss and an increased risk for cardiovascular disease (CVD).

Vasomotor symptoms

VMS, including hot flashes and night sweats, are the most common symptoms during the menopausal transition and postmenopause. A hot flash is a sudden sensation of heat that lasts for a few minutes and is often associated with perspiration and sometimes feelings of anxiety. The frequency can range from an average of 1 per day to 1 per hour. VMS occur in up to 80% of women, with frequency of 40% in the early menopausal transition increasing up to 6% to 80% in the late menopausal transition and early postmenopause.[3] The median duration of VMS is 7.4 years with symptoms persisting 4.5 years after the FMP. Women who experience VMS early in the menopausal transition have significantly longer total symptom duration.

Genitourinary symptoms

The genitourinary syndrome of menopause (GSM) is a collection of symptoms caused by changes to labia, vagina, clitoris, urethra, and bladder that happen due to decline in estrogen and subsequent decrease in blood flow. Symptoms can include vulvovaginal dryness, dyspareunia, vulvar or vaginal bleeding, vulvovaginal burning, irritation, or itching, vaginal discharge. About 50% to 70% of women in postmenopause are symptomatic with GSM at least to some degree.[4] GSM develops later in menopausal transition than VMS and usually progressively worsens with longer duration of hypoestrogenism.

Other symptoms

The menopausal transition is associated with new onset of depressed mood even in women with no history of depression,[5] sleep disturbances,[6] subjective cognitive problems,[7] bone loss,[8] and increased risk of CVD.

DISCUSSION
Hormone Therapy Treatment of Vasomotor Symptoms

Hormone therapy (HT) is the most effective for the treatment of menopausal symptoms, with a 70% improvement in frequency and severity of VMS within a few weeks of treatment initiation.[9] The goal of HT is to replace the hormones that a woman's body stops producing during the menopause.

HT comprises estrogen, the "active ingredient," and *in women with an intact uterus*, progesterone is added for protection against endometrial hyperplasia and cancer.[10] This will be referred to as combination HT in this article. For women without a uterus, progesterone is not required. This will be referred to as estrogen-only HT in this article. This is an important clinical distinction because the risks conferred by HT differ based on the presence of progesterone, as will be discussed below.

Hormone therapy indications

HT treats both vasomotor and vaginal symptoms of menopause. HT should be considered as first line in all women with moderate-to-severe VMS that are affecting quality of life who do not have a contraindication. For women with milder VMS or women with a contraindication to HT, nonhormonal pharmacologic treatments or nonpharmacologic treatments for VMS may be considered. These options are discussed in detail in the next section. For women with only genitourinary symptoms of menopause, nonhormonal treatments or local vaginal estrogen therapy is more appropriate initial treatment, as will be discussed below.

Absolute contraindications to HT include pregnancy, either a history of CVD (defined as coronary artery disease or stroke) or active CVD, history of venous thromboembolism (VTE), unexplained vaginal bleeding, acute or decompensated liver disease, history of breast or endometrial cancer, prolonged immobilization, and hypertriglyceridemia (**Box 1**). Relative contraindications to HT include increased risk of breast cancer based on personal characteristics or family history, increased risk of CVD, migraine with aura, and active gallbladder disease.

Hormone therapy risks and benefits. The safety of HT has been the subject of discussion for decades. The Women's Health Initiative (WHI) study was a randomized, prospective, double-blind trial of approximately 27,000 women aged 50 to 79 years of age designed to examine the balance of risk and benefits of postmenopausal HT in healthy women.[11] There were 2 study arms: participants with a uterus were randomized to the use of conjugated equine estrogens (CEEs) with medroxyprogesterone acetate (MPA; "combined HT") or placebo, participants without a uterus were randomized to CEE

Box 1
Contraindications to hormone therapy

Absolute Contraindications
  Pregnancy
  History of cardiovascular disease (coronary artery disease or stroke)
  Acute cardiovascular disease
  History of venous thromboembolism
  Unexplained vaginal bleeding
  Acute or decompensated liver disease
  History of breast cancer
  History of endometrial cancer
  Prolonged immobilization
  Hypertriglyceridemia

Relative Contraindications
  Increased risk of breast cancer
  Increased risk for cardiovascular disease
  Migraine with aura
  Active gallbladder disease

(estrogen-only HT) or placebo. The trial was terminated early due to safety concerns when preliminary results indicated an increased risk of CVD, stroke, VTE and breast cancer among women who used hormones compared with placebo. It is notable that the average age of entry into this study was 63 years, more than a decade after average onset of menopause, and a large proportion of women in both treatment and placebo arms had prior exposure to HT before enrolling in the trial.

Subsequent reanalyses of WHI data have examined the timing of the initiation of HT because it relates to age and onset of menopause on these risks. From these studies has emerged consensus around a "timing hypothesis," in which HT in healthy, younger, and recently menopausal women is safe carries a favorable benefit–risk ratio.[12] More specifically, HT is considered to be safest in women who are within 10 years of menopause onset or younger than 60 years of age.[13] Risk of HT also depends on the type (combination vs estrogen-alone), dose, duration, and route of administration.

Mortality
Importantly, long-term data follow-up from the WHI does not demonstrate any difference in mortality (all-cause, breast cancer, or coronary heart disease [CHD]) between HT users and nonusers.[14,15]

Cardiovascular, stroke, and venous thromboembolism risk
Age and time of the initiation of HT strongly influence the impact of HT on CHD, stroke, and VTE. Women who initiate HT within 10 years of menopause onset carry no increased risk for CHD.[12,14,16] For women who initiate HT more than a decade after menopause do carry an increased risk for CHD but not mortality.[12] Similarly, the risk of stroke and VTE are highest in women treated with HT who are more than a decade from the onset of menopause.

There is no evidence of increased risk of stroke with topical vaginal estrogen therapy for genitourinary symptoms. Transdermal estrogen formulations carry a lower risk of stroke and VTE than do oral formulations, although this has not been demonstrated for CHD risk.[17]

Breast cancer risk
The risk of breast cancer depends on the type and duration of HT. Women without a uterus receiving estrogen-only HT *do not* carry a clinically significant increased risk of

breast cancer. Women with an intact uterus receiving combined HT do carry an increased risk for invasive breast cancer, which increases with duration of therapy but carry *no difference* in breast cancer deaths.[15] Data from the WHI indicate an attributable risk of breast cancer of approximately 1 additional case per 1000 users of combination HT over 1 year. This risk is similar to that associated with drinking 2 alcoholic beverages per day, obesity, and low activity.[18,19]

A recent meta-analysis demonstrated a relative risk for breast cancer among women using combination HT 5 years from age 50 of 1.60 (95% CI 1.52–1.69). This confers an absolute risk increase of 1 in 50 treated with daily progesterone and 1 in 70 with cyclic progesterone use and approximates the risk conferred by having a second-degree relative with breast cancer.[20]

Determining candidacy for hormone therapy

As previously mentioned, HT is the most effective treatment of VMS. In order to determine if HT is appropriate, the following criteria should be met: (1) VMS are moderate-to-severe and affecting quality of life and (2) no contraindications exist (see **Box 1**).[21]

Assuming these are the case, it is important to next complete a cardiovascular risk assessment (in all women) and breast cancer risk assessment (only in women with a uterus who would be receiving combined HT).

- If the woman is aged 60 years or younger and within a decade of menopause onset and at low risk of CVD and breast cancer (if she has a uterus), HT should be recommended.
- If she is distant from menopause onset, aged older than 60 years, or at moderate risk for breast or CVD, shared decision-making is warranted.
- If she is at high baseline risk for breast cancer (and has a uterus) or CVD or at moderate risk and distant from the onset of menopause, it is likely that the risks of HT outweigh benefits and other modalities for treatment should be pursued.

Prescribing hormone therapy

Approach to prescribing. Once the decision has been made to prescribe HT for the treatment of menopausal symptoms, the following questions need to be answered:

- Is progestin needed?
- What route should estrogen be delivered?
- What type and dose of estrogen?
- What is the most appropriate progestin regimen?

Determining if a progestin is needed. The first consideration in prescribing HT is to ascertain if endometrial protection is warranted. Women with an intact uterus should be prescribed a progestin along with an estrogen (combination HT) in order to mitigate the proliferative effect of estrogen on the endometrium, which can increase the risk of endometrial hyperplasia, atypia, and ultimately cancer. Women who do not have a uterus do not require prescription and should be prescribed only an estrogen.[9]

Choosing an estrogen. Estrogen treats vaginal and VMS of menopause. Estradiol and CEEs are most-studied formulations.

Estrogen can be prescribed in an oral, transdermal, and vaginal formulations (**Table 1**). All preparations are equally effective in treating symptoms of menopause. Oral estrogen has a greater effect on the liver due to first past effect; intestinal absorption leads to portal vein estrogen concentrations that are initially higher than those after the transdermal formulations. Because transdermal estrogen carries a lower risk of VTE and stroke than oral estrogen, it is preferred, considering patient preference.[17]

Table 1
Estrogen, progestin, and combination hormone therapy products

Estrogen Formulations			
Route	**Preparation (Brand)**	**Typical Dosing**	**Clinical**
Oral	Conjugated equine estrogen (Premarin)	0.3–1.25 mg/d	
	Micronized estradiol (Estrace)	0.5–2.0 mg/d	
	Esterified estrogen (Menest)	0.3–1.25 mg/d	
Transdermal	Estradiol patch • Weekly (Climara, Menostar) • Twice-weekly (Vivelle-dot, Minivelle, Alora)	0.025–0.1 mg/d	
	Estradiol gel • Elastrin 0.06%, Elestrin 0.06% • Divigel 0.1%	• 0.52–0.75 mg per pump • 0.25–1 mg per pouch	Apply from wrist to shoulder
	Estradiol spray (Evamist)	1.53 mg/spray	Risk to children and pets
Vaginal	Systemic estradiol ring (Femring)	0.05–0.1 mg/d over 3 mo	For treatment of vasomotor symptoms
	Local estradiol ring (Estring)	7.5 mcg/d	For treatment of genitourinary symptoms
	Estradiol tablet (Vagifem, Yuvafem)	10 mcg/tablet applied 2–3 times per week	For treatment of genitourinary symptoms
	Estradiol cream (Estrace)	0.1 mg/g applied 2–3 times per week	For treatment of genitourinary symptoms
	Conjugated equine estrogen cream (Premarin)	0.625 mg/g applied 2–3 times per week	For treatment of genitourinary symptoms
Progestin Formulations			
Oral	Medroxyprogesterone acetate (Provera)	Cyclic: 5–10 mg daily × 12 d Continuous: 1.25–2.5 mg daily	
	Micronized progesterone (Prometrium)	Cyclic: 200 mg daily × 12 d Continuous: 100–200 mg daily	
Intrauterine	Levonorgestrel-releasing (Mirena)		Off-label
Combination Estrogen and Progesterone Formulations			
Oral	Conjugated equine estrogen/ medroxyprogesterone (Prempro)	0.3 mg/1.5 mg, 0.45 mg/ 1.5 mg, 0.625 mg/ 2.5 mg, 0.625 mg/5 mg	Continuous
	Estradiol/norgestimate (Prefest)	1.0 mg/0.09 mg	Cyclic

(*continued on next page*)

Table 1 (*continued*)			
Estrogen Formulations			
Route	**Preparation (Brand)**	**Typical Dosing**	**Clinical**
	Estradiol/norethindrone acetate (Activella, Mimvey)	0.5 mg/0.1 mg, 1.0 mg/ 0.5 mg	Continuous
	Ethinyl estradiol/ norethindrone acetate (Jevantique Lo, Jinteli)	2.5 mcg/0.5 mg, 5 mcg/ 1 mg	Continuous
	Estradiol/drospirenone (Angeliq)	0.5 mg/0.25 mg, 1 mg/ 0.5 mg	Continuous
Transdermal	Estradiol/norethindrone patch (CombiPatch)	0.05 mg/0.14 mg, 0.05 mg/ 0.25 mg twice weekly	
	Estradiol/levonorgestrel (Climara pro)	0.045 mg/0.015 mg weekly	

Transdermal patches are applied to the thighs or between the wrist and shoulder, avoiding the breast tissue. Estrogens can also come in micronized or conjugated formulations, which increase absorption.

Guidelines suggest starting with the lowest dose of estrogen (0.625 mg CEE by mouth daily, 50 mcg estradiol patch applied weekly, or vaginal ring 0.05–0.1 mg estradiol per day exchanged monthly) and titrating upward every 4 weeks until the symptoms are relieved.

Prescribing clinicians should also be aware of medication interactions with estrogen therapy. Oral estrogen, but not transdermal, increases thyroid-binding globulin and, as a result, women prescribed levothyroxine may require dose-increases. Similarly, estrogen increases sex hormone-binding globulin, leading to a decrease in free testosterone levels. This may be an important consideration in women being treated for sexual dysfunction and/or low libido, who may prefer transdermal preparations. Anticonvulsants (ie, carbamazepine, phenytoin) increase hepatic metabolism of estrogen and women prescribed these medications may require increased dosages to achieve symptom relief.[22]

Custom compounded bioidentical hormones are no more effective than Food and Drug Administration (FDA) approved preparations and are not quality-controlled. Given a lack of safety data, oversight, and the risk of inconsistent dosing and/or product impurity, these are not recommended in lieu of commercial preparations.[23]

Choosing a progesterone. Progesterone, a necessary component of menopause HT in women with a uterus, also comes in oral and transdermal preparations.

Progestogen can be dosed cyclically or in a continuous regimen. Cyclic regimens result in monthly withdrawal bleeding, which may limit acceptability of this regimen. Commonly prescribed cyclic regimen includes MPA 5 to 10 mg daily or 200 mg micronized progesterone 12 days per month. Continuous regimens eventually lead to amenorrhea in most. Commonly prescribed continuous regimens include MPA 1.25 to 2.5 mg daily or 100 to 200 mg daily. The main drawback to continuous regimens is irregular bleeding soon after therapy is started, which may last for months.

Common side effects of oral progesterone therapy include bloating and mood changes.

Levonorgestrel-containing intrauterine devices (IUDs) can be combined with estrogen formulations to provide endometrial protection but is not FDA-approved for this indication.

Recommended monitoring for patients prescribed hormone therapy

Women newly prescribed HT should be reevaluated within 4 to 6 weeks. If symptom burden is not adequately controlled, the dosage should be augmented. If VMS do not respond to maximum recommended dosing of HT, treatment should be discontinued.

Common side effects include breast tenderness, low-grade nausea, or uterine bleeding early after HT initiation. Any woman reporting a change in bleeding pattern, heavy or persistent bleeding, or spotting (eg, >12 months in a woman who is prescribed combination HT) should be evaluated for structural causes with a pelvic examination and screened for endometrial cancer with transvaginal ultrasonography and/or endometrial biopsy.

Stopping hormone therapy

Because of long-term risks (eg, stroke, VTE, CAD, breast cancer), HT should be prescribed for the shortest possible period and the lowest effective dose.

For women with a uterus who are prescribed combination HT, the risk of breast cancer becomes clinically significant at approximately 5 years on-treatment and increases in a dose-dependent fashion thereafter. Because the risk for breast cancer increases in a dose-dependent fashion thereafter, it is reasonable to trial discontinuing HT after 5 years of use.[13,20] If severe VMS persist, it would be reasonable to trial a nonhormonal treatment (eg, selective serotonin reuptake inhibitor [SSRI]/serotonin norepinephrine reuptake inhibitors [SNRI] or gabapentin) or to engage in shared decision regarding risk and benefits of continued HT treatment.

As a reminder, for women with a hysterectomy who are using estrogen only HT, the risk of breast cancer is lower. In this case, it is rather the risk of stroke and VTE that should drive a shared discussion related to the risks and benefits of ongoing treatment after 10 years of use or at age 60.

If the decision is made to stop HT, existing data do not support increased tolerability of gradual taper as compared with an abrupt discontinuation of therapy.[24] If a taper is preferred, it is reasonable to reduce the dosage of estrogen over weeks to months as tolerated. If VMS persist, nonhormonal pharmacotherapy and/or complementary-alternative medication strategies may be considered.

Nonhormonal Pharmacologic Treatment of Vasomotor Symptoms

Although HT is the most effective treatment of VMS, there is a variety of nonhormonal pharmacologic treatment options for women who are not candidates for HT or who chose not to take it. In this article, we have included all such therapies with level I or level II evidence as graded by the North American Menopause Society (NAMS) where level I evidence is based on high-quality randomized control trials and systematic reviews of level I studies and level II is based on lesser quality RCTs, systematic reviews of level II studies, or level I studies with inconsistent results.[25] The medications used for nonhormonal treatment of VMS are summarized in **Table 2**.

No clear recommendations can be given for efficacy of one nonhormonal prescription therapy over another because there are no high quality head-to-head comparison efficacy trials. The choice of medication should be based on patient preference, comorbid conditions, and side effect profile.

Selective serotonin reuptake inhibitors (SSRIs) and serotonin norepinephrine reuptake inhibitors (SNRIs)

The SSRIs paroxetine, citalopram, and escitalopram and the selective SNRIs venlafaxine and desvenlafaxine have all been shown to reduce VMS in randomized controlled trials and systematic reviews with Level I and II evidence.[25–32] Reduction in hot flashes varies from 25% to 69%. The mechanism of action is not known

Table 2
Nonhormonal pharmacologic therapies for vasomotor symptoms

Medication	Dose	Level of Evidence[a]	Clinical Considerations
Paroxetine salt	7.5 mg daily	I	Single fixed dose Approved by Food and Drug Administration for treatment of vasomotor symptoms May be more expensive than other options
Paroxetine Citalopram Escitalopram Desvenlafaxine Venlafaxine	10–25 mg daily 10–20 mg daily 10–20 mg daily 100–150 mg daily 37.5–150 mg daily	I to II	Start lowest dose and titrate to effect Good choice for women with concurrent anxiety or depression
Gabapentin	900–2400 mg daily in divided doses	I	Start lowest dose and titrate to effect Side effects include drowsiness and dizziness Good choice for women with concurrent sleep disruptions from vasomotor symptoms
Clonidine	Oral: 0.1–1 mg daily in divided doses Transdermal patch: 0.1–0.3 mg/d	II	Start lowest dose and titrate to effect Less effective than other nonhormonal pharmacologic therapies Side effects including hypotension, dizziness, headache, dry mouth, constipation

[a] Level of evidence is as graded by the North American Menopause Society.[25]

although hot flashes have been linked to imbalance in serotonin. The onset of action of the SSRIs and SNRIs is faster than when using these medications for the treatment of mood disorders, usually within 2 weeks. It is recommended to initiate at the lowest dose and titrate to effect.

Paroxetine salt is the only nonhormonal medication that has received FDA approval for the treatment of VMS and is used at a fixed dose of 7.5 mg. However, this formulation may be more expensive and is not covered by many insurers. Paroxetine should be avoided in women taking tamoxifen due to inhibition of CYP2D6, which converts tamoxifen to its active metabolite.

Using SSRIs and SNRIs to treat VMS may be most useful in women with concurrent depression or anxiety where these medications may have additional benefit.

Gabapentin
Gabapentin, an antiepileptic medication, has been shown to reduce VMS in randomized controlled trials at 900 to 2400 mg/d in divided doses with Level I evidence.[33,34] Higher doses of gabapentin can be as effective as HT but the effectiveness of higher doses is limited by increased side effects such as dizziness, drowsiness, and headache.[35] Using gabapentin to treat VMS may be most useful in women with concurrent sleep disturbances or other indications for gabapentin such as diabetic neuropathy or postherpetic neuralgia.

Clonidine

Clonidine, a centrally acting alpha 2 adrenergic antagonist, has been shown to reduce VMS compared with placebo with Level II evidence but is less effective than the SSRIs, SNRIs, and gabapentin.[31,36] Both the oral and transdermal formulations can be used. The use of clonidine may be limited by side effects including hypotension, dizziness, headache, dry mouth, constipation.

Nonpharmacological Treatment of Vasomotor Symptoms

Between 50% and 75% of postmenopausal women use complementary and alternative therapies for the management of menopausal symptoms.[37] The safety and efficacy of most of these therapies are not well established and interpretation of the available data has been difficult given the small size and short duration of many studies. However, given the prevalence of usage, it is important to know how to counsel patient regarding their use. The nonpharmacologic therapies for the treatment of VMS that have level I or II evidence to support their use as graded by NAMS include cognitive behavioral therapy, clinical hypnosis, mindfulness-based stress reduction, stellate ganglion block, weight loss, and soy isoflavones (**Table 3**).

There are many therapies that are commonly used but do not have robust evidence to support their use. These therapies include lifestyle changes such as avoiding triggers, exercise, and yoga, supplements such as black cohosh, flaxseed, and primrose oil, and other therapies such as acupuncture and chiropractic intervention. We suggest recommending against these therapies because they are unlikely to be beneficial in alleviating VMS.

Mind–body techniques: cognitive behavioral therapy, clinical hypnosis, and mindfulness-based stress reduction

Cognitive behavioral therapy,[38,39] clinical hypnosis,[40] and mindfulness-based stress reduction[41] have all some supporting evidence that they reduce VMS severity and/or frequency. All 3 of these mind–body techniques are likely to be risk-free therapies; however, there may be barriers such as availability of credentialed providers, cost, and time commitment.

Stellate ganglion block

Stellate ganglion block, which involves image-guided injection of a local anesthetic into the stellate ganglion in the anterior cervical spine, is commonly used for pain management. There are some small pilot trials with promising results for the treatment of severe VMS but more studies are needed.[42] Adverse events including seizures and bleeding are very rare.

Table 3 Nonpharmacologic therapies for vasomotor symptoms	
Therapy	**Level of Evidence[a]**
Cognitive behavioral therapy	I
Clinical hypnosis	I
Mindfulness-based stress reduction	II
Stellate ganglion block	II
Weight loss	II
Soy isoflavones	II

[a] Level of evidence is as graded by the North American Menopause Society.[25]

Weight loss
Weight loss may help reduce hot flashes, which was shown by a trial in overweight and obese women randomized to a 6-month long intensive behavioral weight loss intervention or a structured health education program.[43]

Soy isoflavones
Isoflavones are a class of phytochemicals that bind to estrogen receptors. Two types of isoflavones, genistein and daidzein, are found in soybeans, chickpeas, and lentils and are the most potent of the isoflavones. A meta-analysis of trials in women receiving soy isoflavones showed a decrease in the frequency of VMS.[44] Soy isoflavones, either through dietary soy or though supplements, may be a reasonable option for women who are interested in trying them as long as there is no history of soy allergy or intolerance.

Treatment of Genitourinary Symptoms

Treatment of GSM is discussed in detail in another article in this series. Briefly, vaginal moisturizers and lubricants are available without a prescription and provide relief for most women with mild GSM symptoms. Low-dose vaginal estrogen, vaginal dehydroepiandrosterone, and systemic HT for women with concurrent VMS are effective treatments for women with moderate or severe GSM symptoms or women who do not respond to moisturizers and lubricants.

SUMMARY

Menopause, defined as the point in time 12 months after a woman's FMP, reflects the loss of ovarian follicular function with resulting decreased estrogen concentration. Menopause occurs at a median age of 51. During the menopausal transition and postmenopause, woman can experience a variety of symptoms including VMS, genitourinary symptoms, and changes in mood, sleep, and cognition. HT is considered first-line for women with moderate-to-severe VMS who are early in the menopausal transition and do not have a contraindication. HT is composed of estrogen, the "active ingredient," and in women with an intact uterus, progesterone is added for protection against endometrial hyperplasia and cancer. Nonhormonal pharmacologic treatments, such as SSRIs, SNRIs and gabapentin, and nonpharmacologic treatments, such as cognitive behavioral therapy and clinical hypnosis, are also available for the treatment of menopause-related symptoms for women who prefer to avoid hormones or who have a contraindication to HT.

CLINICS CARE POINTS

- Menopause, which occurs at a median age of 51, is diagnosed after 12 months of amenorrhea and does not require laboratory evaluation in women older than age 45.

- In women younger than age 45 or who have baseline menstrual cycle abnormalities, a FSH of greater than 25 IU/L is consistent with menopause.

- VMS, including hot flashes and night sweats, occur in 80% of women and persist for a median of 7 years.

- HT, which includes estrogen as the "active ingredient" and progesterone for endometrial protection only in women with an intact uterus, is the most effective treatment of moderate-to-severe VMS.

- HT has the best risk/benefit ratio in women who are early in the menopausal transition and have low risks for CHD and breast cancer.
- As a result of long-term risks of HT (eg, stroke, VTE, CAD, breast cancer), it should be prescribed for the shortest possible period and the lowest effective dose.
- Nonhormonal pharmacologic treatments, such as SSRIs, SNRIs and gabapentin, and nonpharmacologic treatments, such as cognitive behavioral therapy and clinical hypnosis, are available for the treatment of menopause-related symptoms for women who prefer to avoid hormones or who have a contraindication to HT.
- Clinicians should consider their patients' individual risks and personal preferences when recommending hormonal or nonhormonal treatment of menopause-related symptoms.

DISCLOSURE

The authors have no commercial or financial conflicts of interest.

REFERENCES

1. McKinlay SM, Brambilla DJ, Posner JG. The normal menopause transition. Maturitas 1992;14(2):103–15.
2. Harlow SD, Gass M, Hall JE, et al. Executive summary of the Stages of Reproductive Aging Workshop + 10: addressing the unfinished agenda of staging reproductive aging. J Clin Endocrinol Metab 2012;97(4):1159–68.
3. Tepper PG, Brooks MM, Randolph JF Jr, et al. Characterizing the trajectories of vasomotor symptoms across the menopausal transition. Menopause 2016; 23(10):1067–74.
4. Moral E, Delgado JL, Carmona F, et al. Genitourinary syndrome of menopause. Prevalence and quality of life in Spanish postmenopausal women. The GENISSE study. Climacteric 2018;21(2):167–73.
5. Avis NE, Brambilla D, McKinlay SM, et al. A longitudinal analysis of the association between menopause and depression. Results from the Massachusetts Women's Health Study. Ann Epidemiol 1994;4(3):214–20.
6. Kravitz HM, Ganz PA, Bromberger J, et al. Sleep difficulty in women at midlife: a community survey of sleep and the menopausal transition. Menopause 2003; 10(1):19–28.
7. Sullivan Mitchell E, Fugate Woods N. Midlife women's attributions about perceived memory changes: observations from the Seattle Midlife Women's Health Study. J Womens Health Gend Based Med 2001;10(4):351–62.
8. Greendale GA, Sowers M, Han W, et al. Bone mineral density loss in relation to the final menstrual period in a multiethnic cohort: results from the Study of Women's Health Across the Nation (SWAN). J Bone Miner Res 2012;27(1):111–8.
9. Nelson HD, Haney E, Humphrey L, et al. Management of menopause-related symptoms. Evid Rep Technol Assess (Summ) 2005;120:1–6. Available at: https://www.ncbi.nlm.nih.gov/pubmed/15910013.
10. Furness S, Roberts H, Marjoribanks J, et al. Hormone therapy in postmenopausal women and risk of endometrial hyperplasia. Cochrane Database Syst Rev 2012; 8:CD000402.
11. Rossouw JE, Anderson GL, Prentice RL, et al. Risks and benefits of estrogen plus progestin in healthy postmenopausal women: principal results From the Women's Health Initiative randomized controlled trial. JAMA 2002;288(3): 321–33.

12. Rossouw JE, Prentice RL, Manson JE, et al. Postmenopausal hormone therapy and risk of cardiovascular disease by age and years since menopause. JAMA 2007;297(13):1465–77.
13. The NHTPSAP. The 2017 hormone therapy position statement of The North American Menopause Society. Menopause 2017;24(7):728–53.
14. Manson JE, Aragaki AK, Rossouw JE, et al. Menopausal Hormone Therapy and Long-term All-Cause and Cause-Specific Mortality: The Women's Health Initiative Randomized Trials. JAMA 2017;318(10):927–38.
15. Chlebowski RT, Anderson GL, Aragaki AK, et al. Association of Menopausal Hormone Therapy With Breast Cancer Incidence and Mortality During Long-term Follow-up of the Women's Health Initiative Randomized Clinical Trials. JAMA 2020;324(4):369–80.
16. Boardman HM, Hartley L, Eisinga A, et al. Hormone therapy for preventing cardiovascular disease in post-menopausal women. Cochrane Database Syst Rev 2015;(3):CD002229. https://doi.org/10.1002/14651858.CD002229.pub4.
17. Vinogradova Y, Coupland C, Hippisley-Cox J. Use of hormone replacement therapy and risk of venous thromboembolism: nested case-control studies using the QResearch and CPRD databases. BMJ 2019;364:k4810.
18. Chen WY, Manson JE, Hankinson SE, et al. Unopposed estrogen therapy and the risk of invasive breast cancer. Arch Intern Med 2006;166(9):1027–32.
19. Manson JE, Chlebowski RT, Stefanick ML, et al. Menopausal hormone therapy and health outcomes during the intervention and extended poststopping phases of the Women's Health Initiative randomized trials. JAMA 2013;310(13):1353–68.
20. Collaborative Group on Hormonal Factors in Breast C. Type and timing of menopausal hormone therapy and breast cancer risk: individual participant meta-analysis of the worldwide epidemiological evidence. Lancet 2019;394(10204):1159–68.
21. Shifren JL, Crandall CJ, Manson JE. Menopausal Hormone Therapy. JAMA 2019;321(24):2458–9.
22. Mattson RH, Cramer JA, Darney PD, et al. Use of oral contraceptives by women with epilepsy. JAMA 1986;256(2):238–40. Available at: https://www.ncbi.nlm.nih.gov/pubmed/3723710.
23. Pinkerton JV, Faubion SS, Kaunitz AM, et al. The National Academies of Science, Engineering, and Medicine (NASEM) Report on Compounded Bioidentical Hormone Therapy. Menopause 2020;27(11):1199–201.
24. Haskell SG, Bean-Mayberry B, Gordon K. Discontinuing postmenopausal hormone therapy: an observational study of tapering versus quitting cold turkey: is there a difference in recurrence of menopausal symptoms? Menopause 2009;16(3):494–9.
25. North American Menopause S. The North American Menopause Society Statement on Continuing Use of Systemic Hormone Therapy After Age 65. Menopause 2015;22(7):693.
26. Stearns V, Beebe KL, Iyengar M, et al. Paroxetine controlled release in the treatment of menopausal hot flashes: a randomized controlled trial. JAMA 2003;289(21):2827–34.
27. Barton DL, LaVasseur BI, Sloan JA, et al. Phase III, placebo-controlled trial of three doses of citalopram for the treatment of hot flashes: NCCTG trial N05C9. J Clin Oncol 2010;28(20):3278–83.
28. Freeman EW, Guthrie KA, Caan B, et al. Efficacy of escitalopram for hot flashes in healthy menopausal women: a randomized controlled trial. JAMA 2011;305(3):267–74.

29. Loprinzi CL, Kugler JW, Sloan JA, et al. Venlafaxine in management of hot flashes in survivors of breast cancer: a randomised controlled trial. Lancet 2000; 356(9247):2059–63.

30. Pinkerton JV, Constantine G, Hwang E, et al. Desvenlafaxine compared with placebo for treatment of menopausal vasomotor symptoms: a 12-week, multicenter, parallel-group, randomized, double-blind, placebo-controlled efficacy trial. Menopause 2013;20(1):28–37.

31. Rada G, Capurro D, Pantoja T, et al. Non-hormonal interventions for hot flushes in women with a history of breast cancer. Cochrane Database Syst Rev 2010;9: CD004923.

32. Shams T, Firwana B, Habib F, et al. SSRIs for hot flashes: a systematic review and meta-analysis of randomized trials. J Gen Intern Med 2014;29(1):204–13.

33. Brown JN, Wright BR. Use of gabapentin in patients experiencing hot flashes. Pharmacotherapy 2009;29(1):74–81.

34. Hayes LP, Carroll DG, Kelley KW. Use of gabapentin for the management of natural or surgical menopausal hot flashes. Ann Pharmacother 2011;45(3):388–94.

35. Reddy SY, Warner H, Guttuso T Jr, et al. Gabapentin, estrogen, and placebo for treating hot flushes: a randomized controlled trial. Obstet Gynecol 2006; 108(1):41–8.

36. Pandya KJ, Raubertas RF, Flynn PJ, et al. Oral clonidine in postmenopausal patients with breast cancer experiencing tamoxifen-induced hot flashes: a University of Rochester Cancer Center Community Clinical Oncology Program study. Ann Intern Med 2000;132(10):788–93.

37. Newton KM, Buist DS, Keenan NL, et al. Use of alternative therapies for menopause symptoms: results of a population-based survey. Obstet Gynecol 2002; 100(1):18–25.

38. Mann E, Smith M, Hellier J, et al. A randomised controlled trial of a cognitive behavioural intervention for women who have menopausal symptoms following breast cancer treatment (MENOS 1): trial protocol. BMC Cancer 2011;11:44.

39. Ayers B, Smith M, Hellier J, et al. Effectiveness of group and self-help cognitive behavior therapy in reducing problematic menopausal hot flushes and night sweats (MENOS 2): a randomized controlled trial. Menopause 2012;19(7): 749–59.

40. Elkins GR, Fisher WI, Johnson AK, et al. Clinical hypnosis in the treatment of postmenopausal hot flashes: a randomized controlled trial. Menopause 2013;20(3): 291–8.

41. Carmody JF, Crawford S, Salmoirago-Blotcher E, et al. Mindfulness training for coping with hot flashes: results of a randomized trial. Menopause 2011;18(6): 611–20.

42. Walega DR, Rubin LH, Banuvar S, et al. Effects of stellate ganglion block on vasomotor symptoms: findings from a randomized controlled clinical trial in postmenopausal women. Menopause 2014;21(8):807–14.

43. Huang AJ, Subak LL, Wing R, et al. An intensive behavioral weight loss intervention and hot flushes in women. Arch Intern Med 2010;170(13):1161–7.

44. Franco OH, Chowdhury R, Troup J, et al. Use of Plant-Based Therapies and Menopausal Symptoms: A Systematic Review and Meta-analysis. JAMA 2016; 315(23):2554–63.

Osteoporosis

Vidya Gopinath, MD

KEYWORDS

- Osteoporosis • Menopause • Bone density • Bisphosphonates • Bone fracture
- Osteopenia • Falls • Hip fracture

KEY POINTS

- Osteoporosis is the most common bone disease in adults and is associated with significant morbidity and mortality. A woman's risk of dying from a hip fracture exceeds that of breast cancer, uterine cancer, and ovarian cancer combined.
- Screening rates of eligible patients are low and vary by sociodemographic characteristics. Fewer than one in four privately insured women are screened for osteoporosis. All women above the age of 65 years and women under the age of 65 years and men with risk factors should also be screened.
- If osteoporosis is treated after a patient's first fragility fracture, the likelihood of another fragility fracture within the year is halved. Rates of treatment of osteoporosis after fragility fractures remain low.
- Two widely publicized adverse effects associated with bisphosphonates have contributed to a sharp decline in their use for osteoporosis despite their first-line indication and rarity of those adverse effects.

Abbreviations	
BMD	bone mineral density
DXA	dual-energy x-ray absorptiometry
FRAX	fracture Risk Assessment Tool
MOF	major osteoporotic fracture
USPSTF	US Preventive Services Task Force
NAMS	North American Menopause Society
ONJ	osteonecrosis of the jaw
FDA	Food and Drug Administration

INTRODUCTION
Definitions

Osteoporosis

Osteoporosis is the most common bone disease affecting humans. It is a chronic, progressive bone disease characterized by decreased bone mineral density (BMD),

Warren Alpert Medical School of Brown University, Rhode Island Hospital, 593 Eddy St, Jane Brown Ground, Suite 0100, Providence, RI 02903, USA
E-mail address: Vidya.Gopinath@Lifespan.org

Med Clin N Am 107 (2023) 213–225
https://doi.org/10.1016/j.mcna.2022.10.013
0025-7125/23/© 2022 Elsevier Inc. All rights reserved.

abnormal bone microarchitecture, and bone fragility which results in an increased risk of fracture.

Dual-energy x-ray absorptiometry
The World Health Organization uses a quantitative definition of osteoporosis based on bone density. Dual-energy x-ray absorptiometry (DXA) is considered the "gold standard" for measuring bone density. The guidelines recommend assessment of bone density is performed at the femoral neck region of the proximal femur or the lumbar spine. Measurements of bone density greater than 2.5 standard deviations below a young adult female reference mean ("T score") are diagnostic of osteoporosis for postmenopausal women. Low bone mass or osteopenia is bone density between 1 and 2.5 standard deviations below the young adult female reference mean. Individuals with low bone mass are not necessarily at high risk for fracture; however, it is a risk fracture for the development of osteoporosis.

Fragility or osteoporotic fracture
The presence of radiographic osteoporosis along with a fragility fracture is considered severe or established osteoporosis. A fragility fracture, also known as an osteoporotic fracture or low-trauma fracture, is one that occurs with minimal or no trauma, such as a fall from standing height or less, and would not normally result in a fracture.[1] The most common sites of fragility fractures are the distal forearm (wrist), proximal femur (hip), and vertebrae.[1]

Fracture Risk Assessment Tool. The University of Sheffield developed the Fracture Risk Assessment Tool (FRAX), a web-based 12 question tool which estimates the 10-year probability of hip fracture and major osteoporotic fracture (MOF). The FRAX

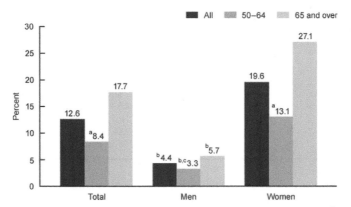

Fig. 1. Prevalence of osteoporosis among adults age 50 and over, by sex and age: United States, 2017-2018. *Source*: CDC.[a] Significantly different from adults aged 65 and over.[b] Significantly different from women.[c] Estimate potentially unreliable due to relative confidence interval width greater than 130%. Notes: Osteoporosis is defined as occurring at the femur neck or lumbar spine or both. Estimates for adults aged 50 and over were age adjusted by the direct method to the 2000 US Census population using age groups 50 to 64 and 65 and over. Crude estimates are 12.0% for total, 4.2% for men, and 18.8% for women. The age-adjusted prevalence of osteoporosis at the femur neck only is 6.3%, lumbar spine only is 4.3%, and both are 2.0%. Access data table for **Fig. 1** at: https://www.cdc.gov/nchs/data/databriefd/db405-tables-508.pdf#1. (Neda Sarafrazi, Ph.D., Edwina A. Wambogo, Ph.D., M.S., M.P.H., R.D., and John A. Shepherd, Ph.D, Osteoporosis or Low Bone Mass in Older Adults: United States, 2017-2018. NCHS Data Brief, No. 405, March 2021.)

tool uses readily clinical data including alcohol use, parental history of hip fracture, and if available, femoral neck BMD. It is the most commonly used FRAX. The tool is country and ethnicity-specific. There are four ethnicity options in the United States: White, Black, Hispanic, and Asian American. Like any risk assessment tool, there are a number of limitations. It underestimates the risk of fracture in people with diabetes, high-dose steroid exposure, a family history of non-hip fragility fractures. The tool was designed to predict fracture risk, not BMD.

Background: Epidemiology/pathophysiology. In the United States, an estimated 10.2 million adults above the age of 50 years have osteoporosis, and an additional 43.3 million have low bone mass.[2] Among women above the age of 65 years, the prevalence of osteoporosis is above 27% (**Fig. 1**).[2] Data from the National Health and Nutrition Examination Survey in 2017 to 2018 demonstrated an increase in the prevalence of osteoporosis in women from 14.0% to 19.6% during the preceding decade.[2] The prevalence of osteoporosis in adults over 50 years during that same decade increased from 9.4% to 12.6%.[2] No change was seen in the prevalence of low bone mass (**Fig. 2**). The prevalence of low bone mass at either the femur neck or lumbar spine or both is 43.1% in adults aged 50 years and over and 47.5% in adults aged 65 years and over.[2]

Osteoporosis can affect individuals of any sex, age, or ethnicity. However, it is three-fold more common in women, particularly non-Hispanic white women and Asian women, with 71% of osteoporotic fractures occurring in women.[3] Peak bone mass is reached around age 30 years, and women have a lower peak bone mass than men. Bone tissue is maintained by bone remodeling; osteoclasts resorb old bone, and

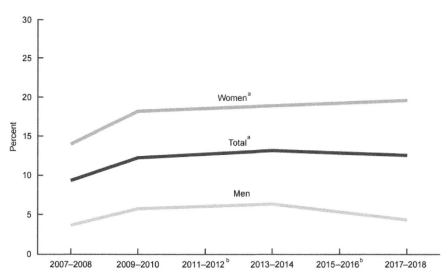

Fig. 2. Trends in age-adjusted prevalence of osteoporosis among adults aged 50 and over, by sex: United States, 2007-2008 through 2017-2018. *Source*: CDC.[a] Significant increasing linear trend.[b] Data not available. Notes: Osteoporosis is defined as occurring at the femur neck or lumbar spine or both. Percentages are age adjusted by the direct method to the 2000 projected. The US Census population using age groups 50 to 64 and 65 and over. Access data table for Figure 3 at: https://www.cdc.gov/nchs/data/databriefs/db405-tables-508.pdf#3. (Neda Sarafrazi, Ph.D., Edwina A. Wambogo, Ph.D., M.S., M.P.H., R.D., and John A. Shepherd, Ph.D, Osteoporosis or Low Bone Mass in Older Adults: United States, 2017-2018. NCHS Data Brief, No. 405, March 2021.)

osteoblasts build new bone. Osteocytes comprise the majority of all bone cells and are the mechanosensory cells of the bone. Osteocytes regulate the location and rate of bone remodeling. One of the regulators of osteocyte activity is estrogen. During menopause, decreasing estrogen levels increase the expression of RANK ligand, which activates osteoclasts. During this period, osteoblasts do not build bone at a rate to match the highly active osteoclasts so there is accelerated bone loss. Bone mass is stable in healthy, premenopausal women but beginning 1 to 3 years before menopause and continuing for 5 to 10 years after, the rate of bone loss is about 2% per year.[4] After this period of rapid bone loss, bone density decreases by 0.5% per year; therefore by age 80 years, women have lost an average of 30% of their peak bone mass.[4]

Overall screening rates of eligible patients remain low. An analysis of over 1.6 million women with Medicare insurance found among women aged 50 to 64, 65 to 79, and 80+ years, screening rates were 21.1%, 26.5%, and 12.8%.[5] Only one in four privately insured women over 65 years is screened for osteoporosis for primary prevention.[5] The highest rates of screening are in Hispanic and Asian women and the lowest are in non-Hispanic black women.[5]

If the first fragility fracture is recognized and osteoporosis is treated, the rates of another osteoporotic fracture decrease by half.[1] However, in the first year after a fracture, only 24% of women age 60 years and older receive treatment.[6]

Bisphosphonates are the first-line treatment of osteoporosis for the majority of patients. After a decade of increased prescription of bisphosphonates, there was a dramatic decline in its use between 2008 and 2012. One key cause of this decline was two widely-publicized rare side effects: osteonecrosis of the jaw (ONJ) and atypical femur fractures. The US Food and Drug Administration (FDA) released statements on this association in 2005 and 2007, respectively, though did not recommend safety restrictions in their use. In 2016, the American Society for Bone and Mineral Research released a statement recommending a "drug holiday" after 5 continuous years of bisphosphonate therapy. Sales of oral bisphosphonates increased from 21.3 million prescriptions in 2002 to 31.0 million in 2007 and 2008.[7] In the next 4 years, they decreased by 53% down to 14.7 million in 2012.[7] This trend was also seen in sales of intravenous (IV) bisphosphonates. An ecological analysis of trends in media reports and oral bisphosphonate prescriptions found a significant interaction between patient behavior and popular media rather than between patient behavior and scientific publications.[8] The decline in bisphosphonate prescription was predominantly seen among white women, women with education levels less than high school, and the rural population.[8] During this time, the use of oral bisphosphonates has increased in Asian, Hispanic, and black women.[8] In addition to the safety concerns highlighted by the FDA and questions about optimal duration, the medication, and drug holidays, the Fosamax (alendronate) patent expired in February 2008.

Morbidity and mortality

There are more than 2 million fractures related to osteoporosis annually in the United States.[4] Approximately 40% of women have a fracture related to osteoporosis in their lifetime in the United States.[9] Worldwide, one in three women and one in five men over the age of 50 years will experience an osteoporotic fracture in their lifetime.[10] Age-adjusted rates of fragility fractures are decreasing; however, the incidence of fragility fractures is increasing rapidly due to the increasing population of older adults.[11] Among fragility fractures, hip fractures are associated with the greatest disability and death, and there are more than 300,000 hip fractures per year. Lifetime risk for hip fracture is 17% for White Americans, 14% for Hispanic Americans, and 6% for

Black Americans.[4] The risk of hip fracture increases with age and doubles for each decade after age 50 years.[11] The average age at which a hip fracture occurs is 82, which is relevant given the aging population and the number of adults in the United States over 65 years will double in the next 40 years.[4] After experiencing a hip fracture, 20% to 30% of people die within the year.[3] The surgery carries a 4% mortality risk and the first 3 months afterward confers a 5 to 8-fold increase in all-cause mortality.[11] A woman's risk of dying from a hip fracture exceeds that of breast cancer, uterine cancer, and ovarian cancer combined.[1] Hip fracture almost always requires hospitalization with up to 25% of people requiring some long-term care and 50% have some long-term loss of mobility.[4]

Vertebral fractures are the most common osteoporotic fracture, they are typically diagnosed on imaging, and approximately 75% of them are asymptomatic or cause minimal symptoms. Severe or multiple vertebral fractures can cause back pain, loss of height, kyphosis, and decreased mobility. An existing vertebral fracture increases the risk of subsequent fractures 5 to 7-fold.

Clinical Assessment and Screening

All postmenopausal women should be assessed for their risk of osteoporosis. Clinicians should take into account an individual patient's medical conditions, fixed and modifiable risk factors, and medications (**Table 1**).

The US Preventive Services Task Force (USPSTF) recommends screening for osteoporosis in all women 65 years and older.[3] In postmenopausal women younger than 65 years with at least one risk factor, they recommend determining who should be screened with BMD testing using a clinical risk assessment tool. In addition to FRAX, there are other risk assessment tools including the Osteoporosis Self-Assessment Tool, Osteoporosis Risk Assessment Instrument, Osteoporosis Index of Risk, and the Simple Calculated Osteoporosis Risk Estimation. One approach to determine which postmenopausal women below the age of 65 years should be screened is to use the benchmark 10-year risk of MOF in a 65-year-old white woman, which is 8.4% in the United States.[3]

All leading organizations agree with the USPSTF recommendation to screen all women above the age of 65 years and women under the age of 65 years with risk factors who carry the same risk as a 65-year-old white woman. The American College of Obstetrics and Gynecology specifies women under age of 65 years with FRAX 10-year risk of MOF of 9.3% or higher. The North American Menopause Society (NAMS) includes postmenopausal women with a fragility fracture. The National Institute of Health does not recommend universal screening but BMD only for individuals at high risk for osteoporosis.

Interval for screening

The optimal screening interval is not known. The Choosing Wisely campaign recommends against repeating BMD testing in fewer than 2 years even in high-risk patients as most changes that may be seen are within the measurement of error of DXA scans.[12] In postmenopausal women aged 50 to 64 years with a T-score greater than −1.5, NAMS recommends repeating BMD screening at age 65 years.[4] Data have also indicated that repeat BMD compared with baseline BMD measurement alone does not improve accuracy in predicting subsequence hip or MOFs.[13,14] One approach is to repeat screening based on T-score and risk factors. The recommendation is to repeat BMD every 2 years for individuals with low bone mass (T-score −2.00 to −2.49) or risk factors contributing to ongoing bone loss. Individuals with T-score

Table 1
Clinical assessment and screening

Medical Conditions	Fixed Risk Factors	Modifiable Risk Factors	Medications
Inflammatory diseases (rheumatoid arthritis, inflammatory bowel disease)	Increasing age	Excessive alcohol intake (>4 drinks/day for men and >2 drinks/day for women)	Steroids
Diseases associated with malabsorption: celiac disease, gastrectomy	Female gender	Tobacco use	Aromatase inhibitors
Endocrinopathies: Cushing syndrome, gonadal insufficiency, type 1 and 2 diabetes mellitus	Family history of osteoporosis	Excessive caffeine intake (>2.5 units/day)	Phenytoin
Genetic diseases: osteogenesis imperfecta, thalassemia	Gonadal hormone deficiency in men	Poor nutrition, vitamin D deficiency, and low dietary calcium	Immunosuppressive medications: cyclosporine
Chronic renal disease, chronic liver disease	Postmenopausal state in women	Low body mass index (BMI)	Excess doses of thyroid hormone
Hematologic malignancies	Ethnicity: White or Asian race	Immobility and physical inactivity	Gonadotropin-releasing hormone agonists or antagonists

−1.50 to 1.99 without risk factors would recommend repeat BMD measurement in 3 to 5 years and for T-scores greater than −1.49, recommend repeat in 10 to 15 years.

Secondary Osteoporosis

Up to 30% of postmenopausal women with osteoporosis have a secondary cause.[9] Primary osteoporosis is due to aging and decreased gonadal function. Secondary causes of osteoporosis include medical conditions and medications noted as risk factors for osteoporosis such as rheumatologic diseases and hematologic malignancies.

Laboratory workup

For patients with osteoporosis on BMD, laboratory testing is done to evaluate for common secondary causes and determine appropriateness of therapeutic options. There is controversy about the laboratory workup for individuals found to have osteoporosis on BMD testing who are other asymptomatic. The most common recommended laboratory tests are serum 25-hydroxyvitamin D, creatinine, and thyroid-stimulating hormone. NAMS also recommends a complete blood count, serum calcium, alkaline phosphatase, albumin, and phosphate.

Although markers of bone turnover are used in clinical trials, their routine use in assessment of patients with osteoporosis is not recommended. These including markers of bone resorption (fasting serum C-telopeptide of type I collagen) or bone formation by osteoblasts (bone-specific alkaline phosphatase or serum procollagen type I N-terminal propeptide).[4]

Treatment

Encouraging healthy lifestyle choices such as smoking cessation, a healthy diet and adequate physical activity is important in all postmenopausal women for general and bone health. For individuals with osteoporosis, these general changes do not result in a significant increase in BMD and pharmacologic therapy is recommended to reduce the risk of osteoporotic fractures.

Lifestyle Modifications/Nonpharmacologic Interventions

Smoking and alcohol

Cessation of smoking and limiting alcohol intake is recommended. Women who smoke have twice the prevalence of osteoporosis as nonsmokers. Smoking leads to changes in the microarchitecture of trabecular bone. Alcohol intake above the recommended seven drinks per week is associated with a higher risk of osteoporosis, primarily through dysregulation of calcium and hormone deficiencies.

Physical activity

Immobilization is associated with an increased risk of developing osteoporosis as impact-loading exercises are associated with increased skeletal mass. A Cochrane review found exercise can improve BMD slightly and decrease bone loss compared with a non-exercising control group. They found a small but statistically significant decrease in the likelihood of a fracture.[15] A high-intensity exercise such as jogging has not definitively been shown to be of greater benefit than a lower intensity exercise such as walking, although a systematic review found a tendency to indicate an association between exercise intensity and bone response.[16] Given the variable data, we recommend encouraging exercise that is identified by a patient as sustainable.

In addition to a benefit in BMD, physical activity is associated with a decreased incidence of falls. Exercise programs that target balance, gait, and muscle strength are the most effective way to prevent falls in older adults.

A multidisciplinary approach to fall prevention is also recommended in the management of osteoporosis. Discuss potential hazards in the home and how to fall-proof the home by installing grab bars, removing loose carpets, and so forth. Decreased visual acuity is also associated with falls; therefore, regular vision screenings and wearing glasses when required can decrease the risk of falls. Physical therapy can improve strength and balance and assess individuals for assistive devices such as walking aids.

Calcium and vitamin D

Although calcium and vitamin D intake are critical in the development of healthy bones, the use of calcium and vitamin D supplementation in healthy postmenopausal women is controversial. There is evidence showing calcium and vitamin D supplementation can increase BMD, but their effect on fracture risk is variable. Expert opinion continues to recommend their use in individuals with osteoporosis and to ensure normal calcium and vitamin D levels before starting pharmacologic therapy.

Vitamin D increases absorption of dietary calcium and phosphate. A negative calcium balance results in a rise in parathyroid hormone (PTH) and increases bone resorption. Initiation of bisphosphonates in the setting of vitamin D deficiency can theoretically result in decreased effectiveness of those medications, though supporting data have not been robust. The recommendation for vitamin D supplementation is becoming increasingly controversial as new studies are published. A recent study showed no benefit of vitamin D supplementation on longevity, falls, cancer, or cardiovascular disease.[17] The first large randomized controlled study in the United States on vitamin D supplementation in the general population and older faults was published in July 2022 in the New England Journal of Medicine (NEJM).[18] It demonstrated no decreased risk of fracture including in individuals with low vitamin D or osteoporosis. Many physicians continue to recommend vitamin D supplementation in patients with osteoporosis given the minimal risk of harm. The optimal dose is unknown, and the range of recommended doses from groups is 600 to 1000 IU of vitamin D daily. One study demonstrated an increased risk of first-time falls with fracture with supplementation above 1000 IU daily.[19]

Chronically high levels of vitamin D have been associated with a slight increase in mortality and falls. The level at which vitamin D can cause toxicity is unknown.

Calcium is critical for strengthening bone with calcium hydroxyapatite crystals, and adequate calcium levels are important in maintaining equilibrium with PTH, phosphorus levels, and bone tissue. The recommended daily intake of calcium per the Institute of Health is 1000 to 1200 mg per day. The average dietary calcium intake in postmenopausal women in the United States is 700 to 800 mg daily and 500 mg daily in dairy-free diets. Therefore, many experts recommend reviewing a patient's dietary intake and encouraging increased intake of calcium-rich foods to reach approximately 1200 mg per day. If it is not possible to reach that level with dietary intake, supplements are recommended. The Women's Health Initiative found that women given an additional 1000 mg calcium supplement with a total intake of over 2000 mg/day had a 17% increased risk of kidney stones. There is mixed data on a potential association between calcium supplementation and increased cardiovascular risk. High doses of calcium intake cause GI effects such as bloating, constipation, and dyspepsia.

Pharmacologic treatment

There are three major indications for pharmacologic treatment. The first is patients with osteoporosis by BMD testing. The second is patients with low bone mass by

BMD testing whose 10 year probability of a hip fracture exceeds 3% or MOF exceeds 20% as determined by FRAX. Finally, patients with a fragility fracture. Patients with a hip or spine fracture have a high future risk of a second fracture and a high likelihood of benefit from pharmacologic treatment.

There are two categories of anti-fracture medications. The first is anti-remodeling agents that inhibit bone resorption and, to some extent, bone formation. They can improve BMD and reduce fracture risk but do not repair trabecular structure. Their benefits begin to wane when treatment is stopped. These include bisphosphonates, denosumab, estrogen, and estrogen agonists/antagonists (EAA). Osteoanabolic agents stimulate new bone and can induce large increases in BMD and reduce fracture risk more quickly like PTH receptor agonists.

When deciding among agents, initial fracture risk can guide treatment. For patients at moderate to high risk, a bisphosphonate is a reasonable choice. For patients at very high risk, we recommend consideration of an osteoanabolic drug. One important consideration is that some drugs improve vertebral fracture risk without a change in the risk of hip and nonvertebral fractures.

Bisphosphonates

Bisphosphonates are synthetic analogs of pyrophosphate and bind to bone matrix and impair osteoclast function. They are first-line therapy for the majority of postmenopausal women with osteoporosis. Their use can decrease the risk of vertebral fractures by 41% to 70% over 3 years.[4] Alendronate decreased the risk of spine and hip fractures by 50% over 3 years in patients with osteoporosis at the hip or a history of vertebral fracture. They are contraindicated in individuals with kidney disease with eGFR less than 30 to 35 mL/min. There are oral and intravenous bisphosphonates, and esophageal disorders and bariatric surgery with anastomoses in the upper GI tract are contraindications to the oral formulations. Alendronate, risedronate, and zoledronate reduce the risk of vertebral, hip, and nonvertebral fracture. Ibandronate reduces the risk of vertebral fractures but has not been documented to reduce the risk of nonvertebral fracture. Owing to potential esophageal effects with bisphosphonates, we emphasize the importance of taking the tablet on an empty stomach, first thing in the morning and remaining upright for 30 to 60 min without other oral intake (30 min for alendronate and risedronate, 60 min for ibandronate). The mechanism of the rare side effect of ONJ is impaired bone resorption due to decreased osteoclast activity. Old bone survives beyond its lifespan with decreased vascular perfusion leading to avascular necrosis of the jaw. It occurs in the jaw due to a higher remodeling rate than other bones so it is more sensitive to the effects of bisphosphonates.[20] According to a 2022 update from the American Association of Oral and Maxillofacial Surgeons, the risk of ONJ with bisphosphonates is less than 0.02% to 0.05%, the risk with placebo is 0% to 0.02%.[21] Atypical femur fractures are another well-known rare adverse effect. They are fragility fractures in the subtrochanteric region and along the femoral diaphysis. The incidence of atypical fractures increased as duration of bisphosphonate use increased and rates decreased with time since bisphosphonate discontinuation. One risk factor for atypical femur fracture is Asian ancestry; a large study published in NEJM in August 2020 found that 49% of the patients with atypical femur fracture were Asian despite being 10% of the patient population which confers a rate five to six times higher than other races. The risk of atypical femur fracture increased significantly particularly beyond 5 years. The absolute risk is small compared with other osteoporotic fractures. After 3 years, among white women 149 hip fractures and 541 clinical fractures were prevented and 2 bisphosphonate-associated atypical femur fractures.[22]

The optimal duration of therapy and timing of drug holidays is not definitively known. The Task Force of the American Society Bone and Mineral Research made a statement in September 2015 recommending a drug holiday after 5 years of oral bisphosphonates in women who were not at high fracture risk. A large cohort study published in December 2020 examined women who had completed 5 years of oral bisphosphonate therapy and then discontinued at study entry, discontinued 2 years later or discontinued 5 years later.[23] Patients who continued treatment for 5 additional years had the same hip fracture risk as the group who discontinued treatment at study entry.[23] One strategy for determining if appropriateness of a bisphosphonate holiday is if a patient meets all three criteria: T-score greater than −2.5, no history of prior hip or vertebral fracture and stable BMD since initiation of therapy. After a drug holiday, patients can either restart bisphosphonates or reassess BMD after another 2 years of pharmacologic treatment to determine reinitiation. For higher risk patients who do not meet those criteria, the recommendation is alendronate for 10 years and zoledronate for 6 years, but management at this juncture is controversial.[24]

Denosumab

RANK ligand is the principal stimulator of bone resorption. Denosumab is a monoclonal antibody inhibitor of RANK ligand and is also approved for bone loss in women with breast cancer on aromatase inhibitor therapies and men at high risk of fracture. It is administered as a subcutaneous injection every 6 months. Denosumab treatment over 3 years decreases the risk of vertebral fractures by 68% and hip fractures by 40%.[4] It can be used in patients with impaired renal function. Adverse effects include the increased risk of cellulitis and skin rash, and it may also cause hypocalcemia.

There is no limit to duration of denosumab therapy. Discontinuation of denosumab leads to a rapid decrease in BMD, and there are studies of vertebral fractures occurring 3 to 18 months after stopping denosumab. If it is stopped, therapy with a bisphosphonate should be initiated.

Calcitonin

Salmon calcitonin is a daily intranasal spray approved for women at least 5 years postmenopausal when there are no suitable alternative treatments. It decreases vertebral fractures by 30% but does not reduce the risk of nonvertebral fractures. There is a possible association with certain cancers, although a definitive causal relationship was not demonstrated.

Estrogen therapy/hormone replacement therapy

Estrogen withdrawal around menopause is associated with significant bone loss and the use of estrogen replacement therapy is FDA-approved for the prevention of osteoporosis, though non-estrogen treatments are recommended to be considered if its use is solely for fracture prevention. Women with a uterus require progesterone in addition to estrogen. Five years of hormone therapy reduced vertebral and hip fractures by 34% in the Women's Health Initiative. There are a variety of preparations including oral, transdermal, and transvaginal formulations. Risks include increased risk of venous thromboembolism (VTE), store, coronary artery disease (CAD) with 5 years of treatment. The safety profile is best within 10 years of menopause. Discontinuation of hormone therapy is associated with rapid bone loss.

Conjugated estrogens/bazedoxifene (Duavee) is a conjugated estrogen and selective estrogen receptor modular (SERM). It is approved for moderate to severe vasomotor symptoms and prevention of postmenopausal osteoporosis.

Raloxifene

Raloxifene is an SERM, an EAA. It reduces the incidence of vertebral fractures after 3 years by 30% in patients with a prior vertebral fracture and 50% in patients without a history of vertebral fracture; however, it does not reduce the risk of hip or nonvertebral fracture. The major adverse effect is VTE and its use increased VTE risk about three-fold, the same as estrogen therapy, and fatal stroke (HR 1.49).

Parathyroid hormone analogs

PTH levels regulate calcium and bone formation on trabecular and endocortical bone surfaces. Teriparatide and abaloparatide activate the PTH receptor and are administered by daily subcutaneous injections. Teriparatide reduced the risk of vertebral fractures by 65% and nonvertebral fractures by 35%. It is also approved for glucocorticoid-induced osteoporosis and high-risk women. Treatment duration was previously restricted to 24 months due to concerns for an increased risk of osteosarcoma in rat trials but has not been seen in humans, so longer durations can be considered in high-risk patients. When discontinued, alternative agents should be considered to prevent rapid bone loss.

Sclerostin inhibitor (romosozumab)

Romosozumab is a monoclonal antibody to sclerostin that inhibits bone resorption and stimulates bone formation. It reduced the risk of a vertebral fracture by 73% and clinical fractures by 36%, and high risk had significantly fewer fractures compared with alendronate. It is a monthly subcutaneous injection and its use is limited to 1 year. The major adverse effects are an increased risk for cardiovascular disease and stroke.

Special considerations

The anti-fracture benefits of these medications have primarily been studied in postmenopausal women so data on their benefit for glucocorticoid-induced osteoporosis and men are limited.

Goals of therapy

Osteoporosis is a chronic condition and a "treat to target" strategy is recommended. A patient-specific treatment target is generated with close monitoring to achieve that goal. After initiating pharmacologic therapy, a repeat BMD is performed after 2 years or when clinically appropriate. At least annual assessment of patient satisfaction with this regimen should be performed given the high rates of noncompliance with osteoporosis medications; 25% to 30% never start their osteoporosis regimen and 50% do not continue after 1 year.[25]

CLINICS CARE POINTS

- All women older than 65 years of age should be screened for osteoporosis with dual-energy x-ray absorptiometry.
- Women under 65 years of age who have risk factors for osteoporosis should be assessed for their risk of osteoporosis with a tool like the Fracture Risk Assessment Tool.
- Treatment of osteoporosis after fragility fracture results in a dramatic decrease in repeat fragility fracture; therefore, all patients with a fragility fracture should be assessed for pharmacologic treatment.
- Bisphosphonates are first-line treatment and safe and effective for osteoporosis with drug holidays recommended after 3 to 5 years.

DISCLOSURE

I hereby certify that, to the best of my knowledge, no aspect of my current personal or professional circumstance places me in the position of having a conflict of interest with this content.

REFERENCES

1. van Oostwaard M. Osteoporosis and the Nature of Fragility Fracture: An Overview. In: Patient Hertz K, Santy-Tomlinson J, editors. Fragility Fracture Nursing: Holistic Care and Management of the Orthogeriatric. Springer; 2018. p. 1–40.
2. Sarafrazi N. Osteoporosis or low bone mass in older adults: United States, 2017-2018. 2021. https://stacks.cdc.gov/view/cdc/103477. Accessed July 30, 2022.
3. US Preventive Services Task Force. Screening for Osteoporosis to Prevent Fractures: US Preventive Services Task Force Recommendation Statement. JAMA 2018;319:2521–31.
4. Management of osteoporosis in postmenopausal women: the 2021 position statement of The North American Menopause Society. Menopause 2021;28:973–97.
5. Gillespie CW, Morin PE. Trends and Disparities in Osteoporosis Screening Among Women in the United States, 2008-2014. Am J Med 2017;130:306–16.
6. American College of Obstetricians and Gynecologists' Committee on Clinical Practice Guidelines–Gynecology. Osteoporosis Prevention, Screening, and Diagnosis: ACOG Clinical Practice Guideline No. 1. Obstet Gynecol 2021;138: 494–506.
7. Wysowski DK, Greene P. Trends in osteoporosis treatment with oral and intravenous bisphosphonates in the United States, 2002-2012. Bone 2013;57:423–8.
8. Jha S, Wang Z, Laucis N, et al. Trends in Media Reports, Oral Bisphosphonate Prescriptions, and Hip Fractures 1996-2012: An Ecological Analysi. J Bone Miner Res 2015;30:2179–87.
9. Jeremiah MP, Unwin BK, Greenawald MH, et al. Diagnosis and Management of Osteoporosis. Am Fam Physician 2015;92:261–8.
10. Epidemiology of osteoporosis and fragility fractures. 2019. https://www.osteoporosis.foundation/facts-statistics/epidemiology-of-osteoporosis-and-fragility-fractures. Accessed July 30, 2022.
11. Friedman SM, Mendelson DA. Epidemiology of fragility fractures. Clin Geriatr Med 2014;30:175–81.
12. ABIM Foundation. American Coll of Rheumatology - DXA scans every 2 years. Choosing Wisely | Promoting conversations between providers and patients. 2013. https://www.choosingwisely.org/clinician-lists/american-college-rheumatology-routine-repeat-dxa-scans-more-than-once-every-two-years/. Accessed July 30, 2022.
13. Crandall CJ, Larson J, Wright NC, et al. Serial Bone Density Measurement and Incident Fracture Risk Discrimination in Postmenopausal Women. JAMA Intern Med 2020;180:1232–40.
14. Fitzpatrick LA. Secondary causes of osteoporosis. Mayo Clin Proc 2002;77: 453–68.
15. Howe TE, Shea B, Dawson LJ, et al. Exercise for preventing and treating osteoporosis in postmenopausal women. Cochrane Database Syst Rev 2011;(7): CD000333. https://doi.org/10.1002/14651858.CD000333.pub2.
16. Kistler-Fischbacher M, Weeks BK, Beck BR. The effect of exercise intensity on bone in postmenopausal women (part 1): A systematic review. Bone 2021;143: 115696.

17. Manson JE, Cook NR, Lee I-M, et al. Vitamin D Supplements and Prevention of Cancer and Cardiovascular Disease. N Engl J Med 2019;380:33–44.
18. LeBoff MS, Chou SH, Ratliff KA, et al. Supplemental Vitamin D and Incident Fractures in Midlife and Older Adults. N Engl J Med 2022;387:299–309.
19. Wanigatunga AA, Sternberg AL, Blackford AL, et al. The effects of vitamin D supplementation on types of falls. J Am Geriatr Soc 2021;69:2851–64.
20. Gupta M, Gupta N. Bisphosphonate related jaw osteonecrosis. StatPearls Publishing; 2022. StatPearls.
21. Ruggiero SL, Dodson TB, Aghaloo T, et al. American Association of Oral and Maxillofacial Surgeons' Position Paper on Medication-Related Osteonecrosis of the Jaws—2022 Update. J Oral Maxillofac Surg 2022;80:920–43.
22. Black DM, Geiger EJ, Eastell R, et al. Atypical Femur Fracture Risk versus Fragility Fracture Prevention with Bisphosphonates. N Engl J Med 2020;383:743–53.
23. Izano MA, Lo JC, Adams AL, et al. Bisphosphonate Treatment Beyond 5 Years and Hip Fracture Risk in Older Women. JAMA Netw Open 2020;3:e2025190.
24. Das A., Green R., Jones S., et al., Osteoporosis Management: Staying Hip on the Literature. (2022). The National Society for General Internal Medicine (SGIM), conference on April 9th 2022.
25. LeBoff MS, Greenspan SL, Insogna KL, et al. The clinician's guide to prevention and treatment of osteoporosis. Osteoporos Int 2022. https://doi.org/10.1007/s00198-021-05900-y.

Polycystic Ovarian Syndrome

Sneha Shrivastava, MD, MSEd[a],*, Rosemarie L. Conigliaro, MD[b]

KEYWORDS

- Polycystic • Abnormal uterine bleeding • Metabolic syndrome • Hyperandrogenism
- Infertility • Oligo/amenorrhea

KEY POINTS

- Polycystic ovarian syndrome (PCOS) is a metabolic condition.
- PCOS is commonly diagnosed using the Rotterdam criteria, which requires the presence of 2 of 3 criteria: androgen excess, ovulatory dysfunction, and polycystic ovarian morphology.
- The pathogenesis of PCOS is influenced by genetic, hormonal, and environmental factors.
- Patients with PCOS experience a higher incidence of type 2 diabetes, hyperlipidemia, early cardiovascular disease, obstructive sleep apnea, adverse pregnancy outcomes, nonalcoholic fatty liver disease, depression, anxiety, low self-esteem (related to issues of body image as well as potential infertility), suboptimal sexual function, and decreased quality of life.
- Lifestyle intervention (weight loss, dietary modification, and increased exercise) is the first line of treatment.

INTRODUCTION

Polycystic ovarian syndrome (PCOS) is the most common endocrine pathology in females of reproductive age worldwide. The prevalence of PCOS varies between 6% and 13% based on which diagnostic criteria are used: the National Institutes of Health, Rotterdam, or Androgen Excess-PCOS Society.[1]

The Rotterdam criteria, which are the most widely used and accepted, identify 4 phenotypes (**Table 1**). The classic phenotype has hyperandrogenism and abnormal uterine bleeding with (phenotype A) or without (phenotype B) polycystic ovarian morphology on ultrasonography. The "ovulatory phenotype" or phenotype C has features of hyperandrogenism and polycystic ovarian morphology. The

[a] Donald and Barbara Zucker School of Medicine/Northwell, 256-11 Union Turnpike, Glen Oaks, NY 11004, USA; [b] Donald and Barbara Zucker School of Medicine/ Northwell, 225 Community Drive, Lake Sucess, NY 11020, USA
* Corresponding author. Medical Specialities at Glen Oaks, 256-11 Union Turnpike, Glen Oaks, NY 11004.
E-mail address: sshrivastava1@northwell.edu

Med Clin N Am 107 (2023) 227–234
https://doi.org/10.1016/j.mcna.2022.10.004
0025-7125/23/© 2022 Elsevier Inc. All rights reserved.

Table 1			
Polycystic ovarian syndrome phenotypes			
	Clinical Presentation		
Phenotype	**Androgen Excess[a]**	**Ovulatory Dysfunction**	**Polycystic Ovarian Morphology[b]**
A	✔	✔	✔
B	✔	✔	
C	✔		✔
D		✔	✔

[a] Chemical androgen excess can be diagnosed by: • Calculated free testosterone or free androgen index OR. • Calculated bioavailable testosterone OR. • Consider androstenedione or DHEAS if testosterone is normal and high index of suspicion for hyperandrogenism.
[b] Ultrasound criteria: Ultrasonography should be transvaginal and using high resolution. Follicle count per ovary should be greater than or equal to 25 (2–9 mm) or ovarian volume greater than or equal to 10 mL.

nonhyperandrogenic phenotype" or phenotype D has abnormal uterine bleeding and polycystic ovarian morphology.

PATHOPHYSIOLOGY

PCOS is a metabolic condition. Insulin resistance (IR) is a key feature found in patients with PCOS and is tissue sensitive. Skeletal muscle, adipose tissue, and liver lose their sensitivity to insulin, whereas adrenal glands and ovaries remain sensitive. Insulin plays a vital role in androgen production in ovarian theca cells, stimulating ovarian follicle growth, hormone secretion, and ovarian steroidogenesis. In synergy with insulin-like growth factor (IGF)-1 and luteinizing hormone (LH), hyperinsulinemia increases LH-binding sites and the androgen-producing response of LH. IR independently increases the production of androstenedione and testosterone (T). Hyperinsulinemia reduces hepatic sex hormone-binding globulin (SHBG) and increases free T levels in the blood. Hyperinsulinemia also inhibits IGF-1-binding hormone, which leads to increased levels of IGF-1, causing higher production of androgens in theca cells, accelerating granulosa cell apoptosis, and inhibiting folliculogenesis. Collectively these mechanisms contribute to the menstrual irregularities, anovulatory subfertility, and growth of immature follicles seen in PCOS.[2]

Hyperinsulinemia also contributes to PCOS by affecting the pituitary gland and hypothalamus and increasing the production of LH and gonadotropin-releasing hormone. Hyperinsulinemia affects the adipose tissue by increasing adipogenesis and lipogenesis, inhibiting lipolysis, and increasing visceral and subcutaneous fat accumulation.[2]

Hyperandrogenism reduces SHBG levels, leading to a higher free T concentration. In women with PCOS, higher T levels are converted to estrone in adipose tissue. Increased alternation of estrone and estradiol affects follicle growth and increases LH to follicle-stimulating hormone (FSH) ratio, resulting in ovulatory dysfunction.[2]

The pathogenesis of PCOS is complex and influenced by multiple genetic, environmental, and hormonal factors. Obesity, particularly visceral fat accumulation, which is common in patients with PCOS, causes low-grade chronic inflammation, resulting in hyperinsulinemia, insulin resistance, and hyperandrogenism. However, nonobese patients with PCOS may also develop visceral fat accumulation, which is proinflammatory, thus leading to metabolic irregularities.[2]

Saturated fatty acids and vitamin D have been associated with the pathogenesis of PCOS. Saturated fatty acids reduce insulin sensitivity by triggering the inflammatory pathway. Vitamin D deficiency exacerbates PCOS and its comorbidities by decreasing insulin sensitivity in adipose tissue and skeletal muscles, downregulating the antimül-lerian hormone (AMH) promoter, and increasing insulin resistance via a proinflammatory response.[2]

There may exist a correlation between stress and PCOS. Stress is a proinflammatory process. Chronic stress can alter adipocytes, immune cells, inflammatory cytokines, cortisol levels, gluconeogenesis by the liver, insulin levels, AMH, and sex hormone levels, all of which are significant in the pathogenesis of PCOS.[2]

PCOS has been associated with multiple genetic alternations. Nineteen risk gene loci, including *THADA, ESHR, INS-VNTR,* and *DENND1A,* have been identified in the neuroendocrine, metabolic, and reproductive pathways.[3] There is a causal link between PCOS, and genetic variants associated with body mass index (BMI), fasting insulin, menopause timing, depression, and male pattern baldness. In addition to genetic foci, PCOS has also been linked to epigenetic mechanisms (inheritable alternations in the genome without changes in DNA sequence). Patients with PCOS have (1) an increased expression of LH receptor on the theca cell surface, resulting in increased steroidogenesis; (2) an increased gene expression and overproduction of the enzyme (epoxide hydrolase 1 EPHX1), reducing the transformation of T to estradiol[2]; and (3) alterations in granulosa cell receptors affecting hyperandrogenism and ovarian function.

PCOS has a component of transgenerational transmission. Daughters born to mothers with PCOS have a 5-fold higher risk of developing PCOS, possibly due to prenatal androgen excess and early androgen exposure.[3] The known genetic risk alleles account for less than 10% of PCOS heritability, suggesting that other etiologic risk factors play a role in PCOS development.

DIAGNOSIS

PCOS is a syndrome and not a uniform disease process; therefore, there is no single clinical finding or laboratory test that confirms the diagnosis. The 2003 Rotterdam criteria[4] are widely accepted for evaluating patients with possible PCOS; they consist of 3 criteria: (1) oligomenorrhea or amenorrhea, (2) clinical or biochemical evidence of androgen excess, and (3) polycystic ovaries on transvaginal ultrasonography. Patients designated as having PCOS must have 2 of these 3 criteria. Amenorrhea is usually secondary, defined as menstrual cycles of less than 21 or greater than 35 days 3 years postmenarche. Clinical hyperandrogenism includes hirsutism, acne, and male-pattern alopecia.

The advent of improved ultrasound technology has resulted in a change in the ovarian morphology criteria, previously based on ovarian size and weight, and now specifying the actual number and size of cysts/follicles. Ultrasonography should be transvaginal and use high resolution. For a diagnosis of PCOS, patients should have at least 25 small follicles (2 to 9 mm) in the entire ovary. Ovarian size at 10 mL remains the threshold between normal and increased. **Table 2** reviews a complete differential diagnosis and indications for additional testing.

There is incomplete agreement regarding the optimal biochemical test for androgen excess. Unlike total T, the measurement of free T is unaffected by the level of SHBG. There are recommendations for checking either free T or total T or calculation of the androgen index (total T/SHBG $\times$ 100).[4,5] Additional testing includes dehydroepiandrosterone and androstenedione if suspicion is high for an androgen-secreting tumor. There are strong recommendations *not* to pursue testing for AMH, FSH, or insulin levels.[5]

Table 2
Differential diagnosis of polycystic ovarian syndrome

Diagnosis	Testing	Diagnostic Workup[a]
Congenital adrenal hyperplasia (late-onset) (21-hydroxylase deficiency)	17-Hydroxy-progesterone	• 17-Hydroxy-progesterone • ACTH stimulation test • Genetic testing when biochemical tests are borderline and before conception
Androgen-secreting tumor (adrenal or ovarian)	Serum T and DHEA (markedly elevated)	• Total testosterone • DHEAS • 17-Hydroxy-progesterone • Rule out Cushing syndrome (see later) • IGF-1
Cushing syndrome	24-h UFC or overnight DST	Initial screening test • Late-night salivary cortisol (2 measurements) OR 24-h UFC excretion (2 measurements) OR overnight 1 mg DST Confirmatory tests • ACTH • CRH or desmopressin test • Imaging if indicated
Hypogonadotropic hypogonadism	Diagnosis of exclusion	• Serum testosterone • Pituitary hormone levels • GnRH stimulation test • Genetic testing before conception

Abbreviations: ACTH, Adrenocorticotropic Hormone; CRH, Corticotrophin-releasing hormone; DHEA, dehydroepiandrosterone; DHEAS, dehydroepiandrosterone sulfate; DST, dexamethasone suppression test; GnRH, gonadotropin-releasing hormone; TSH, Thyroid stimulating hormone; UFC, urinary free cortisol.
[a] TSH, prolactin, and, when appropriate, pregnancy test should be done on all patients as initial laboratory screening tests.

The diagnostic criteria for hyperandrogenism, initially limited to clinical findings only, were widened to include biochemical evidence of androgen excess to facilitate the diagnosis, because clinical signs of hyperandrogenism are only seen in 60% of patients with PCOS.[6] In addition, despite a universally accepted visual scoring system for assessing hirsutism (Ferriman-Gallway score[7]), hirsutism is difficult to quantitate, varies by race and ethnicity, and may be masked by procedures patients undergo to treat it (shaving, chemical removal or bleaching, electrolysis, laser removal). There are also visual scores for androgenic alopecia (AA) (the Hamilton-Norwood classification system for male pattern AA and the Ludwig grade system for female pattern AA) but none for acne.[7] Acanthosis nigricans may be seen in PCOS because it is a clinical manifestation of IR and may aid in diagnosis.

In the past, serum LH/FSH ratio was used for the diagnosis of PCOS. Because the LH and FSH hormone levels can vary in women with PCOS and their effects on oocyte maturity and fertilization is uncertain and variable, the Rotterdam European Society of Human Reproduction and Embryology/American Society of Reproductive Medicine (ESHRE/ASRM)-sponsored PCOS consensus panel does not recommend the measurement of serum LH and FSH ratios for the clinical diagnosis of PCOS.[8] LH levels are useful in basic science research, and additional studies are needed to clarify the clinical relevance of LH in PCOS, which may also pave the way for LH-related treatment options.

The diagnosis of PCOS in adolescents and perimenopausal women is problematic. In the former, menstrual cycles are often anovulatory for the first several years following menarche. In addition, adolescents often have large polycystic ovaries on ultrasonography, so using this criterion for diagnosis is unreliable.[3] Thus, in the absence of adolescent-specific criteria, anovulation should not be considered until greater than 2 years postmenarche, and ultrasound assessment should be delayed until 8 years postmenarche.[1,3,9] For older women, menstrual cycles may become more regular as they approach perimenopause, and women with PCOS may complete menopause at a later age; thus, the diagnosis may be more challenging to make in women in their postreproductive years.[3,9]

Because PCOS is familial and polygenic, the phenotypic expression will vary based on genetic penetrance and environmental factors. Four distinct phenotypes have been identified (see **Table 1**), although the clinical utility of these designations outside the research setting is unclear.[1] Along with the diagnosis of PCOS, screening for its associated diseases should be undertaken and appropriate treatment initiated (see later discussion). The prevalence of phenotypes varies considerably based on population, race, and ethnicity. Phenotypes A and B are seen frequently in obese women and are associated with more hyperandrogenism, insulin resistance, and worse cardiometabolic profiles. The prevalence of metabolic syndrome prevalence is lowest in phenotype D.[1] The different diagnostic criteria and varying phenotypes may contribute to the difficulty in recognizing and diagnosing this disorder.

CLINICAL IMPLICATIONS AND COMORBIDITIES

The most common abnormalities associated with PCOS are menstrual disorders, infertility, obesity, type 2 diabetes mellitus (T2DM), and the metabolic syndrome.[10]

PCOS has been associated with multiple reproductive comorbidities. Women with PCOS experience higher rates of infertility; they have an increased prevalence of adverse pregnancy outcomes, including gestational hypoglycemia, gestational diabetes, perinatal death, preeclampsia, pregnancy-induced hypertension, preterm delivery, cesarean delivery, and miscarriages.[11]

PCOS is a metabolic and not a gynecologic disease. IR is the critical underlying pathology of PCOS, resulting in a significant (3–7 times) increase in the risk of developing T2DM. IR is independent of obesity but may be worsened by it. Overweight or obese adult and adolescent women with PCOS have significantly higher total cholesterol, low-density lipoprotein, and triglyceride levels and significantly lower high-density lipoprotein levels.[11] Pregnant women with PCOS have higher systolic blood pressure when compared with nonpregnant women with PCOS. It is thought that patients with PCOS may have an increased prevalence of cardiovascular disease (CVD) and are at significantly increased risk for coronary heart disease and stroke; further studies are required to establish this association.[11]

Once the diagnosis of PCOS has been made, patients should be screened regularly for the development of T2DM, obesity, and hyperlipidemia. Again, the optimal screening test for T2DM is not agreed upon because the test with the best sensitivity and specificity, the 2-hour oral glucose tolerance test, is not routinely performed in most offices and is more cumbersome for patients. Fasting blood glucose or HbA_{1c} are acceptable options for most patients.[9] Obtaining insulin levels is not recommended in the evaluation of PCOS.

Patients with PCOS have an increased prevalence of metabolic syndrome and nonalcoholic fatty liver disease (NAFLD). Vitamin D deficiency in patients with PCOS worsens fasting blood glucose and fasting insulin; correcting the vitamin D deficiency improves insulin sensitivity. Patients with PCOS also have lower vitamin D levels, further exacerbating insulin resistance.[11]

PCOS negatively influences the quality of life measured by the health-related quality of life (HRQoL) index.[12] Studies have found that hyperandrogenism, menstruation abnormalities, BMI, and body weight issues have the strongest impact on quality of life.[11] Patients with PCOS have significantly higher depressive and anxiety symptoms scores, along with low self-esteem (related to issues of body image as well as potential infertility) and suboptimal sexual function.

In addition, adult women with PCOS have an increased risk of developing obstructive sleep apnea (OSA) compared with reproductive-age women of similar age. The risk for sleep disturbances in PCOS increases with age and adiposity. OSA in PCOS is associated with worsening metabolic parameters, anxiety, and depression.[13]

Finally, due to the relative excess of estrogen over progesterone and the lack of regular uterine lining shedding seen with regular menses, patients with PCOS have a 2.7 times higher risk for developing endometrial cancer, but not breast or ovarian cancer.[11,14]

MANAGEMENT

The management of patients with PCOS is varied and ultimately dictated by the patient's desired clinical outcomes. These outcomes may include weight loss, regression of hirsutism, regulation of menstrual cycles, and obtainment of pregnancy. In addition, attention should be paid to addressing metabolic risks and abnormalities (which vary by phenotype), lowering the risk of endometrial hyperplasia, and improving mental health. Despite the menstrual irregularly, most women with PCOS become pregnant without medical intervention, so the inclusion of contraception in treatment options should not be dismissed.

For all patients with PCOS, regardless of their clinical goals and preferences, lifestyle interventions should be initiated. Weight loss, dietary modification, and increased exercise should be part of first-line therapy for all patients. These interventions result in decreased androgen levels and IR, with as little as 5% to 10% weight loss resulting in improved CVD risk; the effect of lifestyle changes on ovulatory function, menstrual cycles, and fertility is minimal or uncertain.[15]

For hirsutism, many women use mechanical means, including local hair removal via plucking or shaving, bleaching, electrolysis, laser destruction of the follicles (epilation), and regular, long-term application of an ornithine decarboxylase inhibitor/eflornithine cream.[10] These interventions are usually required even when medications are used to achieve the desired cosmetic effect. Spironolactone, an antiandrogen, is explicitly used to target clinical hyperandrogenism features at doses starting at 50 mg daily and increasing to 100 mg twice daily. Because this drug is a known teratogen, it must be used in combination with a reliable method of contraception.[14] Other antiandrogens that may be used include ketoconazole and flutamide.[10]

Acne may be managed as in any other patient, using topical benzoyl, topical or oral antibiotics, and isotretinoin.[16] The use of combined estrogen/progesterone contraceptives, with or without specific acne treatment, will also improve this clinical manifestation of hyperandrogenism.

Menstrual irregularities can be managed with hormonal contraception—oral combination or progestin-only pills, combination patches, cyclic progesterone, or a progesterone-containing implant or intrauterine device. All these methods will provide endometrial protection, and all except cyclic progesterone will also provide reliable contraception. Only estrogen-containing products will improve hyperandrogenism but may also increase CVD risk via increased risk for venous thromboembolism and adverse effects on cholesterol profiles.[14] Choosing a preparation with a lower dose of ethinylestradiol (30 μg or less) and a progestin with lower androgenic activity (norgestimate, drospirenone) can mitigate some of these effects.[9]

For patients desiring pregnancy, lifestyle modification, especially in women with obesity, may be all that is required. For ovulation induction, letrozole, an aromatase inhibitor, has replaced clomiphene as the first-line treatment, because recent data favor it over clomiphene for live birth and pregnancy rates and reduced time to pregnancy.[17] If letrozole is not available or if the cost is prohibitive, clomiphene is still very effective as a single agent or in combination with metformin. A trial of gonadotrophins may be considered for patients who fail to conceive with these 2 agents. Patients with PCOS who fail to conceive with ovulation induction medications may opt for in vitro fertilization and embryo transfer.

Metformin, a biguanide used in T2DM, has modest effectiveness in improving pregnancy rates in patients with PCOS through its mechanism against IR. Other medications currently being studied that show promise for patients with PCOS are thiazolidinedione, statins, vitamin D, fibroblast growth factor, and glucagonlike peptide (GLP-1) agonists.[10,18]

Bariatric surgery should be considered part of the treatment in morbidly obese patients with PCOS with metabolic syndrome.

SUMMARY

PCOS is a complex, familial, polygenetic metabolic condition. The Rotterdam criteria are commonly used to diagnose PCOS. Lifestyle changes are the first-line treatment of PCOS. Treatment options for menstrual irregularities and hirsutism are based on the clinical goals and preferences of the patient. Along with treating the symptoms of PCOS, it is essential to screen and treat the comorbid conditions commonly associated with PCOS, including T2DM, obesity, NAFLD, hyperlipidemia, OSA, anxiety, depression, infertility, and vitamin D deficiency.

CLINICS CARE POINTS

- PCOS is diagnosed using the Rotterdam criteria.
- Weight loss, dietary modification, and increased exercise is the first-line therapy for all patients.
- The treatment of symptoms, acne, hirsuitism or menstrual irregularities, is based on patients desired clinical outcomes.
- Screen and treat the comorbid conditions commonly associated with PCOS.

DISCLOSURE

The authors do not have any commercial or financial conflicts of interest.

FUNDING SOURCE

No funding sources for all authors.

REFERENCES

1. Neven ACH, Laven J, Teede HJ, et al. A summary on polycystic ovary syndrome: diagnostic criteria, prevalence, clinical manifestations, and management according to the latest international guidelines. Semin Reprod Med 2018;36(1):5–12 (In eng).
2. Sadeghi HM, Adeli I, Calina D, et al. Polycystic ovary syndrome: a comprehensive review of pathogenesis, management, and drug repurposing. Int J Mol Sci 2022;23(2) (In eng).
3. Hoeger KM, Dokras A, Piltonen T. Update on PCOS: consequences, challenges, and guiding treatment. J Clin Endocrinol Metab 2021;106(3):e1071–83 (In eng).
4. Al Wattar BH, Fisher M, Bevington L, et al. Clinical practice guidelines on the diagnosis and management of polycystic ovary syndrome: a systematic review and quality assessment study. J Clin Endocrinol Metab 2021;106(8):2436–46 (In eng).
5. Teede HJ, Misso ML, Costello MF, et al. Recommendations from the international evidence-based guideline for the assessment and management of polycystic ovary syndrome. Fertil Steril 2018;110(3):364–79 (In eng).
6. Barthelmess EK, Naz RK. Polycystic ovary syndrome: current status and future perspective. Front Biosci (Elite Ed 2014;6(1):104–19 (In eng).
7. Yildiz BO, Bolour S, Woods K, et al. Visually scoring hirsutism. Hum Reprod Update 2010;16(1):51–64 (In eng).
8. The Rotterdam EAsPcwg. Revised 2003 consensus on diagnostic criteria and long-term health risks related to polycystic ovary syndrome (PCOS). Hum Reprod 2004;19(1):41–7.
9. Huddleston HG, Dokras A. Diagnosis and Treatment of Polycystic Ovary Syndrome. JAMA 2022;327(3):274–5 (In eng).
10. Bednarska S, Siejka A. The pathogenesis and treatment of polycystic ovary syndrome: What's new? Adv Clin Exp Med 2017;26(2):359–67 (In eng).
11. Gilbert EW, Tay CT, Hiam DS, et al. Comorbidities and complications of polycystic ovary syndrome: An overview of systematic reviews. Clin Endocrinol (Oxf) 2018;89(6):683–99 (In eng).
12. Cronin L, Guyatt G, Griffith L, et al. Development of a health-related quality-of-life questionnaire (PCOSQ) for women with polycystic ovary syndrome (PCOS). J Clin Endocrinol Metab 1998;83(6):1976–87 (In eng).
13. Sam S, Ehrmann DA. Pathogenesis and Consequences of Disordered Sleep in PCOS. Clin Med Insights Reprod Health 2019;13. https://doi.org/10.1177/1179558119871269. 1179558119871269. (In eng).
14. McCartney CR, Marshall JC. CLINICAL PRACTICE. Polycystic Ovary Syndrome. N Engl J Med 2016;375(1):54–64 (In eng).
15. Lim SS, Hutchison SK, Van Ryswyk E, et al. Lifestyle changes in women with polycystic ovary syndrome. Cochrane Database Syst Rev 2019;3(3):Cd007506 (In eng).
16. Conway G, Dewailly D, Diamanti-Kandarakis E, et al. The polycystic ovary syndrome: a position statement from the European Society of Endocrinology. Eur J Endocrinol 2014;171(4):P1–29 (In eng).
17. Wang R, Li W, Bordewijk EM, et al. First-line ovulation induction for polycystic ovary syndrome: an individual participant data meta-analysis. Hum Reprod Update 2019;25(6):717–32 (In eng).
18. Jin P, Xie Y. Treatment strategies for women with polycystic ovary syndrome. Gynecol Endocrinol 2018;34(4):272–7 (In eng).

Abnormal Uterine Bleeding

Elena Lebduska, MD, MS[a], Deidra Beshear, MD[b],
Brielle M. Spataro, MD, MS[c],*

KEYWORDS

- Abnormal uterine bleeding • Heavy menstrual bleeding • Fibroids • Polyps

KEY POINTS

- Abnormal uterine bleeding (AUB) is defined as bleeding coming from the uterus that is abnormal in frequency, duration, volume, and/or regularity.
- Causes of AUB can be classified using PALM-COIEN system. PALM refers to anatomic causes (polyps, adenomyosis, leiomyomas, and malignancy). COIEN refers to nonstructural causes (coagulopathies, ovulatory disorders, iatrogenic, endometrial, and not otherwise classified).
- A comprehensive history and physical should be performed including a bimanual and pelvic examination. All patients should get a pregnancy test and complete blood count (CBC) with platelets.
- Transvaginal ultrasound is usually the imaging of choice in evaluating structural etiologies.
- Medical treatments are based on etiology but can include levonorgestrel intrauterine devices, oral contraceptive pills, tranexamic acid, and nonsteroidal anti-inflammatory drugs. Surgical options vary by patients' desire for future fertility but can include dilation and curettage, endometrial ablation, and hysterectomy.

INTRODUCTION

Abnormal uterine bleeding (AUB) is a common symptom affecting up to a third of premenopausal women leading to office visits with primary care physicians and ob-gyns as well as emergency room visits.[1] Although some women have mild symptoms, others experience significant effects on quality of life, financial losses from decreased work productivity, and poor health outcomes along with significantly increased health care utilization.[1]

Chronic AUB, as defined by the International Federation of Gynecology and Obstetrics (FIGO) classification, includes any bleeding from the uterus that is abnormal in

The authors have no conflicts of interest to disclose.
[a] University of Colorado, UC Heath Internal Medicine - Lowry, 8111 E. Lowry boulevard, Denver, CO 80230, USA; [b] University of Kentucky, 1000 S. Limestone, Lexington, KY 40536, USA; [c] University of Pittsburgh
* Corresponding author. UPMC Shadyside Hospital, North Tower Room 311, 5230 Centre Avenue, Pittsburgh, PA 15232.
E-mail address: spatarob2@upmc.edu

Table 1 Normal parameters of menstruation[3]	
Frequency of Menstruation	**24–38 Days**
Duration	Less than or equal to 8 d
Variation in cycle length	Shortest to longest cycle variation 7–9 d

frequency, duration, volume, and/or regularity that is present the majority of the prior 6 months. Acute AUB is defined as an episode of heavy bleeding that requires immediate attention in the opinion of the treating physician. This can be in the setting of chronic AUB or happen in the absence of preexisting AUB.[2]

Normal menstrual bleeding is defined by bleeding that occurs every 24 to 38 days, lasing less than 8 days, with cycle variation less than 7 to 9 days (**Table 1**). Amenorrhea refers to no bleeding for 3 months in women with regular periods and no bleeding for 6 months for women with irregular periods. Periods happening more than 38 days apart are termed infrequent. Frequent periods occur less than 28 days between cycles. Prolonged menstrual bleeding occurs for greater than 8 days. Irregular periods refer to cycle variation of greater than 8 to 10 days.[2] Intermenstrual bleeding refers to bleeding that occurs between menstrual cycles (**Table 2**). Period volume is determined by patients.[3] Heavy menstrual bleeding is defined as excessive menstrual loss that interferes with physical, social, emotional, or material quality of life.[4] The use of imprecise terms including menorrhagia, metrorrhagia, oligomenorrhea, and dysfunctional uterine bleeding are now discouraged.[2,3]

FIGO also introduced the PALM-COIEN system to classify the causes of AUB in reproductive years. PALM refers to structural causes (polyps, adenomyosis, leiomyomas, and malignancy). COIEN refers to nonstructural causes (coagulopathies, ovulatory disorders, iatrogenic, endometrial, and not otherwise classified)[2] (**Table 3**).

EVALUATION
History and Physical Examination

A thorough history and physical examination are paramount in identifying the etiology of AUB with such a broad differential diagnosis. A medical history should focus on a description of the bleeding pattern, including regularity, duration, frequency, and volume. The patient should be asked about frequency of changing pads/tampons and passage of clots. Although different patients change pads/tampons at different frequencies given personal preference, in general more than two pads in an hour is considered to be a concerning amount of bleeding. Further history should consist of the presence of pain, any underlying bleeding disorders, sexual history, menstrual history, family history with specific attention to bleeding disorders, and an extensive medication review including herbal supplements. Certain bleeding patterns can be associated with specific conditions. Intermenstrual bleeding is more commonly seen with structural abnormalities such as an endometrial polyp or submucosal leiomyoma, whereas irregular bleeding patterns tend to be associated with nonstructural etiologies such as ovulatory dysfunction.[1]

First, it needs to be confirmed that the bleeding is coming from the uterus. Any part of the female genital tract can bleed (cervix, vagina, and vulva).[1] Bleeding may also be from a non-gynecologic source such as the rectum or urethra. A pelvic examination, including inspection, speculum examination, and bimanual will help to discern the actual source of the blood and should be performed in any patient with AUB.[1]

Table 2 Abnormal uterine bleeding patterns[3]	
Amenorrhea	**No Bleeding**
Infrequent periods	Cycles > 38 d
Frequent periods	<24 d
Prolonged	>8 d
Irregular	Shortest to longest cycle variation >8–10 d
Intermenstrual bleeding	Bleeding between cycles

Special attention should also be paid to body mass index (BMI) as one greater than 30 kg/m^2 has been shown to increase risk of endometrial hyperplasia or malignancy fourfold.[5] Hemodynamic stability should be assessed by looking at blood pressure and heart rate. The presence of pallor could indicate anemia. It is important to note dermatologic findings such as acne and hirsutism which may suggest polycystic ovarian syndrome (PCOS) as well as petechiae and ecchymosis that could represent signs of a bleeding disorder. A thorough thyroid examination should be performed to assess for abnormalities.

Laboratory Evaluation

A pregnancy test should be performed as an initial step in the evaluation of AUB. Additional tests should include a complete blood count with platelets and ferritin level. Ferritin can be low even in the setting of normal hemoglobin, indicating iron deficiency. Other workup may include thyroid-stimulating hormone level, prolactin, and cervical cancer screening if not up to date, testing for *Chlamydia trachomatis,* and further testing for coagulopathy if history is suggestive of an underlying bleeding disorder. All patients who are 45 years or older presenting with AUB should undergo endometrial sampling. Women under 45 years of age experiencing AUB with a BMI over 30, a history of unopposed estrogen exposure or failure of medication management should also proceed with endometrial biopsy.[6]

Imaging

Transvaginal ultrasound (TVUS) is the optimal initial imaging test of the uterus to assess AUB. If regular menstrual cycles are present, it is best to perform ultrasonography on days 4 to 6 of the cycle for optimal visualization of the endometrium for structural abnormalities as the endometrial lining is at its thinnest on these days.[7] TVUS is

Table 3 PALM-COIEN classification for causes of abnormal uterine bleeding[2,3]	
P	Polyps
A	Adenomyosis
L	Leiomyoma
M	Malignancy
C	Coagulopathies
O	Ovulatory disorders
E	Endometrial disorders
I	Iatrogenic
N	Not otherwise classified

an important diagnostic tool to exclude the structural abnormalities (PALM) in the PALM-COEIN system. The sensitivity and specificity of TVUS for endometrial pathology are only 56% and 73%, respectively; therefore, if there is not an identifiable cause of AUB on TVUS or visualization is suboptimal, further imaging may be required.[8] Saline infusion sonohysterography (the infusion of sterile saline into the endometrial cavity, whereas transvaginal ultrasonography is performed) is better at detecting intracavitary pathology with sensitivity rates between 94% and 100%.[7,8] The use of MRI is not recommended as a first-line imaging modality for AUB evaluation. MRI may be beneficial, however, for localizing leiomyomas and diagnosing adenomyosis.[8]

Management

In the setting of acute heavy menstrual bleeding of any etiology, patients should be assessed for hemodynamic instability and transfused with blood products as needed. After the patient is hemodynamically stable, options for treatment include intravenous conjugated equine estrogen, oral combined oral contraceptives, oral medroxyprogesterone acetate, and oral or intravenous tranexamic acid. Once the acute episode has resolved, although etiology is being investigated, options for treatment include levonorgestrel intrauterine systems, oral contraceptives, progesterone (oral or intramuscular), tranexamic acid, and nonsteroidal anti-inflammatory drugs (NSAIDs).[9]

Differential Diagnosis

Once a uterine source of the bleeding is confirmed there are a few different ways to approach the cause of the abnormal bleeding. In premenopausal women, this differentiation can be done by first classifying the bleeding as ovulatory versus anovulatory.[10] Ovulatory bleeding refers to bleeding that occurs despite a normal ovulation cycle.[10] Women with ovulatory bleeding may experience very heavy periods or intermenstrual spotting. Examples of ovulatory bleeding include uterine structural issues (fibroids) or a coagulation disorder (Von Willebrand's Disease [vWD]). Anovulatory bleeding refers to bleeding that occurs due to an abnormal hormonal cycle that inhibits regular ovulation. Women with anovulatory bleeding may experience periods that are irregular, infrequent, or absent. Examples of anovulatory bleeding include PCOS and hyperprolactinemia (**Table 4**) and are further discussed in the Ovulatory dysfunction section below.

Menses that are absent, infrequent, or irregular signify anovulation.[10] Most of the cases of anovulation are due to hormonal irregularities. Understanding the interplay of hormones involved in normal female ovulatory cycle is key to evaluate dysregulation.

Table 4	
Differential diagnosis of abnormal uterine bleeding	
Ovulatory	**Anovulatory**
Bleeding disorders	Functional hypothalamic amenorrhea
Structural lesions	Hyperprolactinemia
	Polycystic ovarian syndrome
	Perimenopause
	Medications
	Thyroid hormone dysregulation
	Pregnancy

Normal Hormonal Menstrual Cycle and Physiology

The hypothalamic–pituitary–ovarian (HPO) axis is a regulated feedback loop integral to normal menstruation. Gonadotropin-releasing hormone (GnRH) is produced by the hypothalamus. GnRH pulses stimulate the anterior pituitary to produce luteinizing hormone (LH) and follicle-stimulating hormone (FSH).[11] LH and FSH stimulation cause the ovaries to produce estrogen and progesterone. A variety of other hormones also influence the HPO axis especially prolactin, dopamine, and thyroid. Other factors such as stress and caloric intake can also affect the HPO axis, whereas changes in sex hormone-binding globulin (SHBG) affects bioavailable levels of androgens and to a lesser extent estrogens in the blood.

A normal menstrual cycle can be divided into two parts: a follicular phase and a luteal phase. The follicular phase started on the first day of menses (day 1) and lasts until ovulation occurs (10–14 days later).[11] During the follicular phase, FSH levels rise and a dominant follicle emerges and secretes estrogen. This increase in estrogen during the follicular phase leads to growth of the endometrium (proliferative phase of the endometrium). Initially, estrogen results in negative feedback on LH, but then mid cycle this switches to positive feedback and leads to the LH surge.[11] The LH surge leads to release of the oocyte hours later leading to ovulation. The luteal phase starts after ovulation and is associated with the secretory phase of the endometrium. After ovulation, the dominant follicle becomes the corpus luteum and progesterone (and to a lesser extent) is released. Although estrogen is the dominant hormone during the follicular phase, progesterone is the dominant hormone during the luteal phase and has inhibitory effects on the endometrium. If the oocyte is not fertilized the corpus luteum degenerates and causes a fall in estrogen and progesterone leading to menses.[11]

In patients with AUB caused by anovulatory bleeding no egg is released. As no egg is released, there is no corpus luteum to make progesterone. If there is no progesterone then there is no inhibition of endometrial growth. With no rise in progesterone and therefore no subsequent fall of progesterone, no menses occurs.

PALM-COEIN classification

The FIGO published standardized definitions and classifications for menstrual disorders in 2011. This system, known as PALM-COEIN, classifies AUB in the reproductive-aged, nonpregnant patient into structural (polyp, adenomyosis, leiomyoma, malignancy, and hyperplasia) and nonstructural (coagulopathy, ovulatory dysfunction, endometrial, iatrogenic, not otherwise classified) causes.[12] In conjunction with a complete patient history along with appropriate laboratory evaluation and/or imaging, the PALM-COEIN classification allows for a systematic approach to AUB. The structural etiologies (PALM) require imaging or histopathology for diagnosis.[2]

Structural/PALM

Polyps. AUB may occur in up to 67% of reproductive-aged women with endometrial polyps.[13] The most common presenting symptom is intermenstrual bleeding. The lifetime prevalence of endometrial polyps ranges from 7.8% to 34.9% and seems to increase with age.[14] Polyps are diagnosed with transvaginal ultrasonography, hysteroscopy, or endometrial biopsy; however, some polyps can be visualized protruding through the cervical os on physical examination. Polyps have fewer hormone receptors than typical endometrium, therefore are less responsive to the cyclic changes of menstruation.[15] Most endometrial polyps are benign, with the incidence of malignancy in premenopausal women at 1.7%, up to 5.4% in postmenopausal women.[16,17] Owing to this slight risk of malignancy, polyps are often removed via hysteroscopy and sent for pathologic examination. Polypectomy has been shown to reduce 75% to 100% of AUB in patients with endometrial polyps.[8]

Adenomyosis. Endometrial tissue present in the myometrium is known as adenomyosis. Predicted prevalence rates range from 5% to 70% of women.[18] Risk factors for the development of adenomyosis include multiparity and uterine procedures such as cesarean delivery or endometrial curettage.[19] Many patients with adenomyosis are asymptomatic; however, patients with symptoms report heavy, painful, and/or prolonged menstrual cycles. Physical examination may reveal an enlarged uterus. Diagnosis can be made with transvaginal ultrasonography or MRI. MRI has increased sensitivity (77%) and specificity (89%) for diagnosis of adenomyosis compared with that of ultrasound at 72% sensitivity and 81% specificity.[19] Endometrial biopsy is not useful in the diagnosis of adenomyosis. Medical therapies are the first-line treatments for adenomyosis. Options include suppressive hormonal treatments such as levonorgestrel intrauterine device (LNG IUD), continuous combined oral contraceptive hormones, high-dose progestins, selective estrogen receptor modulators (SERMs), danazol, and temporary use of gonadotropin releasing hormone (GnRH) agonists, with the LNG IUD being the most effective medical therapy for adenomyosis.[20] If medical therapies fail then surgical and interventional techniques are considered. Conservative surgical options require a high degree of skill if preservation of fertility is desired. Both uterine artery embolization (UAE) and MRI-guided focused ultrasound (MgFUS) seem to be promising interventional treatments for adenomyosis, although more comparative data are needed.[21,22] Hysterectomy remains the definitive therapy for adenomyosis when medical treatment or less invasive interventions have failed.

Leiomyomas. Leiomyomas (also called fibroids or myomas) are benign tumors arising from the uterine myometrium. They are the most common pelvic tumors, with an estimated lifetime prevalence of 70% in Caucasian women and 80% in African American women.[23] Prevalence increases with age. Most leiomyomas are asymptomatic, but heavy, painful, or prolonged menstrual bleeding can be present. Larger leiomyomas may be associated with pelvic pressure, urinary frequency, or bowel symptoms. Clinical findings may include an enlarged uterus on physical examination. Pelvic ultrasound is the standard confirmatory test. The FIGO classification of leiomyoma location helps define the relationship of the leiomyomas to the endometrium, myometrium, and uterine serosa.[12] Submucosal leiomyomas are most likely to cause AUB regardless of size.[12] MRI, hysteroscopy, or saline-infusion sonography can be performed if clarification of submucosal leiomyoma location is needed, especially if interventions such as myomectomy, uterine fibroid embolization, or ablation are being considered.

Asymptomatic leiomyomas do not require treatment unless they are associated with fertility concerns. In the case of leiomyomas presenting with AUB alone, medical therapies are very effective. Options may include NSAIDs, tranexamic acid, contraceptive hormones, GnRH agonists, danazol, aromatase inhibitors, and SERMs.[23] NSAIDs suppress prostaglandin production and increases thromboxane A2, increasing platelet aggregation, vasoconstriction and decreasing blood loss. Tranexamic acid blocks plasminogen-binding sites, preventing fibrin and clot degradation.[24] In premenopausal women with heavy menstrual bleeding due to fibroids a combination medication is available. This medication contains three ingredients: relugolix, estradiol, and norethindrone acetate (Myfembree) and can be used for up to 24 months. In patients experiencing bulk symptoms with or without AUB, surgical intervention may be required. If fertility is to be preserved, several uterine-sparing options can be considered. Those procedures include hysteroscopic myomectomy, UAE, MgFUS, or laparoscopic radiofrequency ablation. For submucosal leiomyomas, hysteroscopic myomectomy may be the best option for AUB. Endometrial ablation can be performed in patients with leiomyomas with a normal uterine cavity when fertility is no longer of concern. Hysterectomy may need to be considered if the above treatment options fail.[23]

Malignancy and hyperplasia. The most common symptom of endometrial cancer is AUB; however, malignancy of the vagina or cervix may also cause abnormal bleeding. Therefore, it is important to examine the patient including Pap test screening to eliminate these diagnoses. Endometrial hyperplasia is more common than uterine cancer. In 2015, the WHO classification separated this diagnosis into two groups: hyperplasia without atypia and atypical hyperplasia/endometrial intraepithelial neoplasia (EIN).[6] Long-term unopposed estrogen exposure is the primary risk factor. This includes conditions such as PCOS, obesity, or improper administration of exogenous hormone therapy. Bleeding patterns in patients with endometrial malignancy are highly variable. Imaging alone cannot diagnose these conditions; therefore, endometrial biopsy or endometrial curettage is required for definitive tissue diagnosis.[8] The American College of Obstetricians and Gynecologists recommend that all women with AUB older than 45 years and women younger than 45 years who have additional risk factors for EIN undergo endometrial sampling.[25]

For endometrial hyperplasia without atypia, first-line treatment is LNG IUD. Low-dose oral and injectable progestin is also an acceptable treatment option. Hysterectomy should be reserved for patients who do not want to preserve fertility and who progress to atypia or carcinoma during follow-up, fail to respond to 12 months of medical therapy, or relapse after completion of medical treatment. The preferred treatment of patients with endometrial hyperplasia with atypia is hysterectomy.[26] Treatment of endometrial cancer depends on stage but often consists of hysterectomy, with radiation and chemotherapy, and is beyond the scope of this review.

Coagulopathy. As many as 20% of women with AUB have a bleeding disorder, the most common being vWD.[25] Most coagulopathies are inherited and along with vWD include hemophilia type A (factor VIII deficiency) and type B (factor IX deficiency), platelet dysfunction, and various other factor deficiencies.[27] Coagulopathy should be considered in patients with heavy, prolonged bleeding from an early reproductive age, a history of excessive bruising, gum/dental bleeding, epistaxis, severe surgical bleeding, and/or a family history of a bleeding disorder.[27] If patient's history is suggestive of a bleeding disorder, next steps for evaluation would include a complete blood cell count including platelets, prothrombin time, and activated partial thromboplastin time. Further laboratory testing would be indicated if initial laboratory values are abnormal.[27]

If there is high suspicion for an underlying coagulopathy consultation with a hematologist is recommended and targeted treatment may be an option. Desmopressin intranasally, intravenously, or subcutaneously can be used for vWD. In addition, recombinant factor VIII and von Willebrand factor may also be available and required to control severe hemorrhage. NSAIDs should be avoided in patients with possible coagulopathies.[9]

Surgical treatment options are available for AUB in patients who have a contraindication or are unresponsive to medical therapy. They include dilation and curettage, endometrial ablation, UAE, and hysterectomy. These treatment options are depend on the patients' desires for fertility.[9]

Hormonal Causes

Ovulatory dysfunction

Ovulatory dysfunction should be suspected as an etiology of AUB in women with a history of secondary amenorrhea or when menstrual cycles are spaced more than 38 days apart.[8] Infrequent or absent ovulation during the first few years after menarche and during perimenopause is common and may not indicate underlying pathology. Refer to **Table 4** for the most common causes of anovulation.

Functional hypothalamic amenorrhea

Functional hypothalamic amenorrhea (FHA) refers to absent periods due to suppression of the HPO axis. The suppression of GnRH pulses from the hypothalamus results in lower levels of LH and FSH from the anterior pituitary.[28] Reduced LH and FSH lead to impaired folliculogenesis and a reduced estrogen state. The suppression of the HPO axis can be caused by excessive exercise, weight loss, stress, and disordered eating.[29]

Women should be evaluated for FHA if their menstrual cycle intervals persistently exceed 45 days of they have 3 months of amenorrhea. Diagnosis should be made only after excluding other causes. History should focus on diet, eating disorders, exercise, weight fluctuations, sleep patterns, stressors, mood, menstrual pattern, and substance abuse. Endocrinologic evaluation should include beta human chorionic gonadotropin (HCG), FSH, LH, estradiol, prolactin, and TSH concentrations. If there are signs of hyperandrogenism an androgen panel should be checked.

Patients should be counseled that despite their menstrual irregularities, they could still become pregnant.[28]

Treatment is focused largely on behavioral change whether that is improving nutrition or decreasing exercise or other stressors. Oral contraceptive pills (OCPs) are not recommended for the sole purpose of regaining menses or improving bone mineral density. Transdermal estrogen can be considered to promote bone health.[28]

Hyperprolactinemia

Elevated prolactin levels lead to inhibition of GnRH release and therefore low levels of LH and FSH and reduced folliculogenesis.[30] Common causes of hyperprolactinemia include pituitary tumors, many common medications, renal disease, untreated hypothyroidism, pregnancy, and breast feeding. Common medication classes causing hyperprolactinemia include antipsychotics, anti-emetics, antidepressants, and opiates. Initial workup should include checking serum prolactin levels. If there is no obvious physiologic cause and the patient is not on any medications that could cause high prolactin levels, MRI of the brain must be performed to assess for a prolactinoma.[31] Dopamine is a main regulator of prolactin, and the treatment of hyperprolactinemia involves dopamine agonists.[30]

Polycystic ovarian syndrome

PCOS is the most common endocrinopathy among reproductive-aged women in the United States.[32] It is a complex syndrome with androgen excess and insulin resistance being hypothesized as main components. It is hypothesized that insulin resistance suppresses synthesis of SHBG and increases adrenal and ovarian synthesis of androgens. Higher levels of androgens in the blood prevent ovulation leading to irregular menses and physical signs of hyperandrogenism. Diagnosis is clinical and based on the Rotterdam criteria. Patients must have two of the three criteria: clinical or chemical findings of hyperandrogenism, irregular menses, or polycystic ovaries.[32]

Treatment is based on whether or not fertility is desired. If patients are actively trying to get pregnant first-line treatment to restore ovulation is letrozole and clomiphene.

Metformin can be used to treat metabolic manifestations and underlying insulin resistance; however, it has not been shown to improve fertility. Restoration of menstrual cycle is usually achieved through hormonal contraception, both combined OCPs and LNG IUD. Restoration of ovulation can be improved with weight loss, and lifestyle modification should be considered first-line therapy in patients who are overweight.[32]

Thyroid hormone dysregulation
Both hyper and hypothyroidism can cause AUB. Hypothyroidism can cause heavy and irregular menstrual bleeding and is likely multifactorial affecting: coagulation, HPO axis dysregulation, and SHBG. Hypothyroidism can affect platelet function and the coagulation cascade leading to excess bleeding. Hypothyroidism causes stimulation of thyrotropin-release hormone (TRH) from the hypothalamus. Increased TRH leads to hyperprolactinemia affecting ovulation. Thyroid hormones also affect levels of SHBG.[33] Hypothyroidism causes decreased levels of SHBG and can cause more frequent, heavy bleeding.[33] Although hyperthyroidism has been less linked to anovulation, it can cause lighter and shorter periods due to increased SHBG and reduced bioavailable androgens and estrogens in the blood.[33] Restoring thyroid hormone levels to their normal range in the blood should restore ovulation and improve AUB.

Perimenopause
AUB has a higher prevalence at the extremes of reproductive life: peri-menarche and perimenopause.[2] During late perimenopause, hormonal dysregulation and anovulation are common. A fall in follicle number causes a subsequent increase in FSH and decreased production of estrogen and progesterone. AUB in perimenopause can include shorter or longer cycles, spotting, and lighter or heavier periods. Treatment depends on whether contraception is needed or not. If pregnancy is a concern hormonal contraception can be used (with added benefit of treatment of vasomotor symptoms associated with perimenopause). If contraception is not desired, NSAIDs, tranexamic acid, or uterine ablation are options.

Medications
A variety of classes of medications may affect ovulation. As listed above many of these medications affect prolactin and the HPO axis.

Endometrial
Endometrial disorders of AUB are due to primary dysfunction of endometrial vasoconstriction, infection, or inflammation. This classification of AUB remains a diagnosis of exclusion when a woman has a structurally normal uterus, normal menstrual cycle, and lack of coagulopathy.[2]

Iatrogenic
Multiple pharmacologic therapies may result in AUB. The most common cause of AUB-I is hormonal contraception such as OCPs, or intrauterine, intramuscular, or subdermal contraceptives. Patients can experience amenorrhea, infrequent periods, irregular periods, and/or intermenstrual bleeding. AUB is a main reason why many women may stop their hormonal contraception.[34] Intermenstrual bleeding is common in the first month of OCP use but usually gets better by the third month of use. For patients on OCPs, assessing compliance is the first step in evaluation of AUB.[34] Counseling should be provided if within the first 3 months of therapy. If after the first 3 months bothersome bleeding persists patients can be treated with 800 mg ibuprofen can be used three times a day and/or supplemental estrogen. If there is still no

improvement using an OCP with a higher dose of estrogen up to 35 mcg, or a different progestin may help stabilize the endometrium and lead to less bleeding. Patients can also be offered a different form of contraception like the vaginal ring.

Long-acting progesterone only implants or injections cause irregular menstrual cycles in the majority of patients within the first year and amenorrhea is common. It is important to counsel patients that changes in menstrual cycle while on hormonal contraception do not indicate failure of contraception.

Some other noncontraceptive medications that can lead to AUB include drugs that interfere with sex steroid hormone function or synthesis (SERMs, Aromatase Inhibitors), anticoagulants (heparin, warfarin, and direct oral anticoagulants), antidepressants (tricyclic antidepressants, SSRIs), and antipsychotics. For patients that require anticoagulation, heavier periods are common and affect patients' quality of life. Mainstays of treatment involve long-acting progesterone-based therapies as first line (IUD, implant, or injection).[35] Combined hormonal contraception can also be used if there are no contraindications to estrogen.

Abnormal uterine bleeding not otherwise classified

As defined, this category contains conditions leading to AUB that are poorly defined or rare and do not otherwise fit into the classification system. Included in this category are arteriovenous malformation, myometrial hypertrophy, and cesarean scar defects.[12]

SUMMARY

AUB is a common problem effecting up to a third of women in their reproductive years. The PALM-COIEN classifications describe possible structural and nonstructural etiologies. Evaluation needs to include a comprehensive history with special attention to menstrual history, bleeding history, and a comprehensive physical including both a pelvic and bimanual examination. All patients should get a pregnancy test and a complete blood count (CBC) with platelets. All patients over 45 years of age need to get an endometrial biopsy. TVUS is first-line imaging modalities when structural causes are suspected. Treatment varies based on etiology. Medical options often include hormonal therapy to control bleeding. Surgical options vary based on patients' fertility desires but can include endometrial ablation and hysterectomy.

KEY CLINICAL PEARLS

Abnormal uterine bleeding (AUB) includes any bleeding from the uterus that is abnormal in frequency, duration, volume, and/or regularity that is present the majority of the prior 6 months.

Acute AUB is defined as an episode of heavy bleeding that requires immediate attention in the opinion of the treating physician.

Heavy menstrual bleeding is defined as excessive menstrual loss that interferes with physical, social, emotional, or material quality of life.

The PALM-COIEN system is a way to classify the causes of AUB in reproductive years. PALM refers to structural causes (polyps, adenomyosis, leiomyomas, and malignancy). COIEN refers to nonstructural causes (coagulopathies, ovulatory disorders, iatrogenic, endometrial, and not otherwise classified).

Key components of history include comprehensive menstrual history including duration, regularity, volume, and frequency of bleeding. Special focus should also be given to sexual family history as well as medications and supplements.

Physical examination should be thorough and needs to include a pelvic examination and bimanual. Special attention should also be paid to BMI and vital signs.

Laboratory evaluations include a urine pregnancy test, complete blood count with platelets, and ferritin with further laboratories based on likely etiology.

TVUS is considered the first-line imaging modality.

Treatment is based on underlying etiology. Medical mainstays of treatment include hormonal therapies including LNG IUDs and OCPs as well as NSAIDs. Surgical options include dilation and curettage, endometrial ablation, and hysterectomy. The patients' desire for future fertility needs to be taken into account before surgical interventions.

REFERENCES

1. Wouk N, Helton M. Abnormal Uterine Bleeding in Premenopausal Women. Am Fam Physician 2019;99(7):435–43.
2. Munro MG, Critchley HO, Broder MS, et al, FIGO Working Group on Menstrual Disorders. FIGO classification system (PALM-COEIN) for causes of abnormal uterine bleeding in nongravid women of reproductive age. Int J Gynaecol Obstet 2011;113(1):3–13.
3. Munro MG, Critchley HOD, Fraser IS, FIGO Menstrual Disorders Committee. The two FIGO systems for normal and abnormal uterine bleeding symptoms and classification of causes of abnormal uterine bleeding in the reproductive years: 2018 revisions. Int J Gynaecol Obstet 2018;143(3):393–408, published correction appears in Int J Gynaecol Obstet. 2019 Feb;144(2):237.
4. Marnach ML, Laughlin-Tommaso SK. Evaluation and Management of Abnormal Uterine Bleeding. Mayo Clin Proc 2019;94(2):326–35.
5. Wise MR, Gill P, Lensen S, et al. Body mass index trumps age in decision for endometrial biopsy: cohort study of symptomatic premenopausal women. Am J Obstet Gynecol 2016;215(5):598.e1, 598598.e8.
6. Emons G, Beckmann MW, Schmidt D, et al. Uterus commission of the Gynecological Oncology Working Group (AGO). New WHO Classification of Endometrial Hyperplasias. Geburtshilfe Frauenheilkd 2015;75(2):135–6.
7. Practice bulletin no. 136: management of abnormal uterine bleeding associated with ovulatory dysfunction. Obstet Gynecol 2013;122(1):176–85.
8. Committee on Practice Bulletins—Gynecology. Practice bulletin no. 128: diagnosis of abnormal uterine bleeding in reproductive-aged women. Obstet Gynecol 2012;120(1):197–206.
9. ACOG committee opinion no. 557: Management of acute abnormal uterine bleeding in nonpregnant reproductive-aged women. Obstet Gynecol 2013; 121(4):891–6.
10. Sweet MG, Schmidt-Dalton TA, Weiss PM, et al. Evaluation and management of abnormal uterine bleeding in premenopausal women. Am Fam Physician 2012; 85(1):35–43.
11. Bates GW, Bowling M. Physiology of the female reproductive axis. Periodontol 2000 2013;61(1):89–102.
12. Munro MG. Practical aspects of the two FIGO systems for management of abnormal uterine bleeding in the reproductive years. Best Pract Res Clin Obstet Gynaecol 2017;40:3–22.
13. Golan A, Sagiv R, Berar M, et al. Bipolar electrical energy in physiologic solution–a revolution in operative hysteroscopy. J Am Assoc Gynecol Laparosc 2001;8(2):252–8.
14. Salim S, Won H, Nesbitt-Hawes E, et al. Diagnosis and management of endometrial polyps: a critical review of the literature. J Minim Invasive Gynecol 2011; 18(5):569–81.

15. Clark TJ, Stevenson H. Endometrial Polyps and Abnormal Uterine Bleeding (AUB-P): What is the relationship, how are they diagnosed and how are they treated? Best Pract Res Clin Obstet Gynaecol 2017;40:89–104.

16. Lee SC, Kaunitz AM, Sanchez-Ramos L, et al. The oncogenic potential of endometrial polyps: a systematic review and meta-analysis. Obstet Gynecol 2010; 116(5):1197–205.

17. Ferrazzi E, Zupi E, Leone FP, et al. How often are endometrial polyps malignant in asymptomatic postmenopausal women? A multicenter study. Am J Obstet Gynecol 2009;200(3):235.e1–2356.

18. Dueholm M. Transvaginal ultrasound for diagnosis of adenomyosis: a review. Best Pract Res Clin Obstet Gynaecol 2006;20(4):569–82.

19. Abbott JA. Adenomyosis and Abnormal Uterine Bleeding (AUB-A)-Pathogenesis, diagnosis, and management. Best Pract Res Clin Obstet Gynaecol 2017;40:68–81.

20. Pontis A, D'Alterio MN, Pirarba S, et al. Adenomyosis: a systematic review of medical treatment. Gynecol Endocrinol 2016;32(9):696–700.

21. Ferrari F, Arrigoni F, Miccoli A, et al. Effectiveness of Magnetic Resonance-guided Focused Ultrasound Surgery (MRgFUS) in the uterine adenomyosis treatment: technical approach and MRI evaluation. Radiol Med 2016;121(2):153–61.

22. Smeets AJ, Nijenhuis RJ, Boekkooi PF, et al. Long-term follow-up of uterine artery embolization for symptomatic adenomyosis. Cardiovasc Intervent Radiol 2012; 35(4):815–9.

23. Stewart EA. Clinical practice. Uterine fibroids. N Engl J Med 2015;372(17): 1646–55.

24. Bradley LD, Gueye NA. The medical management of abnormal uterine bleeding in reproductive-aged women. Am J Obstet Gynecol 2016;214(1):31–44.

25. Kadir RA, Economides DL, Sabin CA, et al. Frequency of inherited bleeding disorders in women with menorrhagia. Lancet 1998;351(9101):485–9.

26. Auclair MH, Yong PJ, Salvador S, et al. Guideline No. 390-Classification and Management of Endometrial Hyperplasia. J Obstet Gynaecol Can 2019;41(12): 1789–800 [Erratum in: J Obstet Gynaecol Can. 2020 Oct;42(10):1287. PMID: 31785798].

27. Jamieson MA. Disorders of Menstruation in Adolescent Girls. Pediatr Clin North Am 2015;62(4):943–61.

28. Sophie Gibson ME, Fleming N, Zuijdwijk C, et al. Where Have the Periods Gone? The Evaluation and Management of Functional Hypothalamic Amenorrhea. J Clin Res Pediatr Endocrinol 2020;12(Suppl 1):18–27.

29. Gordon CM. Clinical practice. Functional hypothalamic amenorrhea. N Engl J Med 2010;363(4):365–71.

30. Kaiser UB. Hyperprolactinemia and infertility: new insights. J Clin Invest 2012; 122(10):3467–8.

31. Melmed Shlomo, Casanueva Felipe F, Hoffman Andrew R, et al. Diagnosis and Treatment of Hyperprolactinemia: An Endocrine Society Clinical Practice Guideline. J Clin Endocrinol Metab 2011;96(2):273–88.

32. Williams T, Mortada R, Porter S. Diagnosis and Treatment of Polycystic Ovary Syndrome. Am Fam Physician 2016;94(2):106–13.

33. Doufas AG, Mastorakos G. The hypothalamic-pituitary-thyroid axis and the female reproductive system. Ann N Y Acad Sci 2000;900:65–76.

34. Schrager S. Abnormal uterine bleeding associated with hormonal contraception. Am Fam Physician 2002;65(10):2073–80.

35. Samuelson Bannow B. Management of heavy menstrual bleeding on anticoagulation. Hematol Am Soc Hematol Educ Program 2020;2020(1):533–7.

Contraception

Rachel A. Bonnema, MD, MS

KEYWORDS

• Contraception • Birth control • LARC • Emergency contraception • IUD

KEY POINTS

- Long-acting reversible contraception such as an implant or intrauterine device is safe and extremely effective and should be considered in all women, including nulliparous women.
- Combined estrogen and progesterone methods (eg, pills, patch, and ring) are effective and commonly used, providing excellent cycle control, and can be used in extended-cycle methods for patients who desire fewer than 12 periods per year.
- The use of estrogen has been associated, albeit rarely, with the development of deep vein thrombosis, myocardial infarction, and stroke; estrogen should not be used in smokers older than 35 years and in patients with diabetes with end organ damage, coronary artery disease, migraines with aura, or a known hypercoagulable condition.
- For women with a contraindication to estrogen, progestin-only methods are safe to use.

Nearly half of all pregnancies in the United States are unplanned, a rate substantially higher than that in other highly industrialized regions.[1] Although rates of unintended pregnancy have decreased slightly in all groups studied, large disparities remain. In particular poor, Black, and Hispanic women and girls continued to have much higher rates of unintended pregnancy than Whites and those with higher incomes. In this time in the United States where states are increasingly restricting abortion access, pregnancy prevention becomes of even greater importance for patients. Primary-care physicians (PCPs) need up-to-date knowledge on contraceptive counseling for women to provide the best match between patient and contraceptive method, including appropriate contraceptive counseling for women with particular medical comorbidities. When counseling patients on contraception, options generally fall into long-acting reversible contraception (LARC) and short-acting reversible contraception (SARC). Within the category of SARC, options are further classified by those with combination hormones (estrogen and progesterone) or progestin-only preparations.

Some physicians and providers may feel less comfortable with initiating conversations related to contraception. One approach is using ONE KEY QUESTION (OKQ), developed by the Oregon Foundation for Reproductive Health, advocating screening for pregnancy intention by asking "Would you like to become pregnant in the next

Internal Medicine, University of Texas Southwestern, 5323 Harry Hines Boulevard, Dallas, TX 75390-9126, USA

E-mail address: Rachel.bonnema@utsouthwestern.edu

Med Clin N Am 107 (2023) 247–258
https://doi.org/10.1016/j.mcna.2022.10.005
0025-7125/23/© 2022 Elsevier Inc. All rights reserved.

year?" during all clinic visits.[2] Using this simplistic approach asks patients to consider their wants, rather than plans, to more accurately identify necessary preventive reproductive health services. This equitable method calls on providers to embrace and support the reproductive aspirations of every woman, regardless of social status, and provide a pathway to optimize desired outcomes. OKQ is becoming more widespread as an approach to counseling and has demonstrated high levels of patient satisfaction.[3]

When discussing contraceptive choices with patients, it is important that providers use a patient-centered approach allowing patients to make informed decisions. The only effective contraceptive is one that a patient is willing to use consistently and correctly, and the choice of contraception is ultimately the patient's decision. Providers must educate patients regarding the advantages and disadvantages of each method that is medically appropriate for them, counseling patients on expected side effects as well as expectant management strategies. Discussing a patient's preferences for menstrual frequency and tolerance for scheduled and unscheduled bleeding is important in deciding which contraceptive will best fit a patient's needs. Every effort should be made to remove barriers to initiation, including having no requirement for a pelvic examination or Pap smear before initiation. Using the conversation about contraceptives to also discuss safe sex is ideal.

LONG-ACTING REVERSIBLE CONTRACEPTION

LARC is a term for highly effective and easy-to-use forms of birth control that can last for years at a time and include the intrauterine device (IUD) and the contraceptive implant (**Table 1**). LARCs are frequently recommended as the best birth control method for most women, including teens, because they are highly effective and the LARC remains continuously in place though is immediately reversible with removal.[4] When young women are offered all birth control methods without barriers like cost or clinic access, nearly two-thirds choose LARC over other contraceptives.[5] In addition, LARCs are safe to use immediately postpartum and do not interfere with breastfeeding.[6]

Levonorgestrel Intrauterine System

The levonorgestrel intrauterine system (LNG-IUS) is ideal for those who require highly effective contraception and is particularly beneficial for patients requiring progestin-only contraception. LNG-IUS has been long considered to be reversible sterilization owing to its excellent efficacy in preventing pregnancy and quick return to fertility after removal. There are now multiple formulations of LNG IUS that prevent pregnancy for 3 to 8 years (Skyla, Kyleena, Liletta, Mirena),[7] categorized by the amount of levonorgestrel that they contain: 52 mg in Mirena and Liletta, 19.5 mg in Kyleena, or 13.5 mg in Skyla. Because some formulations of LNG-IUS can now be in place for eight years, the relatively low cost over time is another important factor for patients to consider. Numerous studies have confirmed the effectiveness of the LNG-IUS for reduction of menstrual blood loss in menorrhagia, leiomyomas, and pain caused by endometriosis; Mirena received FDA approval for the indication of menorrhagia and has been shown to decrease menorrhagia for those on anticoagulation. It is now the favored treatment for the management of heavy menstrual bleeding in women on anticoagulation.[8] Insertion of the LNG-IUS requires a trained provider. At the time of placement, cramping and pain may occur; a rare complication of placement is uterine wall rupture.

Table 1
Long-acting reversible contraception

	Intrauterine Device		Implant
	LNG IUD	**Copper IUD**	**Nexplanon**
Duration reversibility	Approved for 3 to 8 y • LNG 52 mg: 8 y • LNG 13.5 mg: 3 y Immediate	Approved for up to 10 years Immediate	3 years Immediate
Typical-use failure rate[a]	0.1% to 0.8%	0.8%	0.1%
Side effects and considerations	All initially cause irregular spotting • LNG 52 mg IUS: ~20% achieve amenorrhea within 1 year • LNG 13.5 mg: spotting more frequent but decreases with longer use	Bleeding and cramping with menses Low risk of ectopic pregnancy Avoid with genital bleeding, cervical cancer, or Wilson's disease	Spotting, unscheduled bleeding, or absence of bleeding
Consider in:	Women with contraindication to estrogen, seizure disorder, hypercoagulable states, menorrhagia, dysmenorrhea, migraine with aura	Women with contraindication to hormones or who desire hormone-free LARC, history of breast cancer Women in need of EC	Women with contraindication to estrogen, seizure disorder, hypercoagulable states, dysmenorrhea, migraine with aura

Abbreviations: EC, emergency contraception; IUD, intrauterine device; LARC, Long-acting Reversible Contraception.
[a] Data from Hatcher RA et al., Contraceptive Technology, 21st ed., New York: Managing Contraception, 2018.

Many will likely develop amenorrhea, though may experience initial irregular bleeding and spotting. If there is no suspicion of another cause for bleeding, reassurance can be provided. There are options to manage the symptoms, though if LNG-IUS was chosen due to a patient's contraindications to estrogen the best option is a five-day course of scheduled nonsteroidal anti-inflammatories such as naproxen 500 mg twice daily. If there is no active thromboembolic disease, another option is tranexamic acid for five days. Finally, if there is no contraindication to estrogen use, a combined hormonal contraceptive or estradiol 0.1 mg patch can be provided for three months.

Copper Intrauterine Device

Currently, the copper IUD (marketed as ParaGard) is the only nonhormonal IUD available in the United States. This is a particularly attractive option for a woman with contraindications to hormone use and is approved for up to 10 years. The mechanism of action for the copper IUD is primarily related to copper ions' toxic effect on sperm motility and viability.[9] Women will continue to have cyclic menses, but may experience an increase in menstrual flow and cramping-type abdominal pain; approximately 10% of users will have the IUD removed for bleeding in the first year of use.

Implant

There is one single-rod subdermal implant available in the United States called Nexplanon that is a highly effective long-term contraceptive containing the progestin etonogestrel (ENG). The rod is implanted in the upper arm and remains active for 3 years. ENG does not cause a hypoestrogenic state and thus is not considered to have any significant effect on bone mineral density (BMD).[10] ENG implantation can be done as a simple procedure by a trained provider under local anesthetic with a preloaded, disposable applicator. Patients experience a quick return to normal cycles after implant removal and there have been no reports of infertility after removal. Similar to other progestin-only forms of contraception, irregular bleeding is the major side effect of the ENG implant. The most common bleeding pattern associated with the implant is infrequent, irregular bleeding. This remains an important counseling point as the highest rate of discontinuation is during the first 8 to 9 months of use, primarily owing to frequent bleeding. If needed, management options for irregular bleeding can be discussed as noted above.

The US Selected Practice Recommendations for Contraceptive Use (US SPR) outline a Quick Start method where providers should consider starting a hormonal contraceptive method at any time, when reasonably certain the patient is not pregnant.[11] The criteria for reasonable certainty of avoiding pregnancy include menses <7 days prior, no unprotected intercourse since last menses, or negative urine pregnancy test. Unless menses occurred <7 days prior women should use a backup method for 7 days. Using this Quick Start, the benefits of starting the contraceptive, in this case the implant, at the time of the initial health care visit likely exceed any risks. Helpful flowcharts for initiating contraceptives can be found at reproductiveaccess.org.[12]

Injectable

Injectable contraception, lasting for months, is generally seen as an intermediate-acting, reversible contraceptive. The intramuscular DMPA injection (Depo-Provera 150 mg) is given every 12 weeks and has a typical-use failure rate of 4%. A lower dose of DMPA (104 mg in Depo-SubQ Provera) has been approved for subcutaneous injection. DMPA suppresses ovulation and thickens cervical mucus, keeping sperm from fertilizing an egg. There are several benefits of DMPA including improvement of pelvic pain in endometriosis and decreased bleeding in women with fibroids. Patients with seizure disorders are particularly good candidates for DMPA injections because, unlike other forms of contraception, the efficacy of DMPA is not affected by enzyme-inducing antiepileptic drugs. Depo-Provera may also decrease seizure frequency, providing additional benefit.

There are possible side effects including initial irregular bleeding and weight gain.[13] Patients considering DMPA should be advised that they are unlikely to experience a regular bleeding pattern during long-term use and should be warned that bleeding might be extremely unpredictable, particularly during the first few months of use. Over time DMPA is more likely to cause amenorrhea. The methods outlined above to manage irregular bleeding may also be used for DMPA users. Weight gain on DMPA is highly variable but black racial background and overweight status have been reported as risk factors. It also has been noted that those with early weight gain on DMPA were at risk for continued excessive weight gain.[14] DMPA reduces serum estradiol levels, which can adversely affect bone health. There is a clear association between DMPA use and decreased BMD; however, data have shown the BMD loss to be reversible with discontinuation of use and there is no increased risk of fracture with use of DMPA. The World Health Organization has recommended that there be no restriction on the use of Depo-Provera in ages 18 to 45. Clinicians should advise patients about the risk for BMD loss but can reassure them about reversibility with discontinuation.[15] Similar to other forms of hormonal contraception, the US SPR describes the benefits of Quick Start for DMPA as likely outweighing risks.[11] The patient should get her DMPA shot every 12 weeks and if she is more than two weeks late, should have a negative pregnancy test before the next shot and use a backup method for the next seven days.

SHORT-ACTING REVERSIBLE CONTRACEPTION
Combined Hormonal Contraception

Combined hormonal contraception (CHC) contains estrogen and a progestin and works primarily by preventing the surge of luteinizing hormone and thereby preventing ovulation. The majority of CHC contain ethinyl estradiol (EE) though a new contraceptive has been approved with a novel endogenous estrogen, estetrol (E4). E4 is naturally produced only by the fetal liver during pregnancy, but can be manufactured from plant-based sources.[16] CHC can be delivered as an oral contraceptive pill (OCP), as a vaginal ring (NuvaRing, Annovera), or as a transdermal patch (Xulane, Twirla). Risks, benefits, side effects, and contraindications of CHC are thought to be largely similar across delivery methods.[17]

There are many noncontraceptive benefits to CHC, including first-line treatment for dysfunctional uterine bleeding, dysmenorrhea, and menorrhagia. Benefits in addition to menstrual control include reduction in the risks for, and symptoms of, endometriosis, ovulatory pain, ovarian cysts, benign breast disease, premenstrual syndrome, and premenstrual dysphoric disorder. CHC also reduces risk of ovarian and endometrial cancers; these risk reductions extend for years after stopping CHC.[10] The most common side effects of CHC are outlined in **Table 2**. The risk of venous thromboembolism (VTE) may be higher in obese patients, smokers, and those who use certain progestins such as desogestrel or drospirenone.[18] This risk is lower, however, than the risk of VTE associated with pregnancy, and the absolute risk of VTE among CHC users remains small. The novel OCP with E4 (Nextstellis) has lower estrogenicity than EE, demonstrated more neutral effects on the liver, and may be associated with reduced VTE risk compared with other CHC.[16]

CHCs can be used safely by those with a range of medical conditions, including well-controlled hypertension, uncomplicated diabetes, migraines *without* aura when less than age 35, and a family history of breast cancer, to name a few.[19] CHC use is contraindicated in patients who have a history of migraine headache with aura at any age, or in those over age 35 with any migraine, owing to elevated risk for stroke. CHC is also contraindicated in patients with diabetes with end organ damage, known cardiovascular disease, and in those who smoke after age 35 years due to elevated risks for cardiovascular disease. Other contraindications include a personal history of breast cancer, an estrogen-dependent tumor, unexplained vaginal bleeding, stroke, known thromboembolic disorder, or known VTE. Use of CHC in postpartum women is restricted in the first six weeks after delivery due to elevated risk of VTE and negative effect on lactation.[19]

Historically women were instructed to wait until the next menses to begin hormonal contraception with the intent to avoid contraceptive use during an undetected pregnancy. "Quick Start", or same-day initiation, is now the recommended approach to reduce barriers to accessing contraception by eliminating unnecessary delays. As outlined above, the US SPR state the benefits of starting CHC at the time of the initial

Table 2
Hormonal contraception

	Combination Estrogen-Progestin				Progestin-Only		
	Traditional OCPs	Extended-Cycle OCPs	Patch	Vaginal Ring	Pill		Injection
Duration Reversibility	Daily pill Immediate	Daily pill Immediate	Weekly for 3 wk, followed by 1 wk no patch Immediate	3 wk followed by 1 wk no ring Immediate	Norethindrone: Daily pill with no hormone-free interval Immediate	Drospirenone: 24 d of hormones, 4 d placebo Immediate	3 months Variable
Typical-use failure rate[a]	7%	7%	7%	7%	7% to 9%		4% to 6%
Side effects[b]	Nausea, headache, breast tenderness, breakthrough bleeding, VTE, stroke, MI	increased unscheduled bleeding	Possible increased risk of VTE compared with OCP	Vaginal discharge	Spotting, unscheduled bleeding, or absence of bleeding (drospirenone may have better menstrual profile)		Spotting, unscheduled bleeding, or absence of bleeding; weight gain, depression, reversible decrease in BMD
Consider in:	Women with dysmenorrhea, menorrhagia, irregular menstrual periods, acne, hirsutism, or polycystic ovary syndrome.	Fewer withdrawal bleeds/yr benefit women with estrogen withdrawal symptoms, endometriosis.	Women who don't want to take a daily pill		Women with contraindication to estrogen, hypercoagulable states, dysmenorrhea, migraine with aura, or breast-feeding.		Women with contraindication to estrogen, seizure disorder, sickle cell disease, hypercoagulable states, dysmenorrhea, migraine with aura, or breast-feeding.

Abbreviations: BMD, bone mineral density; MI, myocardial infarction; OCP, oral contraceptive pill; VTE, venous thromboembolism.
[a] Data from Hatcher RA et al., Contraceptive Technology, 21st ed., New York: Managing Contraception, 2018.
[b] Note: For all combination methods, must have no contraindication to estrogen.

health care visit likely exceed any risks when the provider is reasonably certain the patient is not pregnant.[11]

Combined oral contraceptive pills

There are dozens of formulations of OCPs, which differ by their estrogen dosage (and now type), progestin type and dosage, and hormone delivery schedule. OCPs can be monophasic, where each pill contains the same amount of hormones, or multiphasic, where pills contain different amounts of hormones throughout the monthly cycle. The different formulations offer patients options in cycle length, hormone levels, duration of withdrawal bleeding, and side effect profile. Education should include taking their pill at the same time each day. If a pill is missed, it should be taken as soon as remembered. If 2 days of pills are missed, the regimen includes two pills daily for 2 days in a row with a backup method used. If 3 days of pills are missed, the pill pack should be discarded and a backup method used. At that point, it should be discussed whether to start a new pack or to change contraceptive methods.[17]

For those who desire fewer days of menses or fewer than 12 menses per year, extended-cycle OCP regimens can be offered that offer a placebo week every 4 months or eliminate the placebo week altogether. Extended-cycle regimens have other benefits, including decreased hormone withdrawal symptoms such as headaches, tiredness, bloating, excessive bleeding, or menstrual pain. In addition to estrogen dose and scheduling, it is also important to consider the progestin component, which theoretically may affect libido, weight gain, acne, and hirsutism.[10]

Breakthrough bleeding (BTB) can be experienced with any OCP, and is common in the first three months but declines with time. If BTB persists providers can consider changing to an alternative progestin or estrogen. Third-generation progestogens (ie, norethindrone) may be preferable with regard to BTB. Similarly low-dose EE pills may have more BTB and increasing the EE dose to 30 to 35 mcg may help stabilize the endometrial lining. Finally, a vaginal ring bypasses the issue of variable gastrointestinal absorption and may be an option for women interested in other forms of CHC. There is no evidence that triphasic preparations of OCPs have an advantage in terms of cycle control.[20]

Contraceptive patch

Norelgestromin/EE (Xulane) is a thin transdermal patch delivering a daily dose of 35 μg/d EE and 150 μg/d norelgestromin. Levonorgestrel/EE (Twirla) is a newly approved patch delivering a daily dose of 30 μg/d EE and 120 μg/d levonorgestrel.[21] Both patches are administered similarly: changed weekly for 3 weeks on "patch change day" followed by a patch-free week during which menses occur. Only one patch should be worn at a time, and no more than 7 days should pass during the patch-free week. Both have decreased efficacy in obese women and are contraindicated with body mass index (BMI) > 30 kg/m^2. Most of the noncontraceptive benefits, side effects, cardiovascular risks, and contraindications are similar to those of other forms of CHC, but there may be an increased risk of VTE in patch users compared with users of OCPs though studies are controversial as to the actual increase in risk associated. Of note, the VTE risk associated with patch use is lower than that associated with pregnancy.

Vaginal ring

Contraceptive vaginal rings (CVR) deliver hormones directly through the vaginal epithelium for highly effective contraception without the need for daily dosing. There are currently two CVRs that are US Food and Drug Administration (FDA)-approved for use in the United States.[21] Both rings are highly effective, like other combined hormonal methods, and have excellent cycle control. The vaginal ring has been associated with an increase in leukorrhea, otherwise, its noncontraceptive benefits, side effects, cardiovascular risks, and contraindications are similar to those of other forms of CHC. CVR can remain in the vagina during intercourse.

Etonogestrel/EE (NuvaRing) is a soft plastic ring that is inserted vaginally by the patient, usually for 3 weeks and then removed for 1 week at which time menses occur. A new ring is inserted 7 days after the last was removed even if bleeding is not complete. The ring releases 15 µg of EE and 0.12 mg of ENG daily for 3 to 5 weeks, so it can be kept in longer than 3 weeks for those desiring the benefits of extended-cycling use discussed previously. Each ring releases approximately half the level of hormones as the average OCP without affecting efficacy. If the ring falls out (as occurs rarely), it can be rinsed and reinserted without a change in efficacy. Most find the ring easy to insert and remove and comfortable to retain during intercourse.

A newer ring containing a year's contraception with segesterone acetate (SA) and EE is now available. The SA/EE ring (Annovera) is used for 21 days followed by a 7-day use-free interval for up to 13 consecutive cycles. Continuous use with the same SA/EE ring is still being studied and cannot yet be recommended. The SA/EE ring releases 13 µg of EE and uses a newer non-androgenic progestin making it one of the lowest estrogen dose methods available; it may mean less impact on lipid profile, acne, and weight gain; during counseling, special emphasis should be placed on the increased pregnancy risk for patients who remove the ring for more than 2 h.[21]

PROGESTIN ORAL PILLS

Progestin-only contraceptives are particularly beneficial for those with a contraindication to estrogen because progestin-only methods have decreased medical risks associated including no increased risk of stroke, myocardial infarction, or VTE. All progestin-only methods have a similar method of action: ovulation is variably inhibited, cervical mucus is thickened, and affecting the endometrium. Typical use failure rates are similar to CHC though may be underestimated as many individuals choosing POPs are subfertile (older age or breastfeeding). Unscheduled bleeding and spotting are the most common bleeding patterns and the most frequent cause for discontinuing this contraceptive. POPs can be prescribed immediately postpartum and do not impact lactation.[21]

There are now two progestin-only pills (POPs) available in the United States. Norethindrone pills are taken daily, without a hormone-free interval, and fertility returns immediately on discontinuation. In fact, fertility can return in as little as 3 h after a missed dose; thus patients should be counseled to use a backup method if 3 or more hours late in taking her dose. Given this small window for error, this method should be prescribed only to patients who can adhere closely to a daily pill schedule.

A newer POP contraceptive contains drospirenone 4 mg (Slynd) and is available in a 24-day supply of hormone and a 4-day supply of placebo, allowing for a timed withdrawal bleed.[21] The drospirenone-only pill maintains contraceptive efficacy even with 24-h delayed or missed-pill errors; patients can be counseled to take a missed tablet as soon as remembered if within 24 h or with the next scheduled dose if more than 24 h late. Although intermenstrual bleeding rates are still high, the menstrual profile may be more tolerable compared with the other POP available in the United States.

ON-DEMAND CONTRACEPTION

On-demand contraception includes barrier methods—male and female condoms, vaginal sponges, diaphragms, and cervical caps—as well as chemical barriers (spermicides), which can be used alone or in conjunction with other contraceptive methods. These methods are safe, easily available, inexpensive, and reversible. Barrier methods have the lowest efficacy rates of all contraceptive methods and users should also be counseled these as well as about emergency contraception (EC). Only condom use has been consistently found to protect against sexually transmitted infections (STI) including HIV, and condom use may reduce risks of cervical cancer as well.[21]

Phexxi is a novel pH-buffering spermicide available by prescription only.[21] This comes as a prefilled single-dose applicator of 5 g of gel to be administered intravaginally up to 1 h before each episode of vaginal intercourse. The gel is a vaginal pH regulator that contains lactic acid, citric acid, and potassium bitartrate; these active ingredients maintain the naturally acidic vaginal environment to reduce sperm motility and potentially enhance the vagina's antimicrobial defenses. In contrast to nonoxynol-9-based vaginal contraceptive products, Phexxi has the potential to prevent STI. Early studies have demonstrated decreased risks of chlamydia and gonorrhea and further trials are ongoing. The contraceptive failure rate of Phexxi was 13.7%, and the most frequent side effect was vulvovaginal burning occurring in 20%.[21]

PERMANENT

Permanent birth control methods include vasectomy and female sterilization by various procedures. These methods are highly effective (typical failure rate 0.15% to 0.5%); however, they are permanent.[22] Each sterilization procedure has advantages and disadvantages that should be considered by the patient before choosing which one to use.

EMERGENCY CONTRACEPTION

EC, or postcoital contraception, is used to prevent pregnancy after an unprotected or inadequately protected act of sexual intercourse. Many women are unaware of the existence of EC, misunderstand its use and safety, or do not use it when a need arises. Access to EC is particularly important for those having unprotected sex and for those who are using methods with higher failure rates. Familiarity with EC is critical for physicians, particularly in the United States where reliable access to abortion services may be increasingly limited. EC use has not been shown to reduce compliance with other first-line contraceptive methods.[23] FDA-approved methods of EC include oral administration of progestin (levonorgestrel), a selective progesterone receptor modulator (ulipristal acetate), or insertion of a copper IUD. EC primarily acts by inhibiting or delaying ovulation and works before implantation; if a fertilized egg has already been implanted, EC will not work. All EC options can be used within 5 days of intercourse with varying efficacy; EC pills are most effective when taken in the first 12 h but have gradually decreasing effectiveness for up to 120 h after intercourse.

The most accessible form of EC in the United States contains levonorgestrel only (Plan B One Step) and is over the counter without age restrictions; ulipristal (ella) requires a prescription. Body weight influences the effectiveness of oral EC, levonorgestrel EC may be less effective in women with a BMI >25 kg/m^2, ulipristal may be less effective in women with a BMI >35 kg/m^2. Most people who take EC pills have no adverse effects, some may experience nausea, vomiting, headache, or dizziness for a short time after taking the pills. Patients should be counseled that they may have spotting and their next period may be heavier than typical or may come a few days early or late. No particular treatment needs to occur, the next cycle generally returns to normal.

The copper IUD is the most effective form of EC, with nearly 100% reported efficacy, and is not impacted by body weight. Thus, for women with a BMI >25 kg/m^2, the copper IUD and ulipristal are preferred as first-line options. However, for women who cannot or will not use an IUD or ulipristal, less effective EC options should be provided to minimize risk of unintended pregnancy.[23] Notably, there is no medical condition in which oral EC is contraindicated.[19] The LNG IUD has been investigated for use as EC and in one recent study was noninferior to the copper IUD.[24] Based on this study many family planning clinics in the United States are using the LNG IUD as EC as women may prefer the eventual amenorrhea associated with use.

SUMMARY

In the setting of high rates of unintended pregnancies in the United States, and decreased access to abortion, an understanding of contraception and EC are essential for PCPs. LARC-first counseling is the recommended approach while maintaining patient-centered style as the best contraception is one that a patient is willing to use regularly.

CLINICS CARE POINTS

- A woman is eligible for same day initiation of contraception if her period was <1 week ago, she has not had unprotected sex since her last period, or if she has had sex but has a negative pregnancy test.
- When quick start intiation of contraception is chosen, a back up method is needed for 7 days.
- Any monophasic combined oral contraceptive pill can be utilized as extended cycling method by having patients take only active pills, skipping placebo pills, for 3 pill packs. Patients should be counseled about possibility of breakthrough bleeding.
- Ulipristal should be the favored emergency contraceptive pill for most patients.

DISCLOSURE

The author has no commercial or financial conflicts of interest.

REFERENCES

1. Finer LB, Zolna MR. Declines in unintended pregnancy in the United States, 2008-2011. N Engl J Med 2016;374(9):843–52. https://doi.org/10.1056/NEJMsa1506575. PMID: 26962904; PMCID: PMC4861155.
2. Allen D, Hunter MS, Wood S, et al. One Key Question®: First Things First in Reproductive Health. Matern Child Health J 2017;21:387–92. https://doi.org/10.1007/s10995-017-2283-2.
3. Song B, White VanGompel E, Wang C, et al. Effects of clinic-level implementation of One Key Question® on reproductive health counseling and patient satisfaction. Contraception 2021;103(1):6–12. https://doi.org/10.1016/j.contraception.2020.10.018.
4. Winner B, Peipert JF, Zhao Q, et al. Effectiveness of long-acting reversible contraception. N Engl J Med 2012;366(21):1998–2007.
5. Mestad R, Secura G, Allsworth JE, et al. Acceptance of long-acting reversible contraceptive methods by adolescent participants in the contraceptive CHOICE

project. Contraception 2011;84(5):493–8. https://doi.org/10.1016/j.contraception.2011.03.001. Epub 2011 Apr 27. PMID: 22018123; PMCID: PMC3505875.

6. American College of Obstetricians and Gynecologists' Committee on Obstetric Practice. Committee opinion No. 670: immediate postpartum long-acting reversible contraception. Obstet Gynecol 2016;128(2):e32–7. https://doi.org/10.1097/AOG.0000000000001587. PMID: 27454734.

7. Jensen JT, Lukkari-Lax E, Schulze A, et al. Contraceptive efficacy and safety of 52mg LNG-IUS for up to 8 years: findings from the Mirena Extension Trial. Am J Obstet Gynecol 2022. https://doi.org/10.1016/j.ajog.2022.09.007. XX:x.exex.ex [e-pub].

8. Samuelson Bannow B. Management of heavy menstrual bleeding on anticoagulation. Hematology Am Soc Hematol Educ Program 2020;2020(1):533–7. https://doi.org/10.1182/hematology.2020000138. PMID: 33275699; PMCID: PMC7727540.

9. Hsia JK, Creinin MD. Intrauterine contraception. Semin Reprod Med 2016;34:175–82.

10. Spencer AL, Bonnema RA, McNamara MC. Helping women choose appropriate hormonal contraception: update on risks, benefits, and indications. Am J Med 2009;122:497–506.

11. Curtis KM, Jatlaoui TC, Tepper NK, et al. U.S. selected practice recommendations for contraceptive use, 2016. MMWR Recomm Rep 2016;65(4):1–66. https://doi.org/10.15585/mmwr.rr6504a1. PMID: 27467319.

12. Available at: https://www.reproductiveaccess.org/contraception/.

13. Dianat S, Fox E, Ahrens KA, et al. Side effects and health benefits of depot medroxyprogesterone acetate: a systematic review. Obstet Gynecol 2019;133(2):332–41. https://doi.org/10.1097/AOG.0000000000003089.

14. Bonny AE, Secic M, Cromer B. Early weight gain related to later weight gain in adolescents on depot medroxyprogesterone acetate. Obstet Gynecol 2011;117(4):793–7. https://doi.org/10.1097/AOG.0b013e31820f387c.

15. Lanza LL, McQuay LJ, Rothman KJ, et al. Use of depot medroxyprogesterone acetate contraception and incidence of bone fracture. Obstet Gynecol 2013;121:593–600.

16. Lee A, Syed YY. Estetrol/drospirenone: a review in oral contraception. Drugs 2022;82(10):1117–25. https://doi.org/10.1007/s40265-022-01738-8. Epub 2022 Jul 4. [Erratum appears in: Drugs. 2022 Aug;82(12):1341. PMID: 35781795; PMCID: PMC9363382].

17. Petitti DB. Combination estrogen-progestin oral contraceptives. N Engl J Med 2003;349:1443–50.

18. Parkin L, Sharples K, Hernandez RK, et al. Risk of venous thromboembolism in users of oral contraceptives containing drospirenone or levonorgestrel: nested case control study based on UK General Practice Research Database. BMJ 2011;342:d2139. https://doi.org/10.1136/bmj.d2139.

19. Curtis KM, Tepper NK, Jatlaoui TC, et al. U.S. Medical eligibility criteria for contraceptive use. MMWR Recomm Rep 2016;65(No. RR-3):1–104. https://doi.org/10.15585/mmwr.rr6503a1.

20. Foran T. The management of irregular bleeding in women using contraception. Aust Fam Physician 2017;46(10):717–20. PMID: 29036769.

21. Baker CC, Chen MJ. New contraception update - Annovera, Phexxi, Slynd, and Twirla. Curr Obstet Gynecol Rep 2022;11(1):21–7. https://doi.org/10.1007/s13669-021-00321-4. Epub 2022 Jan 6. PMID: 35795653; PMCID: PMC9255890.

22. Trussell J, Aiken ARA, Micks E, et al. Efficacy, safety, and personal considerations. In: Hatcher RA, Nelson AL, Trussell J, et al, editors. Contraceptive technology. 21st edition. New York: Ayer Company Publishers, Inc.; 2018.
23. Practice bulletin No. 152: emergency contraception. Obstet Gynecol 2015;126(3):
e1–11. https://doi.org/10.1097/AOG.0000000000001047. PMID: 26287787.
24. Turok DK, Gero A, Simmons RG, et al. Levonorgestrel vs. copper intrauterine devices for emergency contraception. N Engl J Med 2021;384(4):335–44. https://
doi.org/10.1056/NEJMoa2022141. PMID: 33503342; PMCID: PMC7983017.

Cervical Cancer Screening

Katherine Gavinski, MD, MPH[a],*, Deborah DiNardo, MD, MS[b]

KEYWORDS

- Cervical cancer • Screening • Human papillomavirus • Pap smear • Co-testing
- Primary HPV testing

KEY POINTS

- Most national organizations recommend starting cervical cancer screening at age 21 and stopping at age 65, provided adequate prior testing.
- Current guidelines endorse the use of cytology only, co-testing, or primary human papilloma virus testing for cervical cancer screening.
- Clinicians should have adequate understanding of what testing strategies they have available to them and how they can be used.
- Management of abnormal cervical cancer screening results has transitioned to a risk-based decision tool that can incorporate multiple protective and risk-enhancing factors.

INTRODUCTION

Primary care providers are uniquely poised to prevent, screen, and diagnose cervical cancer. What started with the Papanicalaou smear in the 1940s,[1] has evolved into multiple modalities to assess for disease and more accurate estimates of patients' risk of cancer. Advances in understanding of the natural evolution of cervical cancer and virus-associated risk factors have improved diagnostic accuracy and ultimately rates of cervical cancer diagnosis. Multiple established organizations currently publish cervical cancer screening guidelines including the United States Preventative Services Task Force (USPSTF), American Cancer Society (ACS), American Society for Colposcopy and Cervical Pathology (ASCCP), American Society for Clinical Pathology (ASCP), the American College of Obstetricians and Gynecologists (ACOG), and the American College of Physicians (ACP). This article aims to describe the current understanding of cervical cancer pathogenesis, review available screening modalities, outline and compare leading guideline recommendations for screening and management, and anticipate future changes in cervical cancer screening.

The authors have no financial disclosures, affiliations, or conflicts of interest to report.
[a] University of Pittsburgh Medical Center, 3459 Fifth Avenue, 9 South, Pittsburgh, PA 15213, USA; [b] VA Pittsburgh Healthcare System, University Drive C, Pittsburgh, PA, 15240, USA
* Corresponding author.
E-mail address: gavinskikr@upmc.edu

Med Clin N Am 107 (2023) 259–269
https://doi.org/10.1016/j.mcna.2022.10.006
0025-7125/23/© 2022 Elsevier Inc. All rights reserved.

medical.theclinics.com

Epidemiology

In 2022, the National Cancer Institute estimates that 14,100 new cases of cervical cancer will be diagnosed in the United States.[2] There will be approximately 4,280 deaths secondary to cervical cancer, which will comprise 0.7% of all new cancer diagnoses and 0.7% of all cancer deaths.[2] Though cervical cancer incidence and death rate consistently declined from the mid-1970s to the mid-2000s, the incidence has stabilized in the last decade[3] and the 5-year survival has remained steady approximately 66.7%.[2] Disparities in survival among US women of different races have also been described. Five-year cervical cancer survival is 67% for white females, but only 56% for black females, with black females having higher rates of advanced disease at diagnosis.[4] Cervical cancer screening has proven to provide significant benefits in detecting earlier stages of the disease and reducing cervical cancer mortality; however, the stagnant rates of 5-year survival and gross disparities in survival by race indicate the need for renewed efforts in cervical cancer screening.

Pathogenesis

Cervical cancer is caused by human papillomavirus (HPV) infection. HPV is associated with cervical, anal, penile, and head and neck cancers. HPV infection has a strong association with invasive cervical cancer, with HPV strains 16 and 18 causing the vast majority of cases.[5] Risk factors for HPV-associated cervical cancer include early onset sexual activity, multiple and high-risk sexual partners, history of sexually transmitted infections, history of neoplasia/cancer, and immunosuppression.[6] Although the lifetime risk of HPV acquisition in the United States is upwards of 85%,[7] most HPV infections do not progress to cancer. In fact, most females clear HPV infections within 2 years.[8] Development of cancer requires persistent infections and progression to precancer and invasive cancer over the course of years.[9] Given this, cervical cancer pathogenesis has a uniquely long latency period in which screening has the potential to detect infection and early cancer. However, given the high rate of spontaneous HPV clearance, screening also has the potential to cause undue harm in testing and treatment of lesions that may never progress. Cervical cancer screening must balance the detection of preventable disease without over-diagnosis of clinically insignificant infections.

Definitions

Cervical cancer screening, by definition, takes place in patients who are asymptomatic and deemed to be of average risk. ACP defines patients as an average risk if they have no history of precancerous lesions or cervical cancer, are not immunocompromised, and have no history of exposure to diethylstilbestrol (DES).[10]

Testing

There are multiple testing options in the United States that are US Food and Drug Administration (FDA)-approved for cervical cancer screening. These include cytology, cytology with HPV testing (also known as "co-testing"), and primary HPV testing. Previous recommendations included cytology and co-testing options for cervical cancer screening. Primary HPV testing has only recently become available and incorporated as a guideline-based option for screening. Importantly, primary HPV testing requires the utilization of a validated primary HPV test and availability of reflex cytology.

DISCUSSION
When to Start Screening?

All major medical organizations agree that cervical cancer screening should not begin before age 21. This is because young patients have high rates of HPV infection[15] without a similarly high incidence of cervical cancer.[16] Screening starting at age 21 decreases the risk of colposcopy and more invasive diagnostic procedures without an appreciable increase in the risk of cervical cancer diagnosis.[11] The newest recommendations from the ACS are the first to recommend delaying initiation of cervical cancer screening until patients are 25 years old[12] (**Table 1**).

How Frequently (and with What Test) Should Screening Be Performed?

The majority of medical organizations endorse screening from age 21 to 29 with cytology alone every 3 years.[10,11,13,14] From age 30 to 65 years old, screening can continue with cervical cytology alone every 3 years, co-testing every 5 years, or primary HPV testing every 5 years.[10,11,13,14] ACS, ASCCP, and ACOG all note a preference for co-testing over cytology in patients between the ages of 30 to 65.[14,17] USPSTF, ASCCP, ACOG, and ACP continue to recognize cytology as a reasonable means of screening in all age groups, particularly when HPV testing is not readily available. In contrast, the ACS recommends that screening be done preferentially with primary HPV testing every 5 years.[12]

When Should Screening Stop?

All organizations agree that screening for cervical cancer should stop at age 65 if the patient has met the criteria for cessation.[10–14] These criteria are similar among all organizations: patients must have had adequate screening within 10 years of cessation, with the most recent testing in the last 5 years.[10–14] Adequate screening includes three consecutive negative cytology tests, two consecutive negative co-tests, or two consecutive negative primary HPV tests.[10–14] Screening should continue in patients of average risk until all conditions are met. Screening should be discontinued for patients with limited life expectancy, regardless of age.

Who Should Not Be Screened?

Women who have had a hysterectomy with removal of cervix, with no history of high-grade precancerous lesions or cervical cancer, should not be screened for cervical cancer.[10,11,14] Screening, in general, does not apply to women who have a history of cervical cancer.[11] These women require ongoing surveillance after treatment, with recommendations for HPV or co-testing every 3 years for at least 25 years after diagnosis.[18] Surveillance can continue at 3-year intervals beyond 25 years if the patient continues to have reasonable life expectancy such that they would benefit from additional tests and treatment of any positive results.[18]

Does Vaccination Change Screening Recommendations?

At this time, no major organization has differing recommendations based on HPV-vaccination status.

Who Is High Risk for Cervical Cancer and How Should They Be Screened?

Cervical cancer screening recommendations differ for patients deemed to be at higher risk. These populations include women with a history of a precancerous lesion (CIN 2 or CIN 3), history of cervical cancer, human immunodeficiency virus (HIV) infection, history of exposure to DES in utero, and current immunocompromised state.[10,19]

Table 1
Screening recommendations

	USPSTF 2018[11]	ACS 2020[12]	ASCCP 2021[13]	ACOG 2021[14]	ACP 2015[10]
<21	No screening	No screening < 25 yo	No screening	No screening < 25 yo	No screening
21 to 29	Cytology alone every 3 years	25 to 65 yo	Cytology alone every 3 years	a25 to 65 yo	Cytology alone every 3 years
30 to 65	Cytology alone every 3 years OR Primary HPV testing every 5 years OR Co-testing every 5 years	Primary HPV testing every 5 years (preferred) OR Co-testing every 5 years OR Cytology alone every 3 years (less preferred)	Cytology alone every 3 years OR Primary HPV testing every 5 years OR Co-testing every 5 years	Primary HPV testing every 5 years	Cytology alone every 3 years OR Co-testing every 5 years
>65	Stop if adequate screening completed	Stop if adequate screening completed	Stop if adequate screening completed	Stop if adequate screening completed	Stop if adequate screening completed

a Can consider primary HPV testing every 5 years starting at 25 years old.

A recent review suggested that patients with solid organ transplant, hematopoietic stem cell transplant, systemic lupus erythematosus, inflammatory bowel disease and rheumatoid arthritis on immunosuppressive medications should all be treated as immunocompromised states, and therefore at higher risk for cervical cancer.[20] Current screening recommendations for this population are based on the guidelines for HIV-positive women, for which there is more data to support recommendations.[18,20] Of note, patients with inflammatory bowel disease and rheumatoid arthritis not on immunosuppressive medications should be screened according to the average risk screening guidelines.[20]

Both the Infectious Diseases Society of America (IDSA), with the Centers for Disease Control (CDC) and Prevention and National Institutes of Health, and the ASCCP have worked to generate recommendations for cervical cancer screening for women living with HIV.[18,21] The IDSA/CDC guidelines recommend HIV-positive women start screening at age 21 with cytology-only testing.[21] The ASCCP recommends that screening for immunocompromised women, including those with HIV, start within 1 year of first insertional sexual activity.[18] Both organizations recommend cytology testing be repeated annually thereafter for 3 years.[18,21] If all three tests are negative, cytology can be continued every 3 years, similar to women of average risk.[18,21] Co-testing is not recommended in immunocompromised women under 30 years old.[18,21] Women over the age of 30 can continue screening with cytology alone or co-testing every 3 years, provided initial testing is negative.[18,21] Screening in immunocompromised women should continue throughout their lifetime.[18,21]

Management of abnormal results

Recent recommendations from the ASCCP marked a shift in the management of abnormal testing results from a test result-based strategy to risk-based management.[18] The estimation of risk is largely based on HPV infection status, and as such, screening with co-testing or primary HPV testing is preferred over cytology surveillance.[18] Owing to this heavy reliance on HPV status, the ASCCP stresses the importance of having the lab capabilities to run further tests, including cytology, on primary HPV samples.[18] Overall, these guidelines decrease the amount of invasive sampling by treating detected abnormalities according to their respective risks of developing into cervical cancer.

Personalized risk assessment for each patient can be made through use of the ASCCP management guidelines (available via web-based and mobile applications), with inputs including demographics, the clinical situation, current test results, and with an option to provide previous screening results.[18] These data are used to calculate an individualized risk of CIN3+, which is then compared with the predetermined evidence-based "clinical action thresholds" to provide guidance regarding next steps.[18] *Immediate* risk for CIN3+ is calculated first.[18] If the immediate CIN3+ risk is greater than 4%, immediate further testing or treatment is recommended as outlined in **Table 2**.[18] If the *immediate* CIN3+ risk is less than 4%, the *5-year risk* of CIN3+ is used to determine the appropriate interval for surveillance.[18] Surveillance should be done with an HPV-based testing strategy, either primary HPV testing or co-testing.[18]

Special Populations

Management of abnormal results in pregnancy and in women under age 25 have special considerations, which can be accessed through the 2019 ASCCP guidelines.[18]

Table 2
Clinical action thresholds and corresponding clinical actions

Immediate CIN3+ Risk	Clinical Action
4% to 24%	Colposcopy recommended
25% to 59%	Expedited treatment or colposcopy acceptable
60% to 100%	Expedited treatment preferred

Five-Year CIN3+ Risk	Clinical Action
<0.15%	Surveillance, return in 5 years
0.15% to 0.54%	Surveillance, return in 3 years
≥0.55%	Surveillance, return in 1 year

Management of rare cytology results

The 2019 management guidelines also address less-common findings including atypical glandular cells, unsatisfactory cytology, absent transformation zone, and benign endometrial cells.

When atypical glandular cells or adenocarcinoma in situ are seen on cytology, colposcopy should be performed, regardless of HPV result.[18] Endocervical sampling should be done concomitantly.[18] Patients should also have endometrial sampling if they are over 35 years old, or less than 35 years old and at increased risk for endometrial neoplasia.[18]

Unsatisfactory cytology with negative HPV or unknown HPV status should have a repeat, age-appropriate, screening within 2 to 4 months.[18] When HPV is positive, management varies from a repeat in 2 to 4 months to referral for colposcopy, which is recommended in all cases when HPV 16 or 18 is present.[18]

When absent transformation zone is reported, follow-up recommendations are based on age and screening modality. Women from 21 to 29 years old and women over age 30 with negative HPV should continue routine screening.[18] Women over 30 who did not have HPV testing can undergo repeat cytology in 3 years or immediate testing for HPV, with next steps dictated by HPV status.[18]

Finally, benign endometrial cells, endometrial stromal cells, or histiocytes in asymptomatic premenopausal women do not require further evaluation.[18] Endometrial biopsy is, however, recommended for benign endometrial cells for postmenopausal patients.[18]

FUTURE DIRECTIONS

With the emergence of primary HPV-based screening as an available (and according to some guidelines, preferred) screening strategy, significant work remains for broad implementation of this strategy within the United States. Most current guidelines continue to recommend three possible screening strategies (cytology alone every 3 years, co-testing every 5 years, primary HPV screening every 5 years), because in many cases the necessary infrastructure is not in place to fully support successful application of primary HPV screening. One important aspect, the need for evidence-based and clear algorithms for the management of positive and negative results, is now satisfied through the availability of the 2019 ASCCP risk-based management guidelines.[18] However, use of the specific HPV tests that are FDA-approved for primary HPV screening and ability to perform HPV genotyping and reflex cytology are all also required for successful and broad-based implementation. Currently, only two HPV tests are FDA-approved for use in primary HPV screening.[22] Furthermore, clinicians may not be aware of which HPV test is being used, or whether a particular laboratory is set up to perform reflex cytology on a specimen sent for primary HPV screening. For these reasons, clinicians should proceed with caution before individual adoption of a primary-HPV screening strategy. As a first step, practitioners must become familiar with which strategies are supported by their local institution and lab systems.

Ongoing efforts in the United States should also focus on addressing disparities in cervical cancer screening uptake and associated inequalities in cervical cancer incidence and mortality.[3] Screening with self-collection of HPV specimens has been investigated as a means of increasing access predominantly outside the United States, and has been found to have similar sensitivity and to increase screening rates compared with provider-collected specimens.[23] In addition, early data in the United States have documented that self-collection strategies are acceptable[24–27] and have been associated with increased screening rates in ethnic minority women.[28] Although self-collection strategies show incredible promise, they are not currently recommended in any US guidelines. Some providers may choose to offer self-collection on an individual, off-guideline basis to patients who are unable or unwilling to undergo provider sample collection. Ongoing investigations within the United States will be required to identify how self-collection can be applied more broadly to increase access to screening and reduce disparities in care.

Finally, a growing body of evidence has documented the impact of HPV vaccination on risk for HPV infection, for pre-cancerous cervical lesions, and more recently, for invasive cervical cancer.[29–39] Although HPV vaccination status is not yet incorporated as an input into the ASCCP individual patient risk estimation tool, the tool was intentionally designed to be able to incorporate additional risk influencers (such as vaccination status) as data evolves.[18] Practitioners should continue to prioritize HPV vaccination for all eligible individuals, and in the future, may be able to more precisely estimate individual risk for cervical cancer according to vaccination status.

SUMMARY

Advancements in the understanding of the pathogenesis of cervical cancer including the pivotal role of HPV infection, along with improved testing capability, have led to the rapid evolution of US screening guidelines. Regardless of screening strategy being used, practitioners can now perform an individualized risk assessment using the 2019 ASCCP risk tool to inform management of abnormal results. Primary HPV-based screening is now recommended as a screening strategy by multiple organizations, but in many cases, the necessary infrastructure is not yet in place to fully support a successful application. Broad scale efforts to further develop and support recommended screening programs that increase access and reduce disparities in cervical cancer screening are needed.

CLINICS CARE POINTS

- Cervical cancer screening should begin at age 21.
- Cytology, co-testing, and primary HPV testing can all be utilized, but clinicians should be attentive to what testing they have access to and differences in guidelines for testing intervals.

- The ASCCP risk-based decision tool allows for rapid, accurate assessment of patient risk for cervical cancer and clear guidance on next steps for patient management, including repeat testing and testing intervals.

CASES

- Title: Management of Unsatisfactory Cytology results
- Presentation: A 49-year-old woman undergoes routine cervical cancer screening with co-testing. Her last screening was 5 years ago and resulted in normal cytology and negative testing for high-risk HPV. Results from this exam are reported as unsatisfactory cytology and negative testing for high-risk HPV.
- Clinical Questions: What is the appropriate next step in management?
- Discussion: When cytology or co-testing results with "unsatisfactory cytology," the ASCCP algorithm[18] makes recommendations for management based on HPV status. Of note, when HPV testing is not available or when the HPV results as negative, as was the case for this patient, the patient should be asked to return for repeat age-based screening in 2 to 4 months.
- Title: Deciding when to stop screening
- Presentation: A 65-year-old woman with a medical history of hypertension undergoes routine cervical cancer screening with co-testing. Results are reported as "ASCUS, high-risk HPV negative." Her two most recent screening exams were 5 and 10 years ago respectively, both reported as negative cytology and negative high-risk HPV.
- Clinical Questions: Should she return for another pap exam in the future?
- Discussion: All current US guidelines recommend that it is appropriate to stop screening at the age of 65. Importantly, however, a woman must have adequate recent normal screening results, defined by three negative cytology specimens or two negative co-tests within the last 10 years, and the most recent test in the last 5 years. Because this patient's most recent result is not normal, guidelines recommend that she continue screening until the described criteria are met.[18]

REFERENCES

1. Vilos GA. The history of the Papanicolaou smear and the odyssey of George and Andromache Papanicolaou. Obstet Gynecol 1998;91(3):479–83.
2.. SEER Cancer Stat Facts: Cervical Cancer. National Cancer Institute. https://seer. cancer.gov/statfacts/html/cervix.html. Accessed June 27, 2022.
3. Cancer Facts & Figures. American Cancer Society. 2022. https://www.cancer.org/ content/dam/cancer-org/research/cancer-facts-and-statistics/annual-cancer-facts-and-figures/2022/2022-cancer-facts-and-figures.pdf. Accessed June 30, 2022.
4. Siegel RL, Miller KD, Fuchs HE, et al. Cancer statistics, 2022. CA Cancer J Clin 2022;72(1):7–33.
5. de Sanjose S, Quint WG, Alemany L, et al. Human papillomavirus genotype attribution in invasive cervical cancer: a retrospective cross-sectional worldwide study. Lancet Oncol 2010;11(11):1048–56.
6. Frumovitz M. Invasive cervical cancer: epidemiology, risk factors, clinical manifestations, and diagnosis. In: Dizon BGDS, editor. UpToDate. 2022. https://www.uptodate. com/contents/invasive-cervical-cancer-epidemiology-risk-factors-clinical-manifestations-and-diagnosis?sectionName=EPIDEMIOLOGY&search=cervical%20cancer%20

pathogenesis&topicRef=8314&anchor=H3&source=see_link#references. Accessed July 4, 2022.

7. Chesson HW, Dunne EF, Hariri S, et al. The estimated lifetime probability of acquiring human papillomavirus in the United States. Sex Transm Dis 2014; 41(11):660–4.
8. Plummer M, Schiffman M, Castle PE, et al. A 2-year prospective study of human papillomavirus persistence among women with a cytological diagnosis of atypical squamous cells of undetermined significance or low-grade squamous intraepithelial lesion. J Infect Dis 2007;195(11):1582–9.
9. Schiffman M, Castle PE, Jeronimo J, et al. Human papillomavirus and cervical cancer. Lancet 2007;370(9590):890–907.
10. Sawaya GF, Kulasingam S, Denberg TD, et al. Clinical Guidelines Committee of American College of P. Cervical Cancer Screening in Average-Risk Women: Best Practice Advice From the Clinical Guidelines Committee of the American College of Physicians. Ann Intern Med 2015;162(12):851–9.
11. USPST Force, Curry SJ, Krist AH, et al. Screening for Cervical Cancer: US Preventive Services Task Force Recommendation Statement. JAMA 2018;320(7): 674–86.
12. Fontham ETH, Wolf AMD, Church TR, et al. Cervical cancer screening for individuals at average risk: 2020 guideline update from the American Cancer Society. CA Cancer J Clin 2020;70(5):321–46.
13. Marcus JZ, Cason P, Downs LS Jr, et al. The ASCCP Cervical Cancer Screening Task Force Endorsement and Opinion on the American Cancer Society Updated Cervical Cancer Screening Guidelines. J Low Genit Tract Dis 2021;25(3): 187–91.
14. Updated Cervical Cancer Screening Guidelines. The American College of Obstetricians and Gynecologists. Practice Advisory Web site. 2021. https://www.acog.org/clinical/clinical-guidance/practice-advisory/articles/2021/04/updated-cervical-cancer-screening-guidelines. Accessed July 4, 2022.
15. Dunne EF, Unger ER, Sternberg M, et al. Prevalence of HPV infection among females in the United States. JAMA 2007;297(8):813–9.
16. Group USCSW. U.S. Cancer Statistics Data Visualizations Tool, based on 2021 submission data (1999-2019). 2022. https://www.cdc.gov/cancer/dataviz. Accessed July 11, 2022.
17. Saslow D, Solomon D, Lawson HW, et al. American Cancer Society, American Society for Colposcopy and Cervical Pathology, and American Society for Clinical Pathology screening guidelines for the prevention and early detection of cervical cancer. J Low Genit Tract Dis 2012;16(3):175–204.
18. Perkins RB, Guido RS, Castle PE, et al. 2019 ASCCP Risk-Based Management Consensus Guidelines for Abnormal Cervical Cancer Screening Tests and Cancer Precursors. J Low Genit Tract Dis 2020;24(2):102–31.
19. Practice Bulletin No. 157: Cervical Cancer Screening and Prevention. Obstet Gynecol 2016;127(1):e1–20.
20. Moscicki AB, Flowers L, Huchko MJ, et al. Guidelines for Cervical Cancer Screening in Immunosuppressed Women Without HIV Infection. J Low Genit Tract Dis 2019;23(2):87–101.
21. Panel on Guidelines for the Prevention and Treatment of Opportunistic Infections in Adults and Adolescents with HIV. Guidelines for the Prevention and Treatment of Opportunistic Infections in Adults and Adolescents with HIV. National Institutes of Health, Centers for Disease Control and Prevention, HIV Medicine Association, and Infectious Diseases Society of America. Available

at: https://clinicalinfo.hiv.gov/en/guidelines/adult-and-adolescent-opportunistic-infection. Accessed July 11, 2022.

22. Salazar KL, Duhon DJ, Olsen R, et al. A review of the FDA-approved molecular testing platforms for human papillomavirus. J Am Soc Cytopathol 2019;8(5): 284–92.

23. Arbyn M, Smith SB, Temin S, et al. Detecting cervical precancer and reaching underscreened women by using HPV testing on self samples: updated meta-analyses. BMJ 2018;363:k4823.

24. Barbee L, Kobetz E, Menard J, et al. Assessing the acceptability of self-sampling for HPV among Haitian immigrant women: CBPR in action. Cancer Causes Control 2010;21(3):421–31.

25. Castle PE, Rausa A, Walls T, et al. Comparative community outreach to increase cervical cancer screening in the Mississippi Delta. Prev Med 2011; 52(6):452–5.

26. Ilangovan K, Kobetz E, Koru-Sengul T, et al. Acceptability and Feasibility of Human Papilloma Virus Self-Sampling for Cervical Cancer Screening. J Womens Health (Larchmt) 2016;25(9):944–51.

27. Sewali B, Okuyemi KS, Askhir A, et al. Cervical cancer screening with clinic-based Pap test versus home HPV test among Somali immigrant women in Minnesota: a pilot randomized controlled trial. Cancer Med 2015;4(4):620–31.

28. Carrasquillo O, Seay J, Amofah A, et al. HPV Self-Sampling for Cervical Cancer Screening Among Ethnic Minority Women in South Florida: a Randomized Trial. J Gen Intern Med 2018;33(7):1077–83.

29. Arbyn M, Xu L, Simoens C, et al. Prophylactic vaccination against human papillomaviruses to prevent cervical cancer and its precursors. Cochrane Database Syst Rev 2018;5:CD009069.

30. Paavonen J, Naud P, Salmeron J, et al. Efficacy of human papillomavirus (HPV)-16/18 AS04-adjuvanted vaccine against cervical infection and precancer caused by oncogenic HPV types (PATRICIA): final analysis of a double-blind, randomised study in young women. Lancet 2009;374(9686):301–14.

31. Group FIS. Quadrivalent vaccine against human papillomavirus to prevent high-grade cervical lesions. N Engl J Med 2007;356(19):1915–27.

32. Drolet M, Benard E, Perez N, et al, Group HPVVIS. Population-level impact and herd effects following the introduction of human papillomavirus vaccination programmes: updated systematic review and meta-analysis. Lancet 2019; 394(10197):497–509.

33. Garland SM, Kjaer SK, Munoz N, et al. Impact and Effectiveness of the Quadrivalent Human Papillomavirus Vaccine: A Systematic Review of 10 Years of Real-world Experience. Clin Infect Dis 2016;63(4):519–27.

34. Silverberg MJ, Leyden WA, Lam JO, et al. Effectiveness of catch-up human papillomavirus vaccination on incident cervical neoplasia in a US health-care setting: a population-based case-control study. Lancet Child Adolesc Health 2018;2(10): 707–14.

35. Herweijer E, Sundstrom K, Ploner A, et al. Quadrivalent HPV vaccine effectiveness against high-grade cervical lesions by age at vaccination: A population-based study. Int J Cancer 2016;138(12):2867–74.

36. Herweijer E, Sundstrom K, Ploner A, et al. Erratum: quadrivalent HPV vaccine effectiveness against high-grade cervical lesions by age at vaccination: a population-based study. Int J Cancer 2017;141(1):E1–4.

37. Leval A, Herweijer E, Ploner A, et al. Quadrivalent human papillomavirus vaccine effectiveness: a Swedish national cohort study. J Natl Cancer Inst 2013;105(7): 469–74.
38. Lei J, Ploner A, Elfstrom KM, et al. HPV Vaccination and the Risk of Invasive Cervical Cancer. N Engl J Med 2020;383(14):1340–8.
39. Rosenblum HG, Lewis RM, Gargano JW, et al. Human Papillomavirus Vaccine Impact and Effectiveness Through 12 Years After Vaccine Introduction in the United States, 2003 to 2018. Ann Intern Med 2022;175(7):918–26.

Breast Cancer

Risk Assessment, Screening, and Primary Prevention

Elena Michaels, MD, Rebeca Ortiz Worthington, MD, MS, Jennifer Rusiecki, MD, MS*

KEYWORDS

- Breast cancer • Breast cancer risk • Mammogram • Breast MRI
- Chemoprophylaxis • SERM • Aromatase inhibitors • Prophylactic surgery

KEY POINTS

- All women should be assessed by history for breast cancer risk starting at age 18 years and counseled on breast awareness and lifestyle modifications such as weight loss, physical activity, reduced alcohol consumption, and smoking cessation.
- Women with above-average risk for breast cancer include those with a personal or family history of breast cancer, known genetic mutation, history of chest radiation before age 30, history of high-risk lesions, or dense breast tissue on mammography.
- Risk calculators should be used to identify high-risk patients who would benefit from yearly breast MRI screening and risk-reducing medications.
- High-risk individuals should be referred to breast cancer prevention specialists including an oncologist and genetic counselor who can assist in co-managing screening and prevention.

INTRODUCTION

Approximately one in eight women will be diagnosed with breast cancer in their lifetime. Breast cancer risk increases as women age with the highest rate of new diagnoses at ages 70 to 74 years. It is also a leading cause of death for women in their 40s and is the second most common cause of cancer deaths in women.[1,2] Although non-Hispanic white women have the highest annual average breast cancer incidence rate, hormone receptor-negative cancer is more common among black women, and breast cancer death rates are highest in black patients despite lower incidence rates.[3] This is

Department of Medicine, University of Chicago, 5841 South Maryland Avenue, MC 3051, Chicago, IL 60637, USA
* Corresponding author.
E-mail address: jrusiecki@medicine.bsd.uchicago.edu

Med Clin N Am 107 (2023) 271–284
https://doi.org/10.1016/j.mcna.2022.10.007
0025-7125/23/© 2022 Elsevier Inc. All rights reserved.

medical.theclinics.com

thought to be due in large part to socioeconomic factors as well as later-stage diagnosis of disease.[4]

Breast cancer incidence is rising by approximately 0.5% per year.[2] Studies suggest that over half of all breast cancer diagnoses could be prevented through lifestyle changes and the use of risk-reducing medications and surgery.[5] The use of targeted interventions such as genetic counseling, MRI, chemoprophylaxis, and prophylactic surgery for high-risk patients are notably underutilized.[6] This is likely multi-factorial and due to a combination of insufficient provider training, time constraints, and patient preference.

This review provides an outline of performing a breast cancer risk assessment, how to apply a risk-based approach to screening, and recommendations for breast cancer prevention both for average and high-risk groups. It is our goal that this review will give providers an evidence-based review and the skills needed to use an individualized, risk-based approach to breast cancer screening and prevention.

Risk Assessment

Assessment of an individual patient's risk of developing breast cancer is the first step in developing a personalized prevention and screening strategy. A risk assessment should be performed for patients as young as 18 years old and revisited every 5 years. Key items to elicit during a patient's history include the following: (a) personal or family history of breast or ovarian cancer, breast cancer-associated genetic mutation, or family history of genetic breast cancer syndrome; (b) personal history of chest radiation < 30 years old; (c) personal history of a high-risk breast lesion, breast biopsy, or dense breasts on mammography.[7–9] **Fig. 1** shows a model for approaching risk assessment via history. Based on a risk factor review and, if needed, a risk calculation, providers can assign patients to a risk group (**Table 1**).

Risk Factor Review and Counseling

An individual's risk for developing breast cancer is based on modifiable and nonmodifiable risk factors (**Table 2**). Approximately 40% of breast cancers are due to hormonal or reproductive factors, 40% are attributable to modifiable risk factors, and about 10% are due to known genetic mutations.[10] The degree of conferred risk varies substantially by each factor (see **Table 2**).

Nonmodifiable Risk Factors

Past Medical History: Chest Radiation and Proliferative Breast Lesions.

A history of chest radiation as a child or young adult leads to a 40% lifetime risk of developing breast cancer.[11] These patients should be co-managed with a breast specialist.

All patients with a history of biopsy-proven atypical ductal hyperplasia (ADH), atypical lobular hyperplasia (ALH), or lobular carcinoma in situ (LCIS) are at an increased risk of breast cancer.[5] These lesions should be removed. Ductal carcinoma in situ (DCIS), unlike other proliferative breast lesions, is managed and treated as a noninvasive breast cancer. Non-proliferative lesions such as fibroadenoma, epithelial hyperplasia, intraductal papilloma, and phyllodes tumors do not carry an increased risk of breast cancer.[12]

Genetic Factors and Family History of Cancer

A strong family history of cancer is defined as a first or second-degree family member with:

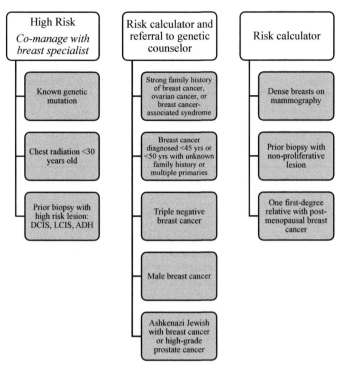

Fig. 1. Risk assessment algorithm. Patients with any of the conditions listed under the "High Risk" box should be comanaged with a breast specialist. Prevention strategies for this group may include prophylactic surgeries, medications, and advanced imaging. Patients with conditions under the "Risk calculation and referral to genetic counselor" box should be offered genetic counseling and based on the results of genetic testing a risk calculation should be performed. For patients that refuse genetic testing, a risk calculation should be performed. For patients with conditions under the "Risk Calculation" box, a risk calculation should be performed. For patients that do not fit into any of these three groupings, a risk calculation is not necessary.

- A known genetic mutation
- Bilateral breast cancer or two or more breast cancer primaries
- Premenopausal breast cancer (<50 years old)
- Ovarian cancer
- Two or more people with breast cancer on the same side of the family
- Male breast cancer, metastatic prostate cancer, or pancreatic cancer

These individuals should be referred to a genetic counselor. Anyone with a personal history of ovarian or pancreatic cancer or 3 or more family members diagnosed with any combination of cancers including breast, pancreatic, or prostate cancer, melanoma, sarcoma, adrenocortical carcinoma, brain tumor, leukemia, gastric, colon, endometrial, thyroid, or kidney cancer, or hamartomatous polyps in the gastrointestinal tract should also be referred per National Comprehensive Cancer Network (NCCN) guidelines.[7,8]

In addition to the above criteria, referral to a genetic counselor is recommended for all women diagnosed with breast cancer under age 45, women diagnosed under 50

Table 1
Risk group

High	Moderate	Average
>20% lifetime calculated risk • Chest radiation • Atypical hyperplasia, DCIS or LCIS • Genetic syndrome • Significant family history[a]	15% to 19% lifetime calculated risk • First-degree family member postmenopausal breast cancer • Dense breast • 3+ hormonal/lifestyle risk factors	<15% lifetime calculated risk • 0 to 3 hormonal/lifestyle risk factors

[a] ≥2 first-degree relatives with breast cancer, or ≥1 relative with premenopausal breast cancer, or male breast cancer.

years old with an unknown family history or multiple breast primaries, triple-negative breast cancer, male breast cancer, and those of Ashkenazi Jewish heritage diagnosed with breast cancer or high-grade prostate cancer.[7]

Genetic factors that increase a patient's risk for developing breast cancer are genetic mutations and hereditary breast and ovarian cancer syndromes. These include

Table 2
Risk factors

Risk Factor Category	Risk Factor	Relative Risk
Non-modifiable	• Personal or family history of known genetic mutation • Personal history of breast cancer • Personal history of ovarian cancer • History of DCIS, LCIS, atypical ductal or lobular hyperplasia • Chest radiation <30 y of age • Hereditary breast and ovarian cancer syndromes (eg, BRCA 1, BRCA 2, and PALB2) • Strong family history of breast cancer	RR >4.0
	• One first-degree relative with postmenopausal breast cancer • Extremely or heterogeneously dense breast tissue • Genetic factors (CHEK2 mutation carrier, Lynch syndrome, Ataxia telangiectasia)	RR 2.1 to 4.0
	• Personal history of melanoma, thyroid cancer, endometrial cancer • History of ≥1 breast biopsies or breast lesion without atypia • Menarche <12 y, menopause >55 y • DES use or exposure • PCOS	RR 1.1 to 2.0
Modifiable	• Hormone therapy within past 5 y • Postmenopausal obesity, inactivity • First live birth ≥30 y, nulliparity • Oral contraceptive use within the past 10 y • Alcohol consumption • Current smoking	RR 1.1 to 2.0

BRCA1, BRCA2, PALB2, CHEK2, Peutz-Jeghers syndrome, Li-Fraumeni syndrome, PTEN hamartoma syndrome, neurofibromatosis 1, and Lynch syndrome.[8]

Modifiable Risk Factors—Lifestyle Counseling

Weight control and physical activity

Postmenopausal overweight or obesity status is associated with an increased risk of breast cancer of 1.03 per 2 kg/m^2 point increase in body mass index (BMI) in postmenopausal women (95% confidence interval [CI] 1.01 to 1.04).[13] In addition, women who experience postmenopausal weight gain can reduce the risk of breast cancer by 8% with every 5 kg/m^2 decrease in BMI.[13]

Several studies have shown that physical activity can reduce cancer risk in postmenopausal women. Any level of physical activity is protective, although a significant reduction in breast cancer risk by 20% was seen in women, regardless of BMI, who performed more than 6.7 metabolic equivalents (MET)-h/wk of physical activity (odds ratio [OR] 0.82, CI 0.7 to 0.92).[14] This is equivalent to a 30-min walk, 4 times a week.

Alcohol

Alcohol consumption of up to 1 to 2 drinks per day is associated with an increased risk of breast cancer. Two cohort studies showed that for every 10 g of alcohol consumed per day, breast cancer risk increased by 10%.[15] Consensus is to limit alcohol use to one drink per day or less and to avoid daily alcohol use.

Modifiable Risk Factors: Hormone and Reproductive Factors

Hormone therapy

The use of hormone therapy (HT) for the treatment of vasomotor symptoms related to menopause has been complicated by the concern about an increased risk of breast cancer. Much of this concern originates from the Women's Health Initiative (WHI), a randomized control trial studying the use of HT in postmenopausal women. The study was terminated early after finding that women who received both estrogen and progestin had a 26% increased incidence of breast cancer (hazard ratio [HR] 1.26; 95% CI, 1.00 to 1.59).[16] This finding partially contributed to changing current prescribing guidelines for postmenopausal HT.

Since the WHI study was published, several prospective, observational studies have shown that estrogen-only HT affects breast cancer risk differently. Most notably, the Nurses' Health Study showed an increase in breast cancer risk for women taking estrogen-only HT starting after 5 years of use and becoming statistically significant after "long-term" use of 20 years or longer (Risk Ratio [RR] 1.42, 95% CI, 1.13 to 1.77).[17] Therefore, NCCN practice guidelines do not recommend against the use of short-term postmenopausal HT of fewer than 5 years duration.[8] However, women and their providers should be aware that there is a small increased breast cancer risk that is more pronounced with progesterone-containing regimens.

Hormone contraceptives

Several studies have shown a small, increased risk of breast cancer from oral contraceptive use. A meta-analysis shows a small but significant increase in breast cancer risk with oral contraceptives (OR 1.15, 95% CI: 1.01 to 1.31, $P = .036$).[18] Conversely, oral contraceptives also have a protective benefit against ovarian and endometrial cancer. The breast cancer risk seen with oral contraception is small and this option should not be withheld from patients based on this risk alone. It is recommended that for women who are concerned specifically about breast cancer risk that providers counsel to limit oral contraceptive use to 5 to 10 years and consider alternative forms of contraception after the age of 40.

Pregnancy and breastfeeding

Counseling on the role of pregnancy in breast cancer risk is complicated. Past pregnancy is not a modifiable risk factor and there are many other factors aside from cancer risk that are considered when planning a pregnancy. Pregnancy under the age of 25 is protective against future breast cancer, whereas women who give birth at or after 30-year-old are at an increased risk of breast cancer. However, nulliparous women have a 2.0 relative risk of breast cancer compared with women who have given birth.[14] In general, it is recommended that women with an elevated risk of breast cancer who wish to become a pregnant plan for pregnancy at a younger age if possible.

For women who give birth, breastfeeding has a protective benefit against breast cancer. A longer duration of breastfeeding is associated with greater risk reduction, although a benefit has been shown within 5 months.[14] Similar to pregnancy, a myriad of factors can affect a woman's ability to breastfeed but it is recommended that providers counsel on the benefits of breastfeeding.

Risk calculation

After reviewing risk factors a calculator should be used for those with a significant family history, personal history of a breast lesion or biopsy, or dense breasts. Risk calculators account for various personal, genetic, family, and hormonal/reproductive factors to estimate an individual's 5-year, 10-year, or lifetime risk for developing breast cancer (**Table 3**). Elevated 5-year risk is used to determine if an individual qualifies for risk reduction medications. Lifetime risk is used to determine whether to offer MRI in addition to mammography for annual screening.[19–22]

Risk-based screening

Screening and early detection of breast cancer is an important tool in improving breast cancer mortality. Mammography remains the preferred option for screening but the timing and duration of screening are less clear with multiple competing guidelines (**Table 4**). Screening decisions should be based on the patient's risk of breast cancer and providers must engage in shared decision-making to determine the appropriate screening plan (**Fig. 2**).

Average risk

The age to initiate screening varies by guideline but there is a consensus that mammogram screening should be initiated by age 50 for average-risk women. It is unclear if screening is appropriate for patients in their 40s. There is a small net benefit of screening from age 40 to 49 (3 deaths avoided per 10,000 women screened for 10 years, compared with 8 to 21 deaths avoided for women age 50 to 75 years).[23] The American Cancer Society (ACS) argues that women age 45 to 50 have a more similar breast cancer risk to those 50 to 54 years old (0.9% vs 1.1% 5-year risk respectively) and that 45 may be a more appropriate starting age.[24] This could be an acceptable option for women who wish to start screening in their 40s.

For patients in their 40s, the risk of early screening must be balanced against the risk of false-positive imaging. Over 10 years of screening, 61% of women in their 40s will have a false-positive mammogram.[25] Moving the screening age from 40 to 50 showed a reduction in false-positive imaging of more than 50%.[23] Patients who have experienced a false-positive mammogram are less likely to return to screening (return to screening within

Table 3
Risk calculators

Calculator	Risk Calculated	Personal History Considered	Family History Considered	Comments and Access
Gail Model or NIH Breast Cancer Risk Assessment Tool (BCRAT)	• 5-y risk • Lifetime risk	• Biopsy history • Reproductive history	First-degree relatives with breast cancer	Widely available Simple Does not consider:LCIS or DCISExtensive family history Increased breast density www.mdcalc.com/gail-modelbreast-cancer-risk or https://bcrisktool.cancer.gov/calculator.html
Breast Cancer Surveillance Consortium (BCSC)	• 5-y risk • 10-y risk	• Breast density • LCIS • Biopsy history	First-degree relatives with breast cancer	Does not consider:Reproductive historyDCIS https://tools.bcsc-scc.org/BC5yearRisk/calculator.htm
International Breast Cancer Intervention Study (IBIS) or Tyrer-Cuzick model	• 5-y risk • 10-y risk • Lifetime risk	• Reproductive history • Menopause • Biopsy history • BRCA testing • Breast density	• ≥2 relatives with cancer • Ashkenazi Jewish heritage • Male breast cancer • Ovarian cancer • Second- or third-degree relatives with breast cancer	Most comprehensivehttps://ibis-risk-calculator.magview.com/ www.ems-trials.org/riskevaluator

5-y risk is used to determine whether a patient should be offered chemoprevention. Lifetime risk is used to determine whether to offer MRI in addition to annual mammography for screening.

Table 4
Screening guidelines for average-risk patients

Guideline	When to Start Screening	Screening for Over Age 45 to 50
USPSTF	• 40 to 49, individualized decision • If screening, biennial	• 50+ biennial screen • Stop at age 75
ACOG	• 40 to 49, individual decision • Annual or biennial based on SDM	• Start screening everyone by 50 • Annual or biennial based on SDM • Start to discuss stopping at age 75
ACS	• 40 to 44 discuss annual screen • 45 to 54 annual screen	• 45 to 54 annual screen • 55+ biennial screen • Stop life expectancy <10 years
ACR	• 40 annual screen	• Annual screen • No upper age cut off

Abbreviations: United States Preventative Services Task Force (USPSTF), American College of Obstetrics and Gynecology (ACOG), American Cancer Society (ACS), American College of Radiology (ACR).

36 months HR 1.36, 95% CI 1.35 to 1.37) and are at higher risk of presenting with late-stage breast cancer (0.4% vs 0.3% for false-positive vs true negative, $P = .001$).[26]

Moving the screening interval from annual to biennial is recommended by the United States Preventative Service Task Force (USPSTF) and the ACS for women in their 50s.[24,27] By moving the screening interval the 80% mortality reduction was maintained but the false-positive test rate dropped from 61.3% to 42%.[23] For average-risk patients a biennial screening model is effective at preventing breast cancer deaths but limits the risk of false-positive imaging.

The decision to stop screening should be based on age, overall life expectancy, and patient screening goals. The USPSTF recommends that screening stop at age 75.[27]

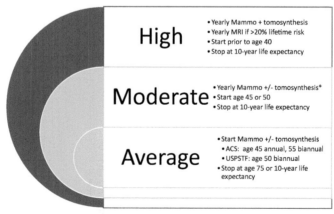

Fig. 2. Risk-based screening recommendations. Based on the patient's risk group an individualized screening strategy should be discussed with the patient. This figure can be used to guide that discussion. [a]Although current guidelines do not recommend supplemental imaging for dense breast tissue, women with extremely dense breasts may benefit from the additions of breast MRI or ultrasound given the limitations of tomosynthesis in this population. A risk calculation can be used to guide this decision.

The ACS recommends screening until the patient's life expectancy is less than 10 years.[24] This is an individual decision that requires shared decision-making between the patient and provider.

Our recommendation for screening average-risk patients is to start the discussion between age 40 and 45. Inform patients of the risk of false-positive imaging in early screening and start screening if the patient is comfortable with this risk. Everyone should start screening by age 50 and a biennial approach is appropriate if it aligns with your patient's goals. Discuss stopping screening at age 75 but consider screening until a 10-year life expectancy in otherwise healthy women.

Moderate risk: screening for those with dense breast tissue

Screening guidelines should be adjusted for patients with moderate breast cancer risk. This includes women with dense breasts, a history of a non-proliferative breast lesion, one, first-degree relative with postmenopausal breast cancer, or a calculated 15% to 19% lifetime risk of breast cancer. These patients should start screening with mammography at age 40.

Breast density is the proportion of glandular tissue to fat on a mammogram. Dense breasts confer a higher risk of breast cancer compared with those with normal density (RR 1.29 extremely, 1.23 heterogeneously dense).[23] Dense breasts may also decrease the sensitivity of mammography. Although no major screening guidelines support supplemental screening for dense breast tissue, there is legislation in most states that women must be notified of their breast density status.

Three main supplemental screening options have been proposed for women with dense breast tissue: tomosynthesis, ultrasound, and breast MRI. Tomosynthesis is a mammogram with additional pictures to provide a three-dimensional image of the breast. This option reduces recall rates but it is unclear if this is a useful option for women with extremely dense breasts. Whole breast ultrasound is not a suitable option due to high rates of false positives and unnecessary biopsies. Breast MRI is reserved for those with an more than 20% lifetime risk of breast cancer. All patients with dense breasts should have a risk calculation performed to see if they qualify for breast MRI. The USPSTF 2016 review concluded there is insufficient evidence for supplemental screening in patients with dense breasts.[27]

High risk

Those with a more than 20% lifetime risk of breast cancer are considered high-risk. This includes women with a history of childhood chest radiation, known high-risk genetic mutation, and prior high-risk breast lesions. Patients in this group should have a yearly mammogram. They should also be offered an annual breast MRI in addition to mammography.[22] Ideally, the mammogram and MRI are spaced 6 months apart to effectively screen twice a year. These patients may need to initiate screening before age 40. Mammography can be offered as early as age 30 and MRI at age 25. The recommended age to start screening high-risk individuals depends on each person's criteria for being high-risk and should be managed in conjunction with a breast cancer specialist.

Primary prevention

Counseling on breast cancer prevention and breast awareness should be offered to women in all risk categories. Below is a detailed outline of methods to reduce breast cancer risk.

General Counseling for all Patients

Breast awareness
It is important to counsel women on breast awareness to learn what normal breast tissue feels like. Although routine self-examinations are no longer recommended, women should be encouraged to seek care if they notice lumps, discharge, localized pain, or any other concerning change.

Personalized screening and prevention plan
All patients and providers should develop an individualized screening and prevention plan based on the patient's level of risk. This should include age to initiate screening, frequency of screening, and need for advanced imaging. If appropriate, a risk calculation should be included to guide this discussion. This is should be repeated yearly and updated with changes in personal or family history. All patients should be counseled on modifiable risk factors (see Risk Factor Review and Counseling section).

Additional Options for High-Risk Patients

Risk-reducing medications
The ACS and NCCN recommend the use of risk-reducing medications for women over the age of 35 with a greater than 1.66% 5-year risk of breast cancer and at least a 10-year life expectancy.[20,21] Alternatively, the USPSTF advises using a 3% 5-year risk cutoff as it identifies the patients most likely to benefit from these agents.[6]

There are two selective estrogen receptor modulators (SERMs) approved for breast cancer prevention: tamoxifen and raloxifene (**Table 5**). Tamoxifen has an estrogen antagonist effect in the breast and an estrogen agonist effect on the bones and uterus. Thus, it improves bone density but is also associated with an increased risk of endometrial cancer and should not be used in postmenopausal women with a uterus. Raloxifene blocks the effects of estrogen in the breast and uterus and has a pro-estrogen effect on the bone. The STAR trial directly compared the efficacy of the two SERMs and found that although tamoxifen is superior to raloxifene in breast cancer prevention (RR 1.24, 95% CI 1.05 to 1.47), raloxifene is associated with fewer side effects.[28] SERMs are contraindicated in women with a history of pulmonary embolism or venous thromboembolism, stroke, hypercoagulable state (ie, clotting disorder, recent surgery, immobilization, pregnancy), or breastfeeding.

Table 5
Risk-reducing medications

Class	SERMs		Aromatase Inhibitors
Medications	Tamoxifen	Raloxifene	Exemestane, Anastrozole
Population	Premenopausal or No uterus	Postmenopausal	Postmenopausal
Dose	20 mg daily	60 mg	Exemestane 25 mg daily Anastrazole 1 mg daily
Duration	5 y	5 y	5 y
Side effects	Menopausal symptoms DVT/PE, TIA/CVA		Arthralgias, menopausal symptoms
Other considerations	Improved bone density Endometrial cancer Cataracts	Less effective prevention than tamoxifen	Decreased bone density, baseline DEXA recommended prior to treatment

Although not US Food and Drug Administration (FDA)-approved, the aromatase inhibitors (AIs) anastrozole and exemestane have been studied for breast cancer risk reduction and are recommended for use by NCCN for postmenopausal women (see **Table 5**).[20] Through inhibition of aromatase, AIs block the conversion of androgens to estrogen, which is the main method of estrogen production in post-menopause women. The MAP.3 and IBIS-II trials showed the efficacy of exemestane (HR 0.47, 95% CI 0.27 to 0.79) and anastrozole (HR 0.47, 95% CI 0.32 to 0.68), respectively. No trials are comparing the risk/benefits of AIs to SERMs.[29,30] Common side effects of AIs include osteoporosis, worsening of vasomotor symptoms, and joint pain (see **Table 5**).[31] All postmenopausal women should undergo a baseline bone density assessment before starting medication.[8] The decisions of which agent to start should be based on if the patient has a uterus, menopause status, and bone density.[31]

The recommended duration of medication for breast cancer prevention is a total of 5 years (see **Table 5** for dosing).[8,28–30] Overall, studies show that providers greatly under-utilize medications for chemoprophylaxis despite a clear benefit in high-risk patients.[32,33] Barriers to care include provider knowledge limitations and time constraints as well as patient concerns about adverse effects.[34] Primary care providers, in particular, should be aware of who is eligible for risk-reducing medications and engage in shared decision-making conversations with eligible patients to potentially prevent future disease. Premenopausal women may elect to defer treatment until completion of child-bearing or after menopause.

Prophylactic surgery

Risk-reducing surgery includes prophylactic mastectomy and, for some women, bilateral oophorectomy. Surgery is offered to patients with a lifetime breast cancer risk of more than 50%.[20] This is generally limited to women with a known genetic mutation, strong family history, or prior chest radiation under the age of 30. Most often surgery is performed once childbearing is complete. NCCN recommends multi-disciplinary consultations when considering surgery to discuss the risks and benefits, treatment alternatives, and available reconstruction options.[20]

SUMMARY

Breast cancer is a preventable disease for many people through lifestyle changes, risk-reducing medications, and surgery. Screening and early detection remain important tools in the treatment of breast cancer. All women, regardless of cancer risk, should undergo a breast cancer risk assessment. Women should also be counseled on ways that they can reduce their own cancer risk, including weight loss, exercise, and reduced alcohol intake. Screening decisions should be made using an individual, risk-based approach with all women receiving mammograms by age 50. A risk calculation should be performed on those with a family history of breast cancer, dense breasts, or prior breast biopsy. This calculation should be used to identify patients that qualify for advanced screening imaging, risk-reducing medications, or surgery.

CLINICS CARE POINTS

- A breast cancer risk assessment should be performed for all women starting at age 18. This should include a review of personal and family medical history, as well as a review of modifiable risk factors.
- A breast cancer risk calculation should be performed for patients with a family history of cancers, prior breast biopsies, or dense breasts.

- All women should receive mammography screening by age 50. Higher-risk women may need to begin screening as early as age 25.
- Risk-reduction medications should be offered to all women with a history of ductal carcinoma in situ, lobular carcinoma in situ, or a more than 3% 5-year risk of breast cancer.
- Breast MRI should be offered with mammography to women with a more than 20% lifetime risk of breast cancer.

DISCLOSURE

The authors have nothing to disclose.

REFERENCES

1. Center for Disease Control. Breast Cancer Statistics. Available at: https://www.cdc.gov/cancer/breast/statistics/index.htm. Accessed May 30, 2022.
2. American Cancer Society. Key Statistics for Breast Cancer. Available at: https://www.cancer.org/cancer/breast-cancer/about/how-common-is-breast-cancer.html. Accessed May 30, 2022.
3. DeSantis C, Ma J, Bryan L, et al. Breast cancer statistics, 2013. CA Cancer J Clin 2014;64(1):52–62. https://doi.org/10.3322/caac.21203. Accessed May 30, 2022.
4. Siegel R, Ward E, Brawley O, et al. Cancer statistics, 2011: the impact of eliminating socioeconomic and racial disparities on premature cancer deaths. CA Cancer J Clin 2011;61(4):212–36.
5. Colditz GA, Bohlke K. Priorities for the primary prevention of breast cancer. CA Cancer J Clin 2014;64(3):186–94. https://doi.org/10.3322/caac.21225.
6. Nelson HD, Smith MB, Griffin JC, et al. Use of medications to reduce the risk for primary breast cancer: a systematic review for the US Preventive Services Task Force. Ann Intern Med 2013;158(8):604–14.
7. Owens DK, Davidson KW, Krist AH, et al. Risk assessment, genetic counseling, and genetic testing for BRCA-related cancer: US Preventive Services Task Force recommendation statement. Jama 2019;322(7):652–65.
8. National Comprehensive Cancer Network. NCCN clinical practice guidelines in oncology: genetic/familial high-risk assessment: breast and ovarian, version 1. 2018. Available at: https://www.nccn.org/professionals/physician_gls/pdf/genetics_screening.pdf. Published online October 3, 2017. Accessed March 11, 2018.
9. Nattinger AB, Mitchell JL. Breast cancer screening and prevention. Ann Intern Med 2016;164(11):ITC81.
10. Sprague B, et al. Proportion of invasive breast cancer attributable to risk factors modifiable after menopause. Am J Epidemiol. 168(4. Available at: https://www.ncbi.nlm.nih.gov/pmc/articles/PMC2727276/. Accessed May 30, 2022.
11. Moskowitz CS, Chou JF, Wolden SL, et al. Breast cancer after chest radiation therapy for childhood cancer. J Clin Oncol Off J Am Soc Clin Oncol 2014;32(21):2217–23.
12. Schnitt SJ. Benign breast disease and breast cancer risk: morphology and beyond. Am J Surg Pathol 2003;27(6):836–41.
13. Bernstein, L et al. Lifetime recreational exercise activity and breast cancer risk among black women and white women. J Natl Cancer Inst. 97(22).
14. Marmot M, Atinmo T, Byers T, et al. Food, nutrition, physical activity, and the prevention of cancer: a global perspective. Published online 2007.

15. Chen WY, Rosner B, Hankinson SE, et al. Moderate alcohol consumption during adult life, drinking patterns, and breast cancer risk. Jama 2011;306(17):1884–90.

16. Chlebowski RT, Anderson GL, Gass M, et al. Estrogen plus progestin and breast cancer incidence and mortality in postmenopausal women. Jama 2010;304(15):1684–92.

17. Chen WY, Manson JE, Hankinson SE, et al. Unopposed estrogen therapy and the risk of invasive breast cancer. Arch Intern Med 2006;166(9):1027–32.

18. Barańska A, Błaszczuk A, Kanadys W, et al. Oral contraceptive use and breast cancer risk assessment: a systematic review and meta-analysis of case-control studies, 2009–2020. Cancers 2021;13(22):5654.

19. Owens DK, Davidson KW, Krist AH, et al. Medication use to reduce risk of breast cancer: US Preventive Services Task Force recommendation statement. Jama 2019;322(9):857–67.

20. National Comprehensive Cancer Network. NCCN clinical practice guideline in oncology: breast cancer risk reduction. 2018;Version 2. 2018. Available at: https://www.nccn.org/professionals/physician_gls/PDF/breast_risk.pdf. Accessed August 13, 2018.

21. Visvanathan K, Hurley P, Bantug E, et al. Use of pharmacologic interventions for breast cancer risk reduction: American Society of Clinical Oncology clinical practice guideline. J Clin Oncol 2013;31(23):2942–62.

22. Saslow D, Boetes C, Burke W, et al. American Cancer Society guidelines for breast screening with MRI as an adjunct to mammography. CA Cancer J Clin 2007;57(2):75–89.

23. Mandelblatt JS, Stout NK, Schechter CB, et al. Collaborative modeling of the benefits and harms associated with different US breast cancer screening strategies. Ann Intern Med 2016;164(4):215–25.

24. Oeffinger KC, Fontham ET, Etzioni R, et al. Breast cancer screening for women at average risk: 2015 guideline update from the American Cancer Society. Jama 2015;314(15):1599–614.

25. Nelson HD, Pappas M, Cantor A, et al. Harms of breast cancer screening: systematic review to update the 2009 US Preventive Services Task Force recommendation. Ann Intern Med 2016;164(4):256–67.

26. Dabbous FM, Dolecek TA, Berbaum ML, et al. Impact of a false-positive screening mammogram on subsequent screening behavior and stage at breast cancer diagnosis. Cancer Epidemiol Prev Biomark 2017;26(3):397–403.

27. Siu AL, US Preventive Services Task Force. Screening for breast cancer: US Preventive Services Task Force recommendation statement. Ann Intern Med 2016;164(4):279–96.

28. Vogel VG, Costantino JP, Wickerham DL, et al. Update of the national surgical adjuvant breast and bowel project study of tamoxifen and raloxifene (STAR) P-2 trial: preventing breast cancer. Cancer Prev Res (Phila Pa 2010;3(6):696–706.

29. Goss PE, Ingle JN, Alés-Martínez JE, et al. Exemestane for breast-cancer prevention in postmenopausal women. N Engl J Med 2011;364(25):2381–91.

30. Cuzick J, Sestak I, Forbes JF, et al. Anastrozole for prevention of breast cancer in high-risk postmenopausal women (IBIS-II): an international, double-blind, randomised placebo-controlled trial. The Lancet 2014;383(9922):1041–8.

31. Farkas A, Vanderberg R, Merriam S, et al. Breast cancer chemoprevention: a practical guide for the primary care provider. J Womens Health 2020;29(1):46–56.

32. Waters E, et al. Use of tamoxifen and raloxifene for breast cancer chemoprevention in 2010. Breast Cancer Res Treat. 134(2). Available at: https://www.ncbi.nlm.nih.gov/pmc/articles/PMC3771085/. Accessed May 30, 2022.

33. Crew K. Addressing barriers to uptake of breast cancer chemoprevention for patients and providers. In: American society of clinical oncology educational book. Vol 35. Available at: https://ascopubs.org/doi/10.14694/EdBook_AM.2015.35.e50. Accessed May 30, 2022.

34. Ropka ME, et al. Patient decisions about breast cancer chemoprevention: a systematic review and meta-analysis. J Clin Oncol. 28(18). Available at: https://www.ncbi.nlm.nih.gov/pmc/articles/PMC2903338/#B31. Accessed May 30, 2022.

Updates in Cardiovascular Disease Prevention, Diagnosis, and Treatment in Women

Sarah Jones, MD, MS[a],*, Melissa McNeil, MD, MPH, MACP[b],
Agnes Koczo, MD[c]

KEYWORDS

- Cardiovascular disease • Women's health • Primary prevention
- Spontaneous coronary artery dissection • Microvascular disease

KEY POINTS

- Reproductive and menopause histories identify the cardiovascular disease (CVD) risk enhancers that should be considered for CVD prevention and diagnosis.
- Consideration of a woman's overall cardiometabolic risk affects guideline-directed management of individual cardiovascular risk factors (cholesterol, blood pressure, diabetes). Advances in anti-obesity pharmacology offer a new opportunity for obesity management. Optimization of other cardiovascular risk factors is favored over prescribing aspirin for primary prevention.
- Delayed diagnosis of CVD and lack of guideline-recommended treatment of CVD are disparities in women's cardiovascular care.
- Spontaneous coronary artery dissection and microvascular disease cause CVD more often in women than men. Improvements in cardiovascular imaging to diagnose and ongoing trials for targeted treatment of these CVD etiologies aim to improve women's CVD care.

As cardiovascular disease (CVD) is the leading cause of death in the United States for both women and men, and with 80% of CVD thought to be preventable, atherosclerotic cardiovascular disease (ASCVD) prevention and risk reduction benefit individuals and society.[1] Many patients do not have access to preventive cardiology so primary

[a] Division of General Internal Medicine, University of Pittsburgh Medical Center, Montefiore Hospital, 933 West, 200 Lothrop Street, Pittsburgh, PA 15213, USA; [b] Warren Alpert School of Medicine of Brown University, Rhode Island Hospital, Women's Health, VHA Central Office, 64 Caswell Street, Narragansett, RI 02882, USA; [c] Division of Cardiology, University of Pittsburgh Medical Center, 2350 Terrace Street, Scaife Hall, S-360, Pittsburgh, PA 15213, USA
* Corresponding author.
E-mail address: jonessa3@upmc.edu

Med Clin N Am 107 (2023) 285–298
https://doi.org/10.1016/j.mcna.2022.10.008
0025-7125/23/© 2022 Elsevier Inc. All rights reserved.

care has the unique opportunity to promote and achieve cardiovascular risk reduction for decades before a first cardiovascular event. Women face disparities in prevention, diagnosis, and treatment of CVD which will be discussed in this review.

PREVENTION OF CARDIOVASCULAR DISEASE

As a framework for clinical discussion of ASCVD prevention and risk reduction, the American Heart Association (AHA) recently expanded from Life's Simple 7 to Life's Essential 8 with the addition of sleep as a notable risk factor in the 2022 update.[2]

Life's Essential 8 includes (1) diet, (2) physical activity, (3) nicotine exposure, (4) sleep duration, (5) weight, (6) cholesterol, (7) blood sugar, and (8) blood pressure (BP).[2] Briefly, Life's Essential 8 are defined as outlined below.

1. Diet: Follow a healthy eating pattern.
2. Physical activity: 150 min of moderate-intensity or 75 min of vigorous-intensity exercise are recommended per week with the addition of strength training and flexibility exercises.
3. Nicotine exposure: Plan to quit inhaling nicotine from cigarettes, e-cigarettes, or vaping.
4. Sleep: 7 to 9 h of sleep per night is recommended.
5. Weight: Maintain a healthy weight, body mass index (BMI) <25.
6. Cholesterol: Decrease low-density lipoprotein (LDL) and increase high-density lipoprotein (HDL).
7. Blood sugar: Diagnose and treat prediabetes and diabetes mellitus (DM).
8. Blood pressure: Treat elevated BP to goal, generally <120/80.

More detailed updates for Diet, Weight, Cholesterol, Blood sugar, and BP will follow—highlighting assessment and treatment of these risk factors not as isolated conditions but as part of a patient's cardiometabolic profile, particularly noting the difference in the women's healthcare.

Diet: Mediterranean

The Mediterranean diet remains a widely recognized and recommended dietary pattern given its benefits for cardiovascular events and metabolic risk factors (obesity, lipid disorders, hypertension, DM).[3] Meta-analyses of randomized control trials that included more than 9,000 participants and examined the Mediterranean diet vs varied dietary recommendations showed a more than 30% risk reduction for CVD incidence and myocardial infarction (MI).[3]

The Mediterranean diet centers on fresh and seasonally available vegetables and fruits at each meal accompanied by minimally processed grains or bread. Olive oil is the primary fat rather than butter or lard. Daily consumption of olives, nuts, seeds, and low-fat dairy is common. White meats, fish, legumes, and eggs may each be added a few times per week, whereas red meat and processed meats are eaten sparingly. Wine may be consumed with meals.

We recommend the Mediterranean diet to patients to reduce CVD risk.

Weight: Anti-Obesity Pharmacology

Rates of obesity in the United States continue to rise. More than 40% of women over age 40 having an obese BMI (≥30), and obesity confers a greater risk for CAD in women than men (64% vs 46%).[4,5] Obesity is not a lack of individual willpower, but rather it is as a multi-factorial chronic illness.

For those with overweight BMI ($\geq$25) or obese BMI ($\geq$30), weight loss of even 5% to 10% can confer health benefits. Apart from cardiometabolic benefits, dietary changes may provide modest weight loss of about 5%. Exercise may provide 2% weight loss but is a mainstay of weight maintenance. Bariatric surgical procedures may provide an estimated 25% to 35% weight loss and can provide CVD risk reduction.[6]

Although anti-obesity pharmacotherapy is recommended for those with BMI $\geq$30 or BMI $\geq$27 with obesity-related comorbidities, less than 1% of eligible individuals receive prescriptions.[7] Modest weight loss benefit ($\sim$5–10%), concerns about long-term use (particularly with phentermine), variable insurance coverage, and high medications costs have largely limited wide-spread prescriptions for anti-obesity medications or their component parts (Qysmia [phentermine/topiramate], Contrave [bupropion/naltrexone], Xenical [orlistat], Adipex [phentermine]). Advocacy to address cost and secure Medicare coverage is ongoing.

Recent developments in anti-obesity pharmacology include U.S. Food and Drug Administration (FDA) approval for the glucagon-like peptide-1 receptor agonists (GLP1-RAs) liraglutide (Saxenda) in 2015 and semaglutide (Wegovy) in 2021. The Semaglutide Treatment Effect in People with Obesity (STEP) Trial showed mean weight loss of almost 15% compared with 2.5% in the placebo group in approximately 2000 obese individuals (BMI $\geq$30) or overweight individuals (BMI $\geq$27) with a weight-related comorbidity over 68 weeks.[8] Results of the Semaglutide Effects on Heart Disease and Stroke in Patients with Overweight or Obesity trial to evaluate longer-term cardiovascular outcomes in this population may be available in late 2023.

Tirzepatide, a combination of a glucose-dependent insulinotropic polypeptide (GIP) and GLP1-RA, showed more than 20% weight loss in obese or overweight participants with co-morbidities when taken at the higher doses over the 72-week trial.[9] The weekly injection tirzepatide (Mounjaro) previously received FDA approval for DM Type 2 and is expected to be approved for weight management.

Evidence to support the maintenance use of anti-obesity medications continues to grow. For example, for 327 participants followed after the STEP1 trial, stopping semaglutide resulted in weight regain (two-thirds of the weight lost) over 1 year of follow-up.[10] Weight regain was similarly shown in other populations with discontinuation of other anti-obesity medications.[11]

Of note, all anti-obesity medications are contraindicated in pregnancy and breast-feeding. GLP1-RAs should be discontinued 2 months before trying to conceive.

We recommend (1) addressing weight management with non-stigmatizing language and attitudes, (2) prescribing anti-obesity medications when indicated and affordable, and (3) continuing prescriptions to maintain weight loss.

Cholesterol: Risk Categorization Including Risk Enhancers and Radiographic Risk Assessment (Coronary Artery Calcium Score) and Medication Management

High-intensity statin therapy is recommended for secondary prevention in those with known ASCVD. To determine which patients may benefit from statin therapy for primary prevention, clinical practice guidelines recommend using the ASCVD Pooled Cohort Equation (PCE).[12]

Risk categorization with risk enhancers
The ASCVD PCE is derived from multiple cardiovascular cohorts, is validated in women and men, and uses patient demographics (age, sex, race) and risk factors (BP, cholesterol, DM, and smoking) to estimate the 10-year ASCVD risk.[12] Cardiovascular events affect women about a decade later than men, which is reflected in the risk calculator.

Clinical cholesterol management guidelines were updated in 2018. For 40 to 75 year old patients at low risk, defined as <5% 10 year ASCVD risk, lifestyle discussion to reduce risk factors is advised.[13] For 40 to 75 year old patients at high risk, defined as ≥20% 10 year ASCVD risk, high-intensity statin therapy is recommended.[13] Between these two groups are the "borderline risk" group at 5% to 7.5% 10-year ASCVD risk and the "intermediate risk" group from 7.5% to 20% 10 year ASCVD risk.[13] For these groups, shared decision-making about at least moderate intensity statin therapy is recommended depending on ASCVD Risk Enhancers.[13]

Risk enhancers increase the risk of ASCVD but are not included in the PCE. They include a family history of premature ASCVD, LDL persistently ≥160, chronic kidney disease (CKD), metabolic syndrome, inflammatory diseases (autoimmune disorders, HIV), ethnicity, and women's specific conditions such as preeclampsia, premature menopause, and polycystic ovarian syndrome (PCOS).[13] If uncertainty remains, a coronary artery calcium (CAC) score can be used to further risk stratify patients.[13] CAC is superior to the PCE for risk stratification and performs equally well in women and men.[14,15]

We recommend taking a comprehensive assessment of both traditional and nontraditional risk factors, including a reproductive and menopausal history, to best counsel patients on their 10-year and lifetime ASCVD risk as well as statin therapy and dose.

Radiographic risk assessment

CAC is one radiographic method of evaluating subclinical or asymptomatic ASCVD. Others include carotid intimal wall thickness and arterial-brachial index. On mammography, breast arterial calcification correlates with CAC, and the absence of BAC has an 81% negative predictive value for CAC.[16] When CAC score = 0, the risk of a CVD event in the next 2 to 5 years is 0.1% per year, and statin therapy may be deferred in borderline and intermediate-risk patients.[13,17] However, for patients with diabetes, strong family history of ASCVD, or active smoking, statin therapy is still recommended.[13] For CAC score 1 to 99, statin therapy is favored for patients ≥ age 55.[13] For CAC ≥100, statin therapy is recommended with a ninefold increased risk of coronary heart disease (CHD) and sixfold increased risk of CVD events compared with CAC = 0.[13,18]

We recommend CAC scoring in patients with borderline or intermediate risk who are uncertain about statin therapy or who would benefit from additional risk assessment. We also recommend assessment of alternate imaging including mammography or prior chest CT to identify surrogates for coronary calcium that argue in favor of statin therapy.

Medication management

Meta-analysis of only trials including women show primary prevention with statins reduces the risk of CHD and CVD events.[19,20] However, women are less likely to be prescribed statins as well as more likely to be prescribed lower doses of statins and have poorly controlled dyslipidemia.[21–23] Once statins are prescribed, women are more likely to experience adverse events such as fatigue, subjective myalgias, and subjective nervous system reactions compared with men.[24] As a consequence, they are more likely to switch or stop statin medications than men.[25] Women also report less satisfaction with communication about statin medications than men.[26]

Statin medications have long been contraindicated in pregnancy (former FDA category X) and should be discontinued 1-2 months before trying to conceive or immediately in unintended pregnancy. However, accumulating evidence on statins in pregnancy—including targeted therapy for preeclampsia—recently led the FDA to remove the strongest warning against statins in pregnancy for high risk women.[27]

If maximal statin therapy fails to achieve goal LDL reductions, >50% for high-risk individuals or 30% to 49% for borderline-risk individuals with risk enhancers or intermediate-risk individuals, further LDL lowering medications can be added.[13] For individuals who cannot tolerate statin therapy, particularly those who have an ASCVD equivalent, other LDL-lowering medications including ezetimibe and proprotein convertase subtilisin/kexin type-9 inhibitors are recommended.[13]

We recommend clear and receptive communication with women about statin therapy as well as a willingness to trial multiple statins to find those which are tolerated. Further, we recommend using alternate lipid-lowering agents in women with prior ASCVD events or at the highest risk of future events.

Blood Sugar: Medication Management to Reduce Cardiovascular Disease

In the 2021 Standards of Medical Care in Diabetes, cardiovascular risk reduction is a central consideration for medication selection.[28] Statin therapy is recommended for adults with diabetes aged 40 to 75 years.[13] The American Diabetes Association (ADA) recommends initial management of DM Type 2 with metformin and comprehensive lifestyle changes.[28]

For patients who are at high risk for or have established ASCVD, CKD, or heart failure (HF), the ADA recommends GLP1-RA or sodium-glucose cotransport-2 (SGLT2) inhibitor medications with demonstrated cardiovascular benefit.[28] For ASCVD benefit, GLP1-RAs with FDA approval include dulaglutide, liraglutide, and semaglutide; the SGLT2 inhibitor with FDA approval for CVD risk reduction is empagliflozin.[29,30] In patients with CKD with proteinuria and already on renin-angiotensin system blockade (RASB), SGLT2 inhibitors are recommended to reduce progression to end-stage renal disease and death due to renal cause.[28] For patients with HF, adding SGLT2 inhibitors has been shown to reduce the risk of HF hospitalizations and cardiovascular death.[30]

Of note, the cardiovascular benefits of GLP1-RAs and SGLT2 inhibitors are independent of glycemic control and have been observed for patients without DM so the ADA recommends using them independently of A1C goal.[28] Given their separate mechanisms of action, cardiovascular benefits from the two medication classes may be additive but clinical evidence does not yet support this practice.[31,32]

We recommend (1) screening women at risk for DM, especially with a history of gestational diabetes, preeclampsia, PCOS, or obesity, and (2) utilizing GLP1-RAs and SGLT2 inhibitors for cardiovascular benefits, particularly for patients with high ASCVD risk, CKD, or HF (ie adding these medications to metformin and lifestyle management to achieve goal A1C and even after A1C target is met).

Blood Pressure: Using Atherosclerotic Cardiovascular Disease Risk to Guide Management

In the 2017 AHA/American College of Cardiology (ACC) Guidelines for hypertension, a patient's overall cardiometabolic risk is again used to determine the intensity of therapy.[33]

Normal BP is defined as BP < 120/80 mm Hg and should be reassessed annually.[33] Elevated BP is 120 to 129/<80 mm Hg which can be treated with lifestyle recommendations and reassessed in 3 to 6 months.[33]

Stage 1 hypertension is defined as 130 to 139/80 to 89 mm Hg, and its management depends on a patient's 10 year ASCVD risk from the PCE.[33] If less than 10%, it is treated like elevated BP as above.[33] If greater than 10% or if specific co-morbidities are present (DM, CKD, CKD post renal transplant, HF, stable ischemic heart disease, peripheral arterial disease), it is treated like Stage 2 hypertension (BP $\geq$ 140/90), and anti-hypertensive medication is recommended with reassessment in 1 month.[33] Therapy should be intensified to reach goal of BP <130/80 mm Hg.[33]

Menopause is a risk factor for hypertension, and more than three-quarters of women over 60 develop hypertension.[34] However, hypertension is underdiagnosed and not as well controlled for women compared with men.[35] For reproductive-age women, calcium channel blockers (specifically nifedipine), beta-blockers, and diuretics are preferred initial choices for BP management given the concern for fetal renal development with RASB.

We recommend (1) screening and diagnosing women with hypertension, and (2) treating hypertension to goal to reduce ASCVD risk.

Low-Dose Aspirin for Primary Prevention: Manage Other Cardiovascular Disease Risks Instead

Low-dose aspirin (75 mg per day) remains a mainstay of secondary prevention for those with known ASCVD. However, low-dose aspirin's role in primary prevention has grown more limited as the risks of bleeding have surpassed protection from ASCVD events. Experts attribute this change to better management of other CVD risk factors.[36,37]

In 2018, the RCTs ASPREE, ASCEND, and ARRIVE generally failed to show protection against ASCVD events compared with bleeding risk with the use of low-dose aspirin for primary prevention of CVD for patients ≥70 years in good health, with diabetes, or with ASCVD risk factors respectively.[38–40]

As a result, the USPSTF recommended AGAINST initiating aspirin for primary prevention in adults over the age of 60 years in their 2021 to 2022 guidelines.[37] For those aged 40 to 59 with ≥10% 10-year ASCVD risk, the USPSTF recommended shared decision-making, noting that the benefit of aspirin is small and those without bleeding risks are more likely to benefit.[37] AHA/ACC similarly recommends against aspirin for primary prevention in those over age 70 years or in adults with increased bleeding risk and reserves low-dose aspirin for those aged 40 to 70 years at higher ASCVD risk without increased bleeding risk.[37]

Aspirin is also used in pregnancy to prevent preeclampsia in high-risk individuals. Studies of the potential benefits of aspirin use in the postpartum period to prevent chronic hypertension and cardiac remodeling are ongoing.[41]

We recommend clear communication with patients that aspirin should be continued for secondary prevention. For primary prevention, we optimize other CVD risk factors before recommending low-dose aspirin—and would limit low-dose aspirin for patients unable to tolerate other risk factor management who do not have increased bleeding risk. In general, for patients over age 60 years, we do not initiate low-dose aspirin and discontinue aspirin for primary prevention.

DIAGNOSIS AND TREATMENT OF CARDIOVASCULAR DISEASE

The most important part of evaluating a patient for CVD is the initial inclusion of acute coronary syndrome (ACS) in the differential diagnosis. Although CVD affects women roughly a decade later than their male counterparts, it still is the leading cause of mortality in the United States.

Diagnosis of Acute Coronary Syndrome

Women experience a greater spectrum of ACS symptoms than men. The Prospective Multicenter Imaging Study for Evaluation of Chest Pain trial looked at approximately 10,000 stable outpatients with suspected CAD and found that chest pain is the most experienced symptom among both men and women.[42] However, women more commonly also experience nausea, fatigue, and shortness of breath.[42]

If the acute coronary syndrome is suspected, guidelines recommend obtaining an electrocardiogram (EKG) and interpretation within 10 min.[43] Cardiac troponin I or T remains the most sensitive marker for myocardial injury, and there is no longer a role for creatine kinase-MB in initial diagnosis.[43] More recently, many institutions have introduced high-sensitivity troponin (hs-cTn) for both faster detection and exclusion of myocardial injury.[43] If ACS is suspected, guideline algorithms for ST elevation (STEMI) and non-ST elevation (NSTEMI) should be followed.

We recommend asking about accompanying symptoms during history taking to achieve a more rapid diagnosis and treatment of ACS in women.

Risk stratification

A myriad of risk scores, including the HEART, ADAPT, and GRACE scores, have been published to aid in the decision to pursue further cardiac testing for patients without MI. When utilizing risk scores, it is important to note that sex-specific considerations as well as representations of women in studies may not have been adequate to determine equal efficacy for both men and women.[44]

Traditional risk factors are often weighted in these scores which fail to account for an increasing body of evidence that non-traditional risk factors—which include sex-specific risks such as premature menopause and hypertensive disorders of pregnancy—significantly contribute to future cardiovascular risk. For example, after controlling for traditional risk factors in postmenopausal women, hypertensive disorders of pregnancy and history of low birth weight were independently associated with ASCVD.[45]

For the highest risk patients in which ACS is suspected, cardiology should be consulted for consideration of invasive coronary angiography. For the patients with acute or stable chest pain who are at intermediate risk, current guidelines note this population would benefit most from further non-invasive cardiac testing. In patients deemed low risk in pretest stratification models, there is a class I indication for no cardiovascular imaging.[43]

We recommend taking a comprehensive assessment of both traditional and nontraditional risk factors, including a reproductive and menopausal history, to assess a woman's risk for ACS.

We recommend cardiology consultation for high-risk patients and non-invasive cardiac testing for those at intermediate risk.

Cardiac imaging

In low-risk individuals in which symptoms remain concerning for coronary disease, exercise stress testing is interpretable with a normal baseline EKG. Sensitivity and specificity of detection of obstructive CAD on exercise stress are decreased for women related to inability to achieve maximal exercise requirements and lower baseline QRS voltage; yet, the negative predictive value remains high.[34,46]

In patients with intermediate pretest risk, most stress testing modalities are considered class I recommendations for investigating anginal symptoms. These include functional stress imaging including echocardiography, single-photon emission computed tomography (SPECT), positron emission tomography (PET), and CMR imaging in addition to anatomic modalities, namely coronary computed tomography (CCTA). Of note, in patients under 65 years of age or in patients where obstructive epicardial coronary disease is not suspected, CCTA is recommended over functional stress testing. **Table 1** depicts the most recent ACC/AHA recommendations for deciding which modality to use depending on unique benefits and inherent risks for each.

Table 1
Factors that assist in choosing the right stress test[43]

	Favors Use of CCTA	Favors Use of Stress Imaging
Goal	• Rule out obstructive CAD • Detect nonobstructive CAD	• Ischemia-guided management
Availability and expertise	• High-quality imaging and expert interpretation routinely available	• High-quality imaging and expert interpretation routinely available
Likelihood of obstructive CAD	• Age < 65 y	• Age ≥ 65 y
Prior test results	• Prior functional study inconclusive	• Prior CCTA inconclusive
Other compelling indications	• Anomalous coronary arteries • Require evaluation of aorta or pulmonary arteries	• Suspect scar (especially if PET or stress CMR available) • Suspect coronary microvascular dysfunction (when PET or CMR available)

	Stress Testing Information				
	ETT	Stress Echocardiography	SPECT MPI	PET MPI	Stress CMR MPI
Patient capable of exercise	✔	✔	✔		
Pharmacologic stress indicated		✔	✔	✔	✔
Quantitative				✔	✔
LV dysfunction/scar		✔	✔	✔	✔

Abbreviations: ASCVD, atherosclerotic cardiovascular disease; CAC, coronary artery calcium; CAD, coronary artery disease; CCTA, coronary computed tomography angiography; CMR, cardiovascular magnetic resonance; ETT, exercise tolerance test; LV, left ventricular; MPI, myocardial perfusion imaging; PET, position emission tomography; SPECT, single-photon emission computed tomography.

Many institutions now have the capabilities and expertise to evaluate for both acute and stable chest pain due to epicardial coronary disease (obstructive or non-obstructive) with CCTA. In addition, CCTA can provide additional information noted on standard chest CT imaging including lung parenchyma. A "triple rule-out" protocol can specifically investigate for acute etiologies of chest pain including aortic dissection and pulmonary arterial embolism.[47]

Women are disproportionately impacted by myocardial infarction due to non-obstructive coronary disease (MINOCA), and considering symptoms attributable to microvascular disease (MVD) is important. In addition to investigating epicardial coronary disease, both stress PET imaging and stress CMR imaging can assess for MVD. Both imaging modalities can indirectly quantitate flow and make inferences about microvascular dysfunction by looking at the ratio of peak stress and rest coronary flow in estimating coronary flow reserve. In addition, as noted above, CCTA can be useful in detecting non-obstructive coronary disease.[48]

We recommend consideration of CCTA for women in whom obstructive disease is suspected and stress PET or CMR for women in whom MVD is suspected. Depending on institutional availability and clinician familiarity with imaging, cardiology consultation may be beneficial.

Special considerations in women

In women who are pregnant or breastfeeding, there are important considerations for both radiation and contrast exposure for cardiac testing. In addition, discussing the risks and benefits of options and utilizing radiation risk-minimizing procedures like abdominal shielding or selecting non-radiation testing (stress echocardiography, CMR) is important. Both iodinated contrast, which can cross the placental barrier, and gadolinium are discouraged in pregnant women. Less than 1% of contrast is excreted in breastmilk, so it is not recommended to stop breastfeeding.[49]

Treatment of Acute Coronary Syndrome

Acute and long-term management of ACS/CAD in women is worse for women than men. Women have delayed door-to-procedure (often measured in the cardiology literature as door-to-balloon) times as well as slower transfers for percutaneous coronary interventions from facilities without this expertise. This is attributed to the delayed presentation of women to a medical setting as well as delayed diagnosis of ACS due to greater heterogeneity in presenting symptoms. Following a woman's ACS event, she is less likely to receive guideline-direct medical therapy.[50]

We recommend recognizing disparities in diagnosis and treatment to allow the intentional closure of this gap in care for women.

Myocardial infarction due to non-obstructive coronary disease causing cardiovascular disease in women: spontaneous coronary artery dissection and microvascular disease

Women are more likely to present with myocardial infarction that is not due to epicardial obstructive coronary disease. The umbrella term for the spectrum of etiologies that can present with ACS is termed MINOCA. Depending on the literature, MINOCA account for 6% to 10% of all causes of ACS, and women have 5 times higher odds of MINOCA.[51] While there are many potential etiologies, our discussion will focus on spontaneous coronary artery dissection (SCAD) and MVD given the increased recognition of these two disease pathologies.[52]

Spontaneous coronary artery dissection

Spontaneous coronary artery dissection (SCAD), a nonatherosclerotic and nontraumatic cause of ACS, disproportionately impacts women. Before the formation of large national and international registries, SCAD was thought to be rare. Although it makes up about 4% of all causes of ACS, it is responsible for about 35% of ACS in women <50.[53] Its etiology is still under investigation, though a high proportion of patients have underlying vascular abnormalities, namely fibromuscular dysplasia (FMD). Given the prevalence of underlying FMD in many patients, head-to-pelvis screening is recommended for all patients who have been diagnosed with SCAD.[53]

Despite the growth of large-scale registries, there are no randomized clinical trials to guide therapeutic management for SCAD. SCAD is a non-atherosclerotic process so lipid-lowering therapy is recommended only if otherwise indicated for primary prevention. SCAD can recur in 10% to 30% of patients, and beta-blocker use and hypertension control have been shown to reduce SCAD recurrence in small studies.[54] For conservatively treated SCAD lesions (withoutcoronary bypass grafts or placement of coronary stents), single antiplatelet therapy with aspirin or dual antiplatelet therapy (DAPT) with P2Y12 inhibitors, like clopidogrel, can be used in patients for a short duration of time.[54] Although lacking robust data for the benefit of antiplatelet agents in these patients, emerging data from international registries suggest DAPT is actually associated with increased major adverse cardiac events.[55]

SCAD can be seen with hormonal fluctuation, including pregnancy-associated SCAD (P-SCAD). This typically occurs in the days to weeks postpartum. P-SCAD patients tend to present with more high-risk features including cardiac arrest, cardiogenic shock, and decreased left ventricular function. Although P-SCAD may not be associated with the risk of recurrent SCAD during subsequent pregnancies, the patient should be appropriately counseled about serious sequelae in considering future pregnancies.[56]

Microvascular disease

An understanding of the pathophysiology of MVD, which primarily affects the coronary arterioles, has evolved greatly in the last decade. There are several distinct physiologic mechanisms proposed, including increased circulating nitric oxide synthase depleting levels of this essential vasodilator, as well as innate vascular narrowing from the increased inward remodeling of the coronary arterioles.

Each underlying mechanism may lead to distinct phenotypes, and patients should ideally receive therapy targeted toward pathologic causes for the most effective symptomatic therapy. The CorMicA trial followed about 150 patients with anginal symptoms and non-obstructive epicardial coronary disease who were stratified to etiology-specific medical management as compared with a control group (blinded coronary angiography results) over 1 year. The targeted treatments included beta-blockers for microvascular dysfunction or calcium channel blockers and long-acting nitrates for vasospasm. Targeted treatment provided a significantly better quality of life and symptomatic improvement.[57] Additional trials of targeted therapies for MVD, including WARRIER and MINOCA-BAT, are ongoing.

We recommend further diagnostic imaging (including the non-invasive imaging detailed previously) for women who have persisting symptoms of angina and signs of myocardial injury or infarction presenting as MINOCA, noting MVD and SCAD etiologies are more common in women. For women diagnosed with these underlying causes of CVD, we recommend consideration of targeted therapies and/or cardiology consultation for treatment recommendations. For P-SCAD, we recommend prescribing effective contraception and avoiding future pregnancy until specialist consultation with cardiology and/or maternal–fetal medicine.

Women experience disparities in cardiovascular care across the spectrum of prevention, diagnosis, and treatment. CVD prevention strategies have effective therapies to treat risk factors directly and to reduce risk given broad consideration of a woman's overall cardiometabolic risk. Identifying differences in the underlying causes of CVD in women and improvements in imaging studies to diagnose them offer an opportunity for targeted treatments with aims to decrease women's morbidity and mortality from CVD and to improve women's quality of life.

CLINICS CARE POINTS

- Assess a woman's comprehensive cardiometabolic risk including hypertensive disorders of pregnancy and menopause to guide overall risk factor management.
- Close the gaps in disparities of undertreated hypertension and hyperlipidemia in women. Close the gaps in undertreated obesity, which increases a women's risk for CVD.
- Communicate clearly about continuation of low-dose aspirin for secondary prevention of ASCVD. Identify the role of low-dose aspirin for primary prevention is limited, and discontinue aspirin for primary prvention when indicated.
- Recogize that ACS in women may present later and with less common symptoms than men. Maintain a high suspeciion for ACS to avoid delayed diagnosis and treatment in women.
- Utilize advanced imaging or cardiology consultation to diagnose SCAD and MVD in women.

DISCLOSURE

The authors have no conflicts of interest to disclose.

FUNDING

AK is supported through the Cardiology NIH Training Grant (T32 HL129964). None for SJ.

REFERENCES

1. Force USPST, Bibbins-Domingo K, Grossman DC, et al. Statin use for the primary prevention of cardiovascular disease in adults: US preventive services task force recommendation statement. JAMA 2016;316(19):1997–2007.
2. Association AH. Life's Essential 8. 2022. Available at: https://www.heart.org/en/healthy-living/healthy-lifestyle/lifes-essential-8.
3. Guasch-Ferre M, Willett WC. The Mediterranean diet and health: a comprehensive overview. J Intern Med 2021;290(3):549–66.
4. Hales CMCM, Fryar CD, Ogden CL. Prevalence of obesity among adults and youth: United States, 2015-2016. National Center for Health Statistics 2017; 288:1–7.
5. Garcia M, Mulvagh SL, Merz CN, et al. Cardiovascular disease in women: clinical perspectives. Circ Res 2016;118(8):1273–93.
6. van Veldhuisen SL, Gorter TM, van Woerden G, et al. Bariatric surgery and cardiovascular disease: a systematic review and meta-analysis. Eur Heart J 2022; 43(20):1955–69.
7. Apovian CM, Aronne LJ, Bessesen DH, et al. Pharmacological management of obesity: an endocrine society clinical practice guideline. J Clin Endocrinol Metab 2015;100(2):342–62.
8. Wilding JPH, Batterham RL, Calanna S, et al. Once-weekly semaglutide in adults with overweight or obesity. N Engl J Med 2021;384(11):989–1002.
9. Jastreboff AM, Aronne LJ, Ahmad NN, et al. Tirzepatide once weekly for the treatment of obesity. N Engl J Med 2022;387(3):205–16.
10. Wilding JPH, Batterham RL, Davies M, et al. Weight regain and cardiometabolic effects after withdrawal of semaglutide: The STEP 1 trial extension. Diabetes Obes Metab 2022;24(8):1553–64.
11. Stanford FC. Controversial issues: A practical guide to the use of weight loss medications after bariatric surgery for weight regain or inadequate weight loss. Surg Obes Relat Dis 2019;15(1):128–32.
12. Stone NJ, Robinson JG, Lichtenstein AH, et al. 2013 ACC/AHA guideline on the treatment of blood cholesterol to reduce atherosclerotic cardiovascular risk in adults: a report of the American College of Cardiology/American Heart Association Task Force on Practice Guidelines. J Am Coll Cardiol 2014;63(25 Pt B): 2889–934.
13. Grundy SM, Stone NJ, Bailey AL, et al. 2018 AHA/ACC/AACVPR/AAPA/ABC/ACPM/ADA/AGS/APhA/ASPC/NLA/PCNA Guideline on the Management of Blood Cholesterol: A Report of the American College of Cardiology/American Heart Association Task Force on Clinical Practice Guidelines. J Am Coll Cardiol 2018. https://doi.org/10.1016/j.jacc.2018.11.003.
14. Greenland P, Alpert JS, Beller GA, et al. 2010 ACCF/AHA guideline for assessment of cardiovascular risk in asymptomatic adults: a report of the American

College of Cardiology Foundation/American Heart Association Task Force on Practice Guidelines. J Am Coll Cardiol 2010;56(25):e50–103.

15. Hecht HS, Cronin P, Blaha MJ, et al. 2016 SCCT/STR guidelines for coronary artery calcium scoring of noncontrast noncardiac chest CT scans: A report of the Society of Cardiovascular Computed Tomography and Society of Thoracic Radiology. J Cardiovasc Comput Tomogr 2017;11(1):74–84.

16. Margolies L, Salvatore M, Hecht HS, et al. Digital mammography and screening for coronary artery disease. JACC Cardiovasc Imaging 2016;9(4):350–60.

17. Budoff MJ, Achenbach S, Blumenthal RS, et al. Assessment of coronary artery disease by cardiac computed tomography: a scientific statement from the American Heart Association Committee on Cardiovascular Imaging and Intervention, Council on Cardiovascular Radiology and Intervention, and Committee on Cardiac Imaging, Council on Clinical Cardiology. Circulation 2006;114(16):1761–91.

18. Miedema MD, Duprez DA, Misialek JR, et al. Use of coronary artery calcium testing to guide aspirin utilization for primary prevention: estimates from the multi-ethnic study of atherosclerosis. Circ Cardiovasc Qual Outcomes 2014; 7(3):453–60.

19. Bukkapatnam RN, Gabler NB, Lewis WR. Statins for primary prevention of cardiovascular mortality in women: a systematic review and meta-analysis. *Prev Cardiol* Spring 2010;13(2):84–90.

20. Mora S, Glynn RJ, Hsia J, et al. Statins for the primary prevention of cardiovascular events in women with elevated high-sensitivity C-reactive protein or dyslipidemia: results from the Justification for the Use of Statins in Prevention: An Intervention Trial Evaluating Rosuvastatin (JUPITER) and meta-analysis of women from primary prevention trials. Circ 2010;121(9):1069–77.

21. Moreno-Arellano S, Delgado-de-Mendoza J, Santi-Cano MJ. Sex disparity persists in the prevention of cardiovascular disease in women on statin therapy compared with that in men. Nutr Metab Cardiovasc Dis 2018. https://doi.org/10.1016/j.numecd.2018.03.012.

22. Zhang H, Plutzky J, Shubina M, et al. Drivers of the sex disparity in statin therapy in patients with coronary artery disease: a cohort study. PLoS One 2016;11(5): e0155228.

23. Peters SAE, Colantonio LD, Zhao H, et al. Sex differences in high-intensity statin use following myocardial infarction in the United States. J Am Coll Cardiol 2018; 71(16):1729–37.

24. Moon J, Cohen Sedgh R, Jackevicius CA. Examining the Nocebo Effect of Statins through statin adverse events reported in the food and drug administration adverse event reporting system. Circ Cardiovasc Qual Outcomes 2021;14(1): e007480.

25. Gulati M, Merz CN. New cholesterol guidelines and primary prevention in women. Trends Cardiovasc Med 2015;25(2):84–94.

26. Karalis DG, Wild RA, Maki KC, et al. Gender differences in side effects and attitudes regarding statin use in the Understanding Statin Use in America and Gaps in Patient Education (USAGE) study. J Clin Lipidol 2016;10(4):833–41.

27. Statins FDA. Drug safety communication - FDA requests removal of strongest warning against using cholesterol-lowering statins during pregnancy. 2022. Available at: https://www.fda.gov/safety/medical-product-safety-information/statins-drug-safety-communication-fda-requests-removal-strongest-warning-against-using-cholesterol.

28. American Diabetes A. Standards of medical care in diabetes-2021 abridged for primary care providers. Clin Diabetes 2021;39(1):14–43.

29. Marsico F, Paolillo S, Gargiulo P, et al. Effects of glucagon-like peptide-1 receptor agonists on major cardiovascular events in patients with Type 2 diabetes mellitus with or without established cardiovascular disease: a meta-analysis of randomized controlled trials. Eur Heart J 2020;41(35):3346–58.

30. McGuire DK, Shih WJ, Cosentino F, et al. Association of SGLT2 Inhibitors With Cardiovascular and Kidney Outcomes in Patients With Type 2 Diabetes: A Meta-analysis. JAMA Cardiol 2021;6(2):148–58.

31. Lee MMY, Petrie MC, McMurray JJV, et al. How Do SGLT2 (Sodium-Glucose Co-transporter 2) Inhibitors and GLP-1 (Glucagon-Like Peptide-1) Receptor Agonists Reduce Cardiovascular Outcomes?: Completed and Ongoing Mechanistic Trials. Arterioscler Thromb Vasc Biol 2020;40(3):506–22.

32. Mantsiou C, Karagiannis T, Kakotrichi P, et al. Glucagon-like peptide-1 receptor agonists and sodium-glucose co-transporter-2 inhibitors as combination therapy for type 2 diabetes: A systematic review and meta-analysis. Diabetes Obes Metab 2020;22(10):1857–68.

33. Reboussin DM, Allen NB, Griswold ME, et al. Systematic Review for the 2017 ACC/AHA/AAPA/ABC/ACPM/AGS/APhA/ASH/ASPC/NMA/PCNA Guideline for the Prevention, detection, evaluation, and management of high blood pressure in adults: a report of the american college of cardiology/American Heart association task force on clinical practice guidelines. J Am Coll Cardiol 2017. https://doi.org/10.1016/j.jacc.2017.11.004.

34. McSweeney JC, Rosenfeld AG, Abel WM, et al. Preventing and from the American Heart Association. Circ 2016;133(13):1302–31.

35. Kim JK, Alley D, Seeman T, et al. Recent changes in cardiovascular risk factors among women and men. J Womens Health (Larchmt) 2006;15(6):734–46.

36. Ridker PM. Should aspirin be used for primary prevention in the post-statin era? N Engl J Med 2018;379(16):1572–4.

37. Lloyd-Jones DM. USPSTF report on aspirin for primary prevention. JAMA Cardiol 2022;7(7):667–9.

38. McNeil JJ, Wolfe R, Woods RL, et al. Effect of aspirin on cardiovascular events and bleeding in the healthy elderly. N Engl J Med 2018. https://doi.org/10.1056/NEJMoa1805819.

39. Group ASC. Effects of aspirin for primary prevention in persons with diabetes mellitus. N Engl J Med 2018. https://doi.org/10.1056/NEJMoa1804988.

40. Gaziano JM, Brotons C, Coppolecchia R, et al. Use of aspirin to reduce risk of initial vascular events in patients at moderate risk of cardiovascular disease (ARRIVE): a randomised, double-blind, placebo-controlled trial. Lancet 2018;392(10152):1036–46.

41. Rana S, Lemoine E, Granger JP, et al. Preeclampsia: pathophysiology, challenges, and perspectives. Circ 2019;124(7):1094–112.

42. Canto JG, Rogers WJ, Goldberg RJ, et al. Association of age and sex with myocardial infarction symptom presentation and in-hospital mortality. JAMA 2012;307(8):813–22.

43. Writing Committee M, Gulati M, Levy PD, et al. 2021 AHA/ACC/ASE/CHEST/SAEM/SCCT/SCMR guideline for the evaluation and diagnosis of chest pain: a report of the American College of Cardiology/American Heart Association Joint Committee on Clinical practice guidelines. J Am Coll Cardiol 2021;78(22):e187–285.

44. Bank IEM, de Hoog VC, de Kleijn DPV, et al. Sex-based differences in the performance of the heart score in patients presenting to the emergency department

with acute chest pain. J Am Heart Assoc 2017;6(6). https://doi.org/10.1161/JAHA.116.005373.

45. Sondergaard MM, Hlatky MA, Stefanick ML, et al. Association of adverse pregnancy outcomes with risk of atherosclerotic cardiovascular disease in postmenopausal women. JAMA Cardiol 2020;5(12):1390–8.

46. Kwok Y, Kim C, Grady D, et al. Meta-analysis of exercise testing to detect coronary artery disease in women. Am J Cardiol 1999;83(5):660–6.

47. Gruettner J, Fink C, Walter T, et al. Coronary computed tomography and triple rule out CT in patients with acute chest pain and an intermediate cardiac risk profile. Part 1: impact on patient management. Eur J Radiol 2013;82(1):100–5.

48. Tonet E, Pompei G, Faragasso E, et al. Coronary microvascular dysfunction: PET, CMR and CT assessment. J Clin Med 2021;10(9). https://doi.org/10.3390/jcm10091848.

49. Chapman AR, Anand A, Boeddinghaus J, et al. Comparison of the efficacy and safety of early rule-out pathways for acute myocardial infarction. Circ 2017; 135(17):1586–96.

50. Perdoncin E, Duvernoy C. Treatment of coronary artery disease in women. Methodist Debakey Cardiovasc J 2017;13(4):201–8.

51. Ya'qoub L, Elgendy IY, Pepine CJ. Syndrome of nonobstructive coronary artery diseases: a comprehensive overview of open artery ischemia. Am J Med 2021; 134(11):1321–9.

52. Mukherjee D. Myocardial infarction with nonobstructive coronary arteries: a call for individualized treatment. J Am Heart Assoc 2019;8(14):e013361.

53. Hayes SN, Tweet MS, Adlam D, et al. Spontaneous coronary artery dissection: JACC State-of-the-art review. J Am Coll Cardiol 2020;76(8):961–84.

54. Saw J, Mancini GBJ, Humphries KH. Contemporary review on spontaneous coronary artery dissection. J Am Coll Cardiol 2016;68(3):297–312.

55. Cerrato E, Giacobbe F, Quadri G, et al. Antiplatelet therapy in patients with conservatively managed spontaneous coronary artery dissection from the multicentre DISCO registry. Eur Heart J 2021;42(33):3161–71.

56. Chen S, Merchant M, Mahrer KN, et al. Pregnancy-associated spontaneous coronary artery dissection: clinical characteristics, outcomes, and risk during subsequent pregnancy. J Invasive Cardiol 2021;33(6):E457–66.

57. Ford TJ, Stanley B, Sidik N, et al. 1-Year outcomes of angina management guided by invasive coronary function testing (CorMicA). JACC Cardiovasc Interv 2020; 13(1):33–45.

Infectious Vaginitis, Cervicitis, and Pelvic Inflammatory Disease

Swati Shroff, MD, MS

KEYWORDS

- Vaginitis • Cervicitis • Pelvic inflammatory disease • Bacterial vaginosis
- Vulvovaginal candidiasis • Trichomoniasis • Chlamydia • Gonorrhea

KEY POINTS

- A pelvic examination should be performed for any woman presenting with vaginal discharge to confirm the diagnosis and rule out an upper tract infection.
- Bacterial vaginosis (BV), vulvovaginal candidiasis, and trichomoniasis are the most common causes of vaginitis in premenopausal women.
- BV and vulvovaginal candidal infections only require treatment if symptomatic and do not require partner therapy, whereas treatment and partner therapy is recommended for sexually transmitted illnesses, such as trichomoniasis, chlamydia, and gonorrhea.
- Any woman presenting with signs of pelvic inflammatory disease should be treated empirically.
- Vaginitis may be uncomfortable, but rarely leads to serious long-term consequences, but pelvic inflammatory disease can lead to serious long-term sequelae, including increased risk for ectopic pregnancy, infertility, and chronic pelvic pain.

INTRODUCTION

Vaginal symptoms are one of the most common reasons women consult with physicians and can significantly impact quality of life.[1,2] Differential diagnosis of vaginal discharge includes physiologic discharge, vaginitis, cervicitis, and pelvic inflammatory disease (PID). Physiologic or normal vaginal discharge is typically white or transparent, odorless, mucous and varies with the menstrual cycle. Vaginitis is an inflammation of the vagina, most commonly caused by bacterial vaginosis (BV), vulvovaginal candidiasis (VC), and trichomoniasis infections. Cervicitis is an inflammation of the cervix and typically caused by *Chlamydia trachomatis* and *Neisseria gonorrhoeae*. PID is infection of the female upper genital tract, involving any or all of the uterus, fallopian tubes,

Internal Medicine, Thomas Jefferson University, Jefferson Women's Primary Care, 700 Walnut Street 2nd Floor, Philadelphia, PA 19106, USA
E-mail address: sxs748@jefferson.edu

Med Clin N Am 107 (2023) 299–315
https://doi.org/10.1016/j.mcna.2022.10.009
0025-7125/23/© 2022 Elsevier Inc. All rights reserved.

ovaries, or pelvic peritoneum and usually caused by *C trachomatis*, *N gonorrhoeae*, and BV-associated pathogens.

Epidemiology of Infectious Vaginitis

Vaginitis is the most common gynecologic diagnosis in primary care, and most women have at least one episode of vaginitis in their lifetimes.[3,4] BV, VC, and trichomoniasis account for at least 70% of cases of vaginitis, and these infectious causes of vaginitis will be the focus of this article.[4,5]

The most common cause of vaginitis in reproductive-aged women, BV, accounts for 40% to 50% of cases of vaginitis.[4,6] BV is caused by a shift in the normal vaginal flora, where anaerobic bacterial species such as *Gardnerella vaginalis* replace the inhabitant *Lactobacillus* species in the vagina.[7] Studies show sociodemographic factors (eg, Black or Hispanic, living at or near the federal poverty line), douching, cigarette smoking, and increased body mass index are the risk factors for BV acquisition.[8–13] There is a clear association between sexual activity and BV, but it is uncertain whether this is caused by direct sexual transmission or the effects of sexual activity on *Lactobacillus* vaginal colonization.[14–16]

VC is the second most common infectious cause of vaginitis, accounting for 20% to 25% of cases of vaginitis.[4] *Candida albicans* causes 85% to 95% of VC infections, and *Candida glabrata* causes a majority of the remaining infections.[17] *Candida* does not always result in symptomatic vaginitis, and up to 30% of asymptomatic women may be colonized with *Candida* as part of their normal vaginal flora.[18] Although there are studies suggesting possible anogenital and orogenital transmission of yeast, penile-vaginal transmission is rare, and yeast infections can occur in celibate women.[17] Antibiotics, uncontrolled diabetes, immunosuppression, contraceptive method (eg, oral contraceptive pills, intrauterine devices (IUDs), diaphragm with spermicide) and hormonal changes, such as in pregnancy, are the potential risk factors for yeast infections.[1,4,12,17,19]

Trichomoniasis is the most prevalent nonviral sexually transmitted infection (STI) in the United States and is caused by the *Trichomonas vaginalis* protozoan.[20] Trichomoniasis is transmitted through sexual contact, and risk factors for trichomoniasis and STIs more generally include history of other STIs, unprotected sex, and multiple sexual partners.

Clinical Manifestations of Infectious Vaginitis

Many women with vaginitis caused by BV, VC, or trichomoniasis are asymptomatic. When symptomatic, the most common presenting symptom is vaginal discharge.

BV typically presents with a thin, homogenous, white discharge with a fishy odor, caused by the release of amines from anaerobic bacterial overgrowth. A lack of perceived odor makes BV less likely (likelihood ratio [LR], 0.07; 95% confidence interval [CI], 0.01 to 0.51), and BV does not generally cause pain or pruritis alone.[5]

VC classically presents with a thick, curd-like white discharge without any odor. Describing a "cheesy" discharge increases the likelihood of VC (LR, 2.4; 95% CI, 1.4 to 4.2).[5] VC may be associated with burning, dysuria, dyspareunia, and pruritis. Pruritis may be the only presenting symptom of VC, and a lack of itching makes a diagnosis of VC less likely (range of LRs, 0.18 [95% CI, 0.05 to 0.70] to 0.79 [95% CI, 0.72 to 0.87]).[5] On the examination, the presence of inflammatory signs, such as vulvar erythema and edema, is associated with VC (range of LRs, 2.1 [95% CI, 1.5 to 2.8] to 8.4 [95% CI, 2.3 to 3.1]).[5]

Trichomoniasis often presents with a malodorous, green-yellow, frothy discharge. It may be associated with burning, dysuria, dyspareunia, and less commonly pruritis. On the examination, vulvovaginal erythema and punctate hemorrhages of the vaginal mucosa and cervix may be observed.[13]

Diagnosis of Infectious Vaginitis

Self-diagnosis is generally not reliable and may lead to missing a more serious diagnosis.[5,21] Traditionally, vaginitis is diagnosed with a combination of history, examination, microscopy, measurement of vaginal pH, and the whiff test. On history, providers should characterize the consistency, color, odor, and amount of discharge and evaluate for any associated symptoms, for example, burning, dyspareunia, and pruritis. It is also important to consider non-vaginitis diagnoses (eg, urinary tract infections [UTI], vulvar conditions, cervicitis, and PID) by obtaining a thorough sexual history and assessing for symptoms such as dysuria, lesions, abdominal pain, fevers/chills, and nausea/vomiting. A urine specimen to assess for a UTI and pregnancy and a vaginal/cervical swab to rule out gonorrhea/chlamydia should be considered.[7] A pelvic examination is critical in any patient presenting with vaginal discharge to rule out an upper tract infection.

Vaginal pH in a premenopausal woman ranges from 4 to 4.5, as estrogen stimulates glycogen production which acts as a substrate for lactic acid production by colonizing lactobacilli.[7] Often underutilized, an elevated pH in a premenopausal woman suggests BV or trichomonas and helps exclude yeast. Under microscopy, observers should evaluate wet preps for clue cells (epithelial cells coated with coccobacilli), budding yeast and hyphae, and motile trichomonas (**Figs. 1–3**). Providers should also "whiff" a potassium hydroxide slide for a fishy odor, which is predictive of BV (LR, 3.2 [95% CI, 2.1 to 4.7]).[5] BV can be diagnosed by the presence of three out of four of Amsel criteria, which include a history of thin, homogenous vaginal discharge, vaginal pH greater than 4.5, a positive whiff test, and clue cells on wet prep. The sensitivity and specificity of Amsel criteria are 69% and 93%, respectively.[22] However, a vaginal pH greater than 4.5 and a positive whiff test may be as sensitive as three or more Amsel criteria.[23] Leukocytes are not typically increased in BV on microscopy, unlike in VC and trichomoniasis.[24]

As most primary care offices do not have microscopes on site and providers often lack the experience in evaluating wet mounts, point-of-care rapid antigen and DNA-amplification tests are becoming increasingly used. The BD Affirm VPIII test, a DNA

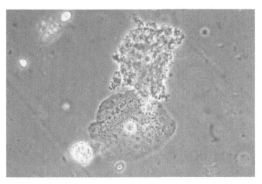

Fig. 1. Bacterial vaginosis. This photomicrograph of a vaginal smear specimen depicts two epithelial cells, a normal cell, and an epithelial cell with its exterior covered by bacteria giving the cell a roughened, stippled appearance known as a "clue cell." (CDC/ M. Rein.)

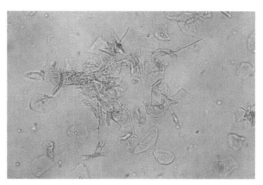

Fig. 2. Vulvovaginal candidiasis. This photomicrograph of a wet mounted vaginal smear specimen, revealed the presence of *C albicans*, which had been extracted from a patient with vaginal candidiasis. (CDC/ Dr. Stuart Brown.)

probe assay, is a more sensitive test for diagnosing BV (sensitivity 95% to 100%), VC (90% to 100%) and trichomonas (90% to 100%) compared with clinical and microscopy criteria commonly used to diagnose vaginitis.[22,25] However, the pitfalls of relying on these newer semi-automated office-based tests are the costs and time required to run the tests and obtain results, resulting in potential treatment delays, compared with immediate diagnosis and treatment recommendations that could be given to a patient with a real-time wet mount diagnosis.[7]

Cultures are not usually used for diagnosing vaginitis as they are costly and delay diagnosis and treatment. However, cultures may have a role for recurrently symptomatic women with negative testing and in women with persistent symptoms after treatment concerning for treatment failure.

Management of Infectious Vaginitis

Women diagnosed with symptomatic BV should be treated; recommended and alternative treatment regimens are listed in **Table 1**.[11] A systematic review found that

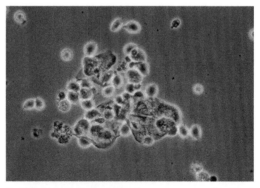

Fig. 3. Trichomoniasis. This photomicrograph of a wet-mounted vaginal discharge specimen reveals numbers of *T vaginalis* protozoan parasites, leading to a diagnosis of trichomoniasis, or "trich," which is a very common sexually transmitted disease (STD) that is caused by infection with *T vaginalis*. Although symptoms of the disease vary, most women and men who have the parasite cannot tell they are infected. (CDC/ Joe Miller)

Table 1
Bacterial vaginosis: treatment regimens

Recommended	Alternative
Metronidazole 500 mg orally twice a day for 7 d	Clindamycin 300 mg orally twice daily for 7 d
Metronidazole gel 0.75%, one full applicator (5 g) intravaginally, once a day for 5 d	Clindamycin ovules[a] 100 mg intravaginally once a bedtime for 3 d
Clindamycin cream[a] 2%, one full applicator (5 g) intravaginally at bedtime for 7 d	Secnidazole 2 g oral granules[b] in a single dose Tinidazole 2 g orally once daily for 2 d Tinidazole 1 g orally once daily for 5 d

[a] Oil-based and may weaken latex or rubber products, for example, condoms.
[b] Oral granules should be sprinkled onto unsweetened apple sauce, yogurt, or pudding before ingestion. A glass of water can be taken after administration to aid in swallowing.
Data from Workowski KA, Bachmann L, Chant P et al. Sexually transmitted diseases treatment guidelines, 2021. MMWR Recommendations and reports: Morbidity and mortality weekly report Recommendations and reports. 2021;70(No 4).

clindamycin and metronidazole had comparable clinical cure rates (91% and 92%, respectively), and confirmed oral and topical preparations also had similar effectiveness.[26] Topical clindamycin was associated with fewer adverse effects than oral metronidazole, such as metallic taste, nausea, and vomiting. However, patients often find oral preparations more convenient, whereas topical preparations are usually more expensive and can breakdown latex (eg, condoms, diaphragms). Previously, patients were advised against drinking alcohol while taking metronidazole to avoid a disulfiram-like reaction (eg, flushing, nausea, vomiting), but since recent research does not confirm an interaction between ethanol and metronidazole, the centers for disease control (CDC) no longer requires abstaining from alcohol while taking metronidazole.[11] The US Food and Drug Administration approved a single dose of secnidazole for the treatment of BV in 2017; however, it is significantly more expensive than other available treatment options. Partner therapy is not recommended for male or female partners of women diagnosed with BV. Pregnant women with symptomatic BV may be treated with the same oral and topical regimens recommended for nonpregnant women with the exception of tinidazole.[11]

Women diagnosed with VC infections should only be treated if symptomatic, as *Candida* may be part of normal vaginal flora. When considering treatment, it is important to differentiate between uncomplicated and complicated VC infections (**Table 2**). Uncomplicated VC infections can be treated with a 1, 3, or 7 day course of a topical

Table 2
Characteristics of uncomplicated versus complicated vulvovaginal candidiasis

Uncomplicated	Complicated
≤ 3 episodes per year	Recurrent VC (≥4 episodes per year)
Mild to moderate symptoms	Moderate to severe symptoms
Probable infection with *C albicans*	Candida species other than *C albicans*
Healthy, nonpregnant woman	Adverse risk factors, for example, pregnancy, poorly controlled diabetes, immunosuppression

Data from Sobel JD. Vulvovaginal candidosis. Lancet (London, England). 2007;369(9577):1961-71.

azole or a single dose of an oral azole. Complicated VC infections should be treated with a 7 to 14 day course of a topical azole or 3 doses of an oral azole separated by 72 hours (day 1, 4, and 7). Oral and topical azoles have comparable cure rates (80% to 90%), although side effects and drug interactions are less of a concern with topical azoles.[11] However, women frequently prefer the convenience of an oral formulation, and oral fluconazole 150 mg is often prescribed.[27] The optimal treatment of non-albicans VC infections is unknown, but the CDC recommends a longer duration (7 to 14 days) of a topical or oral non-fluconazole azole drug (eg, itraconazole).[11,28] For azole-refractory *Candida glabrata* vaginitis, a 2 week course of intravaginal boric acid (600 mg daily) or topical flucytosine may be effective.[1,11,29] However, boric acid may not be available at traditional pharmacies, and most insurance plans will not cover it.[30] It is also important to note boric acid can be lethal if taken orally. Access to flucytosine is typically limited by cost. Low-potency topical corticosteroids may be used for up to 48 hours for severe vulvar inflammation until antifungal medications can take effect. In pregnancy, only topical azole therapies are recommended, as oral therapy may be associated with an increased risk of miscarriage and fetal malformations.[11,12,28] Partner therapy is not recommended for VC infections.

As trichomonas is an STI, unlike BV and VC, treatment is indicated in both asymptomatic and symptomatic women. The CDC recommends metronidazole 500 mg orally twice a day for 7 days for trichomoniasis infections in women, given recent studies demonstrating higher cure rates with a multidose versus single-dose metronidazole treatment regimen.[11,31] Topical antimicrobials are not recommended, as they are unable to achieve therapeutic levels in the urethra and perivaginal glands.[28] An alternative treatment regimen is tinidazole 2 g orally in a single dose, which has similar efficacy but is usually more expensive.[32] For treatment of trichomonas in pregnancy, the preferred treatment is also oral metronidazole 500 mg twice a day for 7 days. Partner therapy is recommended as trichomonas is an STI. Women and their partners should avoid intercourse until they and their sex partners have been treated and symptoms have resolved.[12]

Table 3 summarizes the etiology, symptoms, diagnosis, and treatment of infectious vaginitis.

Follow-Up and Sequelae of Infectious Vaginitis

Recurrent vaginitis is common, and it is important to address risk factors for recurrence.

Approximately 30% of women with BV experience a recurrence of symptoms within 3 months and more than half experience a recurrence within 1 year.[33] Topical metronidazole is the only approved suppressive therapy (nocturnal application 2 nights a week for 6 months) for women with multiple recurrences of BV.[30] It has been hypothesized that a vaginal "biofilm" may lead to BV recurrence, and thus medications, such as vaginal acidifiers, aimed at disrupting the biofilm may reduce BV recurrence. One small uncontrolled, non-randomized study found adding 21 days of intravaginal boric acid (600 mg) therapy followed by twice weekly topical metronidazole for up to 5 months after treatment of the acute BV infection reduced recurrence rates while on treatment, but recurrence after treatment completion increased up to 50% by 36 weeks.[34] Another small randomized trial found that monthly oral metronidazole 2 g plus oral fluconazole 150 mg may reduce the incidence of BV and promote colonization with normal vaginal flora.[35] Patients should be counseled that estrogen-containing contraception, condoms, and smoking cessation may reduce the risk of BV recurrence.[36]

Table 3
Causes, symptoms, diagnosis, and treatment of infectious vaginitis

Type (% prevalence)[a]	Etiology	Symptoms and Signs	Diagnosis	Treatment
Bacterial vaginosis (22% to 50%)	G vaginalis, aneorobic bacteria	• Homogenous, thin, clear/ white/gray, malodorous discharge • Minimal pain • Minimal pruritis	• Amsel's criteria (3+/4): thin, homogenous discharge, positive whiff test, pH > 4.5, clue cells on microscopy • Point-of-care test	• Metronidazole, oral or topical • Clindamycin, topical
Vulvovaginal candidiasis (17% to 39%)	C albicans, C krusei, and C glabrata	• White, thick, odorless discharge • Dyspareunia, dysuria, burning • Frequent pruritis	• NL pH (3.5–4.5) • Budding yeast and hyphae on microscopy • Point-of-care test	• Azoles, oral, or topical
Trichomoniasis (4% to 35%)	T vaginalis	• Green-yellow, frothy discharge • Dyspareunia, dysuria • Minimal pruritis	• pH > 4.5 • Motile trichomonads on microscopy • Point-of-care test	• Metronidazole, oral • Tinidazole, oral

[a] Prevalence per review of studies of symptomatic women presenting in primary care.
Adapted from Shroff S, Ryden J. Vaginitis and Vulvar Conditions. In: Sex- and Gender-Based Women's Health. ; 2020:165-186; and *Data from* Anderson MR, Klink K, Cohrssen A. Evaluation of vaginal complaints. Jama. 2004;291(11):1368-79.

Partner therapy for BV has not been shown to be beneficial in preventing recurrent BV and is not generally recommended.[13,37–39] Although no randomized control studies have specifically evaluated the treatment of female sexual partners, studies have consistently found high rates of concordant BV infections between female sexual partners; therefore some experts consider partner therapy for recurrent infections in this patient population.[7,9,12] Other recommendations such as condom use and proper cleaning of shared sex toys may be beneficial, but have also not been proven to reduce recurrence rates.[13]

Recurrent VC (≥3 episodes in one year) affects up to 5% of women.[40] Non-albicans *Candida* often leads to recurrent VC, and thus cultures should be obtained to confirm the diagnosis in this context. Suppressive weekly azole therapy can be considered for the treatment of recurrent VC with *C albicans*. The Infectious Diseases Society of American recommends 10 to 14 days of induction therapy with a topical or oral azole, followed by oral fluconazole at 150 mg once per week for 6 months.[41] Laboratory monitoring for suppressive azole therapy is not required given the safety profile of low dose fluconazole. Most women will have no reinfections during suppressive therapy, but up to 50% will have a recurrence after therapy is completed.[11]

Up to 17% of women treated for trichomonas may be reinfected within 3 months.[42] A recurrent infection may be caused by the lack of treatment adherence, reinfection from an untreated partner, or less commonly, treatment failure. The CDC recommends rescreening for trichomonas in all sexually active women within 3 months following initial treatment. If there is concern for a persistent infection or reinfection, retesting with culture is the preferred test, but if nucleic acid amplification testing is used, it should not be done before 3 weeks after treatment completion to avoid a false positive from residual nucleic acid.[11] If reinfection is the suspected cause of a recurrent infection, a repeat course of the same treatment regimen is recommended. However, if there is concern for treatment resistant trichomonas, the CDC can offer testing and treatment guidance.[11] A longer course and/or higher dose nitroimidazole treatment regimen (eg, metronidazole or tinidazole 2 g once daily for 7 days) is typically recommended in this scenario.[11]

Both BV and trichomonas may be associated with increased susceptibility to STIs and preterm births, but otherwise, vaginitis is not typically associated with significant long-term sequelae.[43–49] Although some experts support treating asymptomatic BV to reduce STI transmission risk, there is insufficient evidence to support its benefit.[1] Treatment of asymptomatic BV in pregnant women is also controversial because studies have not generally shown a reduction in the incidence of preterm delivery with treatment, although a Cochrane review found that it may reduce preterm delivery in women with a prior history of preterm delivery and current BV.[50,51] The US Preventive Services Task Force (USPSTF) currently recommends against routine BV screening in asymptomatic pregnant women at low risk of preterm delivery.[52] It is unclear whether treatment of trichomonas in pregnancy reduces the risk of preterm birth.[53]

Epidemiology of Infectious Cervicitis and Pelvic Inflammatory Disease

The prevalence of cervicitis and PID are difficult to assess as they are likely underdiagnosed, an unknown number of cases are "silent" or subclinical. PID is often diagnosed during subsequent evaluations for infertility and pelvic pain.[54] Cervicitis may affect up to 40% of patients seen in STI clinics.[55,56] From 1995 to 2001, over 700,000 cases of PID were diagnosed annually in the United States.[57] The highest incidence of both cervicitis and PID is in sexually active women aged 15 to 24.[58,59]

In this article, the author focuses on chlamydia and gonorrhea, the most commonly reported STIs and causes of acute cervicitis and PID in the United States. Over 1.5 million and 600,000 cases of chlamydia and gonorrhea were reported in the United States in 2020, respectively.[60] Risk factors include new sexual partners, multiple sexual partners, young age (<25), inconsistent condom use, and prior history of STIs. In addition, IUDs may slightly increase the risk for PID, but it is primarily limited to the first 20 days after IUD insertion.[61,62]

Clinical Manifestations of Infectious Cervicitis and Pelvic Inflammatory Disease

Most women infected with gonorrhea and chlamydia are asymptomatic.[63] However, when symptomatic, women with cervicitis may complain of vaginal discharge, intermenstrual or postcoital bleeding, dysuria, and dyspareunia. In addition to these symptoms, women with PID may also present with fevers, low back, abdominal and pelvic pain, nausea, and vomiting. Less commonly, women with PID may complain of right upper quadrant pain from perihepatitis (eg, Fitz-Hugh–Curtis syndrome), when there is involvement of the liver capsule, and this presentation of PID may be confused for acute cholecystitis.[62,64]

Diagnosis of Infectious Cervicitis and Pelvic Inflammatory Disease

Both cervicitis and PID are clinical diagnoses requiring pelvic examinations. Cervicitis may be diagnosed by observing either or both of the following signs: (1) purulent or mucopurulent exudate from the endocervix visible grossly or on a swab and/or (2) sustained endocervical bleeding easily induced by gentle passage of a swab through the cervical os, that is, cervical friability.[11,65]

The presentation of PID is widely variable, and a missed diagnosis could result in serious long-term sequelae. Therefore, a presumptive diagnosis of PID should be made when a women at risk for STIs reports pelvic or lower abdominal pain, with no other identified cause of the pain, and has pelvic organ tenderness (ie, cervical motion, uterine or adnexal tenderness) on bimanual examination.[11] Although the sensitivity of pelvic tenderness for PID is over 95%, it has poor specificity.[65] The following additional criteria may improve the specificity of the diagnosis: oral temperature greater than 101 F or 38.3 C, abnormal cervical discharge, cervical friability, abundant white blood cells on microscopy, elevated erythrocyte sedimentation rate or C-reactive protein, and laboratory documentation of cervical infection with N gonorrhoeae or C trachomatis.[11] Endometrial biopsy, imaging, and laparoscopy could allow for a more specific diagnosis of PID or alternative diagnosis to be made. However, these more invasive, expensive diagnostic tools are used sparingly, such as in cases of diagnostic uncertainty or unresponsiveness to therapy, and should not delay treatment.[11,62,66] When compared with laparoscopy, a clinical diagnosis of PID has a positive predictive value ranging from 65% to 90%.[11]

As part of the diagnostic evaluation, it is important to determine the etiology of the cervicitis or PID when possible. When an etiologic organism for cervicitis or PID is identified, it is usually C trachomatis or N gonorrhoeae. For detecting chlamydia and gonorrhea, nucleic acid amplification tests (NAAT) have the highest sensitivity (90%–98% and 90%–95%, respectively) and specificity (98%–100% and 99% to 100%, respectively).[67,68] Although NAAT can be performed on vaginal, endocervical, or urine specimens, as pelvic and bimanual examinations are required for the evaluation of any vaginal discharge to rule out an upper tract infection, provider-collected vaginal or endocervical specimens are usually obtained. If NAAT are unavailable, antigen detection and genetic probe tests may be used with endocervical swabs. Cultures are typically only used when antibiotic resistance is a concern. It is also important to perform an evaluation to rule out other etiologies of the discharge, for example, vaginitis and consider alternative diagnoses, for example, UTI. In women presenting with lower abdominal or pelvic pain, imaging studies may be useful to rule out alternative diagnoses (eg, appendicitis, ectopic pregnancy, endometriosis, ovarian cyst, tub-ovarian abscess), which can be diagnosed in up to a quarter of women thought to have acute PID.[65]

Management of Infectious Cervicitis and Pelvic Inflammatory Disease

If a diagnosis of cervicitis or PID cannot be made by clinical examination, providers should wait for test results to guide treatment.

The recommended treatment for a chlamydial infection (**Table 4**) is doxycycline 100 mg orally twice a day for 7 days, given its superior efficacy compared with azithromycin in treating chlamydial infections in men and rectal chlamydial infections.[11] In case of a doxycycline allergy, azithromycin or levofloxacin may be used instead. In pregnancy or when there is significant concern for nonadherence, azithromycin 1 g orally as a single dose can be used, but posttreatment testing approximately 4 weeks after therapy completion is recommended.[11]

If a diagnosis of gonorrhea is made, single-agent therapy with high-dose ceftriaxone is the preferred treatment (**Table 5**), given concerns for rising gonococcal minimum inhibitory concentrations and often asymptomatic, difficult to treat pharyngeal infections.[11] The routine use of a second agent as in previous CDC guidelines is no longer recommended unless chlamydia coinfection has not been excluded. Pregnant women should be treated with the same recommended regimen. In persons with a history of a penicillin allergy, allergic reactions to third-generation cephalosporins are uncommon.[11] However, in nonpregnant individuals with a history of an Immunoglobulin E (IgE)-mediated penicillin allergy (eg, anaphylaxis), cephalosporins are contraindicated, and dual treatment with single doses of IM gentamycin 240 mg plus oral azithromycin 2 g is recommended.[11]

If a diagnosis of cervicitis can be made by clinical examination, antibiotics to treat chlamydia and gonorrhea should be started empirically for women at increased risk for STIs.[11] For women at lower risk of STIs, deferring treatment until diagnostic test results become available is a reasonable alternative. However, a clinical diagnosis of PID requires immediate empiric treatment to prevent potential long-term sequelae. For PID, providers should assess the severity of symptoms and whether hospitalization for parenteral therapy is required for PID. **Box 1** lists the indications for hospitalization. In women with mild to moderate symptoms, parenteral and oral regimens have demonstrated similar short- and long-term outcomes.[69] Women who do not respond to intramuscular/oral outpatient therapy within 72 hours should be hospitalized.

Table 4 Chlamydia: treatment regimens	
Recommended	**Alternative**
Doxycycline[a] 100 mg orally twice a day for 7 d	Azithromycin 1 g orally in a single dose
	Levofloxacin[a] 500 mg orally once a day for 7 d

[a] Not recommended in pregnancy.

Data from Workowski KA, Bachmann L, Chant P et al. Sexually transmitted diseases treatment guidelines, 2021. MMWR Recommendations and reports: Morbidity and mortality weekly report Recommendations and reports. 2021;70(No 4).

Table 5
Gonorrhea: treatment regimens

Recommended	Alternative[c]
Ceftriaxone 500 mg IM[a]	Gentamicin 240 mg IM in a single dose
If chlamydial infection has not been excluded, treat for chlamydia with doxycycline 100 mg orally 2 times/day for 7 d[b]	PLUS azithromycin 2 mg orally in a single dose or cefixime 800 mg orally in a single dose If chlamydial infection has not been excluded, treat for chlamydia with doxycycline 100 mg orally 2 times/day for 7 d[b]

[a] For persons weighing ≥ 150 kg, 1 g ceftriaxone should be administered.
[b] Not recommended in pregnancy.
[c] If ceftriaxone not available.
Data from Workowski KA, Bachmann L, Chant P et al. Sexually transmitted diseases treatment guidelines, 2021. MMWR Recommendations and reports: Morbidity and mortality weekly report Recommendations and reports. 2021;70(No 4).

The recommended treatment of PID (**Box 2**, **Table 6**) should cover gonorrhea and chlamydia regardless of testing results, as it is possible to have PID without positive endocervical testing.[11] There is controversy surrounding whether the treatment of PID should also cover anaerobic bacteria as it has not been studied in randomized controlled studies.[65] However, given studies have isolated anaerobes in the upper genital tract of women with PID and the significant potential long-term concerns of PID, experts generally recommend covering anaerobic microbes.[11,65] Regardless of disease severity, the recommended treatment duration is 14 days and should result in clinical improvement within 72 hours. In women diagnosed with PID with an IUD, a systematic review found that removal of the IUD usually did not improve outcomes and might delay clinical improvement.[70] Therefore, women with IUDs diagnosed with PID usually do not require IUD removal, although removal may be considered if no clinical improvement occurs within 72 hours of starting treatment.

To minimize disease transmission, women diagnosed with chlamydia, gonorrhea, or trichomoniasis should be instructed to notify sexual partners within the past 60 days and can ask their local health departments for assistance with anonymous partner notification. They should be advised to abstain from sexual activity until completion of therapy or 1 week after a single-dose treatment regimen, partners have been adequately treated, and symptoms have resolved.

Box 1
Indications for hospitalization of patients with pelvic inflammatory disease

Inability to follow or tolerate an outpatient oral medication regimen

No clinical response to oral therapy

Pregnancy

Severe illness, nausea and vomiting, or high fever

Surgical emergencies (eg, appendicitis) cannot be excluded

Tubo-ovarian abscess

Data from Workowski KA, Bachmann L, Chant P et al. Sexually transmitted diseases treatment guidelines, 2021. MMWR Recommendations and reports: Morbidity and mortality weekly report Recommendations and reports. 2021;70(No 4).

Box 2
Intramuscular/oral treatment regimens for pelvic inflammatory disease

Ceftriaxone 500 mg[a] IM

PLUS doxycycline 100 mg orally 2 times/day for 14 d

PLUS metronidazole 500 mg orally 2 times/day for 14 d

Cefoxitin 2 g IM in a single dose

PLUS probenecid 1 g orally administered in a single dose

PLUS doxycycline 100 mg orally 2 times/day for 14 d

PLUS metronidazole 500 mg orally 2 times/day for 14 d

Other parenteral third-generation cephalosporin (eg, ceftizoxime or cefotaxime)

PLUS doxycycline 100 mg orally 2 times/day for 14 d

PLUS metronidazole 500 mg orally 2 times/day for 14 d

[a] For persons weighing $\geq$ 150 kg, 1 g of ceftriaxone should be administered.

Data from Workowski KA, Bachmann L, Chant P et al. Sexually transmitted diseases treatment guidelines, 2021. MMWR Recommendations and reports: Morbidity and mortality weekly report Recommendations and reports. 2021;70(No 4).

Standard partner therapy entails patients informing recent partners of the diagnosis and advising them to seek care. Alternatively, clinicians may provide therapy to the partner without a clinical evaluation by giving written information and a medication or prescription for the partner to the patient, which is referred to as expedited partner therapy (EPT). Studies involving heterosexual men and women with chlamydia and gonorrhea found that EPT led to higher treatment rates and lower risk for persistent or recurrent infections.[11] Therefore, the CDC recommends routinely offering EPT to patients with chlamydia or gonorrhea when the provider has concerns for timely partner evaluation and treatment.[11] The major limitations of using EPT are resistance

Table 6
Parenteral treatment regimens for pelvic inflammatory disease

Recommended[a]	Alternative[a]
Ceftriaxone 1 g IV every 24 h PLUS doxycycline 100 mg orally or IV every 12 h PLUS metronidazole 500 mg orally or IV every 12 h	Ampicillin/sulbactam 3 g IV every 6 h PLUS doxycycline 100 mg orally or IV every 12 h
Cefotetan 2 g IV every 12 h PLUS doxycycline 100 mg orally or IV every 12 h	Clindamycin 900 mg IV every 8 h PLUS gentamicin loading dose IV or IM, followed by maintenance dose every 8 h
Cefoxitin 2 g IV every 6 h PLUS doxycycline 100 mg oral or IV every 12 h	

[a] Transition to oral therapy (doxycycline 100 mg 2 times/day and metronidazole 500 mg 2 times/day) can usually be initiated within 24 to 48 hours after clinical improvement, and should be continued to complete 2 weeks of therapy.

Data from Workowski KA, Bachmann L, Chant P et al. Sexually transmitted diseases treatment guidelines, 2021. MMWR Recommendations and reports: Morbidity and mortality weekly report Recommendations and reports. 2021;70(No 4).

patterns to oral medications for gonorrhea, missed opportunities to assess for other STIs, and state-dependent regulations. The legal status and permissibility of EPT in individual states can be found at https://www.cdc.gov/std/ept.

Both chlamydia and gonorrhea are reportable to health departments, and reporting may be provider- and/or laboratory-based. Clinicians who are unsure of the local reporting requirements should contact their laboratories and local health departments and notify patients that these reports are strictly confidential.

Follow-Up and Sequelae of Infectious Cervicitis and Pelvic Inflammatory Disease

For urogenital chlamydia or gonorrhea treated with either a recommended or alternative treatment regimen, tests-of-cure are not typically required, unless symptoms persist, reinfection is suspected, or in the context of pregnancy. Most posttreatment infections are the result of reinfection rather than evidence of treatment failure.[11] For women with persistent symptoms after treatment and not suspected of having chlamydial reinfection, repeat chlamydial NAATs can be performed 4 weeks after the completion of therapy to avoid false-positive results from residual nonviable organisms.[11] Women with persistent symptoms after the treatment of gonorrhea and not suspected of having reinfection should be evaluated by culture, which potentially allows for an antimicrobial susceptibility assessment, at least 1 week following the completion of therapy. Of note, high prevalence of chlamydia and gonorrhea have been seen in both men and women treated for these STIs during the preceding months. Therefore, the CDC recommends men or women who have been treated for chlamydia or gonorrhea be screened 3 months after treatment or whenever the patient is next present for medical care within 1 year following treatment.[11]

It is important to note that most chlamydial and gonococcal infections are asymptomatic, and an estimated 10% to 20% of women with chlamydial or gonorrheal infections may develop PID if untreated.[66] Owing to scarring and adhesions caused by bacteria-induced tissue damage and host inflammatory and immunologic responses to infection, PID results in an elevated risk for ectopic pregnancy (9%), infertility (20%), and chronic pelvic pain (18%), with increasing risk with number and severity of prior infections.[54,66,71] Although delayed treatment is associated with worse long-term outcomes, even treated PID has an association with these significant reproductive outcomes, highlighting the importance of prevention.[65] The USPSTF recommends screening for both chlamydia and gonorrhea in all sexually active women age 24 years and younger and in older women who are at increased risk for infection and recommends the use of NAATs with urine, endocervical, or vaginal specimens.[72]

CLINICS CARE POINTS

- A pelvic exam should be performed for any woman presenting with vaginal discharge to confirm the diagnosis and rule out an upper tract infection.

- Any woman presenting with signs of pelvic inflammatory disease (PID) should be treated empirically.

- Vaginitis may be uncomfortable, but rarely leads to serious long-term consequences, but PID can lead to serious long-term sequelae, including increased risk for ectopic pregnancy, infertility, and chronic pelvic pain.

- Most chlamydia and gonorrhea infections are asymptomatic, and untreated infections can result in PID. Therefore, the USPSTF recommends screening for both chlamydia and gonorrhea in all sexually active women age 24 years and younger and older women at increased risk.

DISCLOSURE

No disclosures.

REFERENCES

1. Mills BB. Vaginitis: beyond the basics. Obstet Gynecol Clin North Am 2017;44(2): 159–77.
2. Paavonen J, Brunham RC. Bacterial Vaginosis and Desquamative Inflammatory Vaginitis. N Engl J Med 2018;379(23):2246–54.
3. Sobel JD. Vaginitis. N Engl J Med 1997;337(26):1896–903.
4. Paladine HL, Desai UA. Vaginitis : Diagnosis and Treatment. Am Fam Physician 2018;97(5):321–9.
5. Anderson MR, Klink K, Cohrssen A. Evaluation of Vaginal Complaints. JAMA 2004;291(11):1368–79.
6. Koumans EH, Sternberg M, Bruce C, et al. The prevalence of bacterial vaginosis in the United States, 2001-2004; associations with symptoms, sexual behaviors, and reproductive health. Sex Transm Dis 2007;34(11):864–9.
7. Shroff S, Ryden J. Vaginitis and Vulvar Conditions. In: Tilstra S, Kwolek D, Mitchell J, et al, editors. Sex- and Gender-Based Women's Health. 1st ed. Cham, Switzerland: Springer; 2020. p. 165–86.
8. Klebanoff MA, Nansel TR, Brotman RM, et al. Personal hygienic behaviors and bacterial vaginosis. Sex Transm Dis 2010;37(2):94–9.
9. Bradshaw C, Walker S, Vodstrcil L, et al. The Influence of Behaviors and Relationships on the Vaginal Microbiota of Women and Their Female Partners: The WOW Health Study. J Infect Dis 2013;209. https://doi.org/10.1093/infdis/jit664.
10. Smart S, Singal A, Mindel A. Social and sexual risk factors for bacterial vaginosis. Sex Transm Infect 2004;80(1):58–62.
11. Workowski KA, Bachmann LH, Chan PA, et al. Sex Transm Infections Treat Guidel 2021;70:2021.
12. Marnach ML, Wygant JN, Casey PM. Evaluation and Management of Vaginitis. Mayo Clin Proc 2022;97(2):347–58.
13. Nyirjesy P. Management of persistent vaginitis. Obstet Gynecol 2014;124(6): 1135–46.
14. Fethers KA, Fairley CK, Hocking JS, et al. Sexual Risk Factors and Bacterial Vaginosis: A Systematic Review and Meta-Analysis. Clin Infect Dis 2008;47(11): 1426–35.
15. SCHWEBKE JR, RIVERS C, LEE J. Prevalence of Gardnerella vaginalis in Male Sexual Partners of Women With and Without Bacterial Vaginosis. Sex Transm Dis 2009;36(2):92–4. Available at: http://www.jstor.org/stable/44969550.
16. Mitchell C, Manhart LE, Thomas KK, et al. Effect of sexual activity on vaginal colonization with hydrogen peroxide-producing lactobacilli and Gardnerella vaginalis. Sex Transm Dis 2011;38(12):1137–44.
17. Sobel JD. Vulvovaginal candidosis. Lance 2007;369(9577):1961–71.
18. Giraldo P, NOWASKONSKI A, GOMES F, et al. Vaginal Colonization by Candida in Asymptomatic Women With and Without a History of Recurrent Vulvovaginal Candidiasis. Obstet Gynecol 2000;95:413–6.
19. Christine L, Sankey W, Wilson J. Vaginitis and cervicitis. Ann Intern Med 2009; 151(5):ITC3–16. https://doi.org/10.7326/0003-4819-151-5-200909010-01003.
20. Kreisel KM, Spicknall IH, Gargano JW, et al. Sexually Transmitted Infections Among US Women and Men: Prevalence and Incidence Estimates, 2018. Sex

Transm Dis 2021;48(4). Available at: https://journals.lww.com/stdjournal/Fulltext/2021/04000/Sexually_Transmitted_Infections_Among_US_Women_and.2.aspx.

21. Ferris DG, Nyirjesy P, Sobel JD, et al. Over-the-counter antifungal drug misuse associated with patient-diagnosed vulvovaginal candidiasis. Obstet Gynecol 2002;99(3):419–25.

22. Hainer BL, Gibson MV. Vaginitis: Diagnosis and treatment. Am Fam Physician 2011;83(7):807–15.

23. Gutman R, Peipert J, Weitzen S, et al. Evaluation of clinical methods for diagnosing bacterial vaginosis. Obstet Gynecol 2005;105(3):551–6.

24. Frobenius W, Bogdan C. Diagnostic Value of Vaginal Discharge, Wet Mount and Vaginal pH - An Update on the Basics of Gynecologic Infectiology. Geburtshilfe Frauenheilkd 2015;75(4):355–66.

25. Brown HL, Fuller DD, Jasper LT, et al. Clinical evaluation of affirm VPIII in the detection and identification of Trichomonas vaginalis, Gardnerella vaginalis, and Candida species in vaginitis/vaginosis. Infect Dis Obstet Gynecol 2004;12(1):17–21.

26. Oduyebo OOARI, Ogunsola FT. The effects of antimicrobial therapy on bacterial vaginosis in non-pregnant women. Cochrane Database Syst Rev 2009;3. https://doi.org/10.1002/14651858.CD006055.pub2.

27. Watson M, Grimshaw J, Bond C, et al. Oral versus intra-vaginal imidazole and triazole anti-fungal treatment of uncomplicated vulvovaginal candidiasis. Cochrane Database Syst Rev 2001;4.

28. Gioia-Flynt L. Vaginitis. In: Stovall T, Ling F, Zite N, et al. Gynecology for the primary care physician. Philadelphia: Springer; 2008. p. 137-142.

29. Sobel JD, Chaim W, Nagappan V, et al. Treatment of vaginitis caused by Candida glabrata: use of topical boric acid and flucytosine. Am J Obstet Gynecol 2003;189(5):1297–300.

30. Marshall AO. Managing Recurrent Bacterial Vaginosis: Insights for Busy Providers. Sex Med Rev 2015;3(2):88–92.

31. Howe K, Kissinger PJ. Single-Dose Compared With Multidose Metronidazole for the Treatment of Trichomoniasis in Women: A Meta-Analysis. Sex Transm Dis 2017;44(1):29–34.

32. Meites E, Gaydos CA, Hobbs MM, et al. A Review of Evidence-Based Care of Symptomatic Trichomoniasis and Asymptomatic Trichomonas vaginalis Infections. Clin Infect Dis 2015;61(Suppl 8):S837–48.

33. Bradshaw CS, Morton AN, Hocking J, et al. High Recurrence Rates of Bacterial Vaginosis over the Course of 12 Months after Oral Metronidazole Therapy and Factors Associated with Recurrence. J Infect Dis 2006;193(11):1478–86.

34. Reichman O, Akins R, Sobel JD. Boric Acid Addition to Suppressive Antimicrobial Therapy for Recurrent Bacterial Vaginosis. Sex Transm Dis 2009;36(11). Available at: https://journals.lww.com/stdjournal/Fulltext/2009/11000/Boric_Acid_Addition_to_Suppressive_Antimicrobial.13.aspx.

35. McClelland RS, Richardson BA, Hassan WM, et al. Improvement of Vaginal Health for Kenyan Women at Risk for Acquisition of Human Immunodeficiency Virus Type 1: Results of a Randomized Trial. J Infect Dis 2008;197(10):1361–8.

36. Bradshaw CS, Vodstrcil LA, Hocking JS, et al. Recurrence of bacterial vaginosis is significantly associated with posttreatment sexual activities and hormonal contraceptive use. Clin Infect Dis 2013;56(6):777–86.

37. Bradshaw CS, Sobel JD. Current Treatment of Bacterial Vaginosis-Limitations and Need for Innovation. J Infect Dis 2016;214(Suppl 1):S14–20.

38. Mehta SD. Systematic Review of Randomized Trials of Treatment of Male Sexual Partners for Improved Bacteria Vaginosis Outcomes in Women. Sex Transm Dis 2012;39(10). Available at: https://journals.lww.com/stdjournal/Fulltext/2012/10000/Systematic_Review_of_Randomized_Trials_of.15.aspx.

39. Amaya-Guio J, Viveros-Carreño DA, Sierra-Barrios EM, et al. Antibiotic treatment for the sexual partners of women with bacterial vaginosis. Cochrane Database Syst Rev 2016;10. https://doi.org/10.1002/14651858.CD011701.pub2.

40. Denning DW, Kneale M, Sobel JD, et al. Global burden of recurrent vulvovaginal candidiasis: a systematic review. Lancet Infect Dis 2018;18(11):e339–47.

41. Pappas PG, Kauffman CA, Andes DR, et al. Clinical Practice Guideline for the Management of Candidiasis: 2016 Update by the Infectious Diseases Society of America. Clin Infect Dis 2016;62(4):e1–50.

42. Peterman TA, Tian LH, Metcalf CA, et al. High incidence of new sexually transmitted infections in the year following a sexually transmitted infection: A case for rescreening. Ann Intern Med 2006;145(8):564–72.

43. Martin HL Jr, Richardson BA, Nyange PM, et al. Vaginal Lactobacilli, Microbial Flora, and Risk of Human Immunodeficiency Virus Type 1 and Sexually Transmitted Disease Acquisition. J Infect Dis 1999;180(6):1863–8.

44. Myer L, Kuhn L, Stein ZA, et al. Intravaginal practices, bacterial vaginosis, and women's susceptibility to HIV infection: epidemiological evidence and biological mechanisms. Lancet Infect Dis 2005;5(12):786–94.

45. Cohen CR, Lingappa JR, Baeten JM, et al. Bacterial vaginosis associated with increased risk of female-to-male HIV-1 transmission: a prospective cohort analysis among African couples. PLoS Med 2012;9(6):e1001251.

46. Hay PE, Lamont RF, Taylor-Robinson D, et al. Abnormal bacterial colonisation of the genital tract and subsequent preterm delivery and late miscarriage. BMJ 1994;308(6924):295–8.

47. Klebanoff MA, Hillier SL, Nugent RP, et al. Is bacterial vaginosis a stronger risk factor for preterm birth when it is diagnosed earlier in gestation? Am J Obstet Gynecol 2005;192(2):470–7.

48. Mann JR, McDermott S, Gill T. Sexually transmitted infection is associated with increased risk of preterm birth in South Carolina women insured by Medicaid. J Matern Neonatal Med 2010;23(6):563–8.

49. McClelland RS, Sangaré L, Hassan WM, et al. Infection with Trichomonas vaginalis Increases the Risk of HIV-1 Acquisition. J Infect Dis 2007;195(5):698–702.

50. Brocklehurst PGAHE, Milan SJ. Antibiotics for treating bacterial vaginosis in pregnancy. Cochrane Database Syst Rev 2013;1.

51. Thinkhamrop J, Hofmeyr GJ, Adetoro O, et al. Antibiotic prophylaxis during the second and third trimester to reduce adverse pregnancy outcomes and morbidity. Cochrane Database Syst Rev 2015;6. https://doi.org/10.1002/14651858.CD002250.pub3.

52. Calonge N, Petitti DB, DeWitt TG, et al. Screening for bacterial vaginosis in pregnancy to prevent preterm delivery: U.S. Preventive Services Task Force recommendation statement. Ann Intern Med 2008;148(3):214–9.

53. Gülmezoglu AM, Azhar M. Interventions for trichomoniasis in pregnancy. Cochrane Database Syst Rev 2011;5. https://doi.org/10.1002/14651858.CD000220.pub2.

54. Bartz D. Pelvic Inflammatory Disease. In: Stovall T, Ling F, Zite N, et al, editors. Gynecology for the Primary Care Physician. Philadelphia: Springer; 2008. p. 67–74.

55. Marrazzo JM, Martin DH. Management of Women with Cervicitis. Clin Infect Dis 2007;44(Supplement_3):S102–10.
56. Manhart LE, Critchlow CW, Holmes KK, et al. Mucopurulent Cervicitis and Mycoplasma genitalium. J Infect Dis 2003;187(4):650–7.
57. Sutton MY, Sternberg M, Zaidi A, et al. Trends in Pelvic Inflammatory Disease Hospital Discharges and Ambulatory Visits, United States, 1985–2001. Sex Transm Dis 2005;32(12). Available at: https://journals.lww.com/stdjournal/Fulltext/2005/12000/Trends_in_Pelvic_Inflammatory_Disease_Hospital.12.aspx.
58. Satterwhite CL, Torrone E, Meites E, et al. Sexually Transmitted Infections Among US Women and Men: Prevalence and Incidence Estimates, 2008. Sex Transm Dis 2013;40(3). Available at: https://journals.lww.com/stdjournal/Fulltext/2013/03000/Sexually_Transmitted_Infections_Among_US_Women_and.1.aspx.
59. Jennings LKKD. Pelvic inflammatory disease. StatPearls Publishing; 2022. Available at: https://www.ncbi.nlm.nih.gov/books/NBK499959/. Accessed June 7, 2022.
60. CDC. Sexually Transmitted Disease Surveillance 2020: National Overview. 2022. Available at: https://www.cdc.gov/std/statistics/2020/overview.htm#Chlamydia. Accessed June 6, 2022.
61. Grimes DA. Intrauterine device and upper-genital-tract infection. Lancet 2000; 356(9234):1013–9.
62. Curry A, Williams T, Penny ML. Pelvic inflammatory disease: Diagnosis, management, and prevention. Am Fam Physician 2019;100(6):357–64.
63. Zakher B, Cantor AG, Pappas M, et al. Screening for Gonorrhea and Chlamydia: An Update for the U.S. Preventive Services Task Force. Ann Intern Med 2014. https://doi.org/10.7326/M14-1022.
64. Piton S, Marie E, Parmentier J. [Chlamydia trachomatis perihepatitis (Fitz Hugh-Curtis syndrome). Apropos of 20 cases]. J Gynecol Obstet Biol Reprod (Paris) 1990;19 4:447–54.
65. Brunham RC, Gottlieb SL, Paavonen J. Pelvic Inflammatory Disease. N Engl J Med 2015;372(21):2039–48.
66. Gradison M. Pelvic inflammatory disease. Am Fam Physician 2012;85(8):791–6.
67. Van Dyck E, Ieven M, Pattyn S, et al. Detection of Chlamydia trachomatis and Neisseria gonorrhoeae by enzyme immunoassay, culture, and three nucleic acid amplification tests. J Clin Microbiol 2001;39(5):1751–6.
68. Prevention C for DC and. Recommendations for the laboratory-based detection of Chlamydia trachomatis and Neisseria gonorrhoeae–2014. MMWR Recomm Rep Morb Mortal Wkly Rep Recomm Rep 2014;63(RR-02):1–19. Available at: https://pubmed.ncbi.nlm.nih.gov/24622331.
69. Ness RB, Soper DE, Holley RL, et al. Effectiveness of inpatient and outpatient treatment strategies for women with pelvic inflammatory disease: Results from the pelvic inflammatory disease evaluation and clinical health (peach) randomized trial. Am J Obstet Gynecol 2002;186(5):929–37.
70. Tepper NK, Steenland MW, Gaffield ME, et al. Retention of intrauterine devices in women who acquire pelvic inflammatory disease: a systematic review. Contraception 2013;87(5):655–60.
71. Haggerty CL, Gottlieb SL, Taylor BD, et al. Risk of sequelae after Chlamydia trachomatis genital infection in women. J Infect Dis 2010;201(Suppl 2):S134–55.
72. USPST Force. Screening for Chlamydia and Gonorrhea: US Preventive Services Task Force Recommendation Statement. JAMA 2021;326(10):949–56.

Structural Gynecological Disease

Fibroids, Endometriosis, Ovarian Cysts

Amy H. Farkas, MD, MS[a],*, Hannah Abumusa, MD[b],
Brianna Rossiter, MD, MS[b]

KEYWORDS

- Structural gynecological disease • Fibroids • Endometriosis • Ovarian cyst

KEY POINTS

- Fibroids, endometriosis, and ovarian cysts are common.
- Fibroids can present with heavy vaginal bleeding, pain, or pressure sensations and are managed symptomatically.
- Endometriosis can result in chronic cyclical pelvic pain and can be managed with nonsteroidal medication, contraceptives, or surgical resection.
- Ovarian cysts are often diagnosed incidentally and frequently can be managed expectantly given the overall low risk for malignancy.

Benign structural gynecological disease including fibroids, endometriosis, and ovarian cysts are common pathologic conditions particularly among reproductive-aged women. These pathologic conditions can be asymptomatic or present with symptoms such as pelvic pain, abnormal uterine bleeding, and infertility. This article will address the epidemiology, clinical presentation, diagnostic evaluation, and management of each of these conditions.

UTERINE FIBROIDS
Epidemiology/Risk Factors/Pathophysiology

Uterine leiomyomas, more commonly known as fibroids or myomas, are the most common neoplasm of the uterus.[1] Although benign, fibroids are symptomatic and can cause large impacts on a woman's quality of life (QOL). Fibroids originate from smooth muscle cells and fibroblasts of the myometrium. Because fibroids differ in

a Division of General Internal Medicine, Medical College of Wisconsin, Milwaukee VA Medical Center, 5000 West National Avenue, Milwaukee, WI 53295, USA; b Division of General Internal Medicine, University of Pittsburgh School of Medicine, UPMC VAPT, VA Pittsburgh Healthcare System, 4100 Allequippa Street, Pittsburgh, PA 15240, USA
* Corresponding author.
E-mail address: ahfarkas@mcw.edu

Med Clin N Am 107 (2023) 317–328
https://doi.org/10.1016/j.mcna.2022.10.010
0025-7125/23/Published by Elsevier Inc.

medical.theclinics.com

size, shape, and location to the endometrial and serosal surfaces, a standardized nomenclature system for fibroids was developed by the International Federation of Gynecology and Obstetrics FIGO.[2] Fibroids can be embedded in the myometrium or pedunculated, and be either submucosal, intramural or subserosal. Some fibroids are transmural and extend from serosal to mucosal surfaces (**Table 1**).

Fibroids are thought to originate from mutations in uterine myocytes with gonadal steroid hormones influencing pathogenesis.[3] Later menarche and increasing parity decrease the risk of developing fibroids[4,5] demonstrating fibroids' responsiveness to the effects of estrogen and progesterone. Additional risk factors include obesity[6] and genetics,[7] with higher BMI and known family history, conferring a higher risk of fibroid formation.

The prevalence of fibroids is challenging to determine given that leiomyomas can be asymptomatic. Estimated cumulative incidence of fibroids by age 50 range as high as greater than 80% for Black women and nearly 70% for white women.[1] Incidence increases with reproductive age. Likely for many reasons, including but not limited to familial predisposition, social determinants of health and systemic racism, Black women are disproportionately affected by fibroids[8] in terms of symptom severity and impacts on QOL.[9] Further, Black women are more likely be managed with surgical versus nonsurgical treatments, with higher rates of postoperative complications.[10]

The prevalence of fibroids in pregnancy is challenging to determine given the heterogeneity of available studies; however, a 2009 prospective cohort found prevalence to be as high as 10%.[11]

Clinical presentation/symptoms

Fibroids are common and may never cause symptoms. However, when fibroids do cause symptoms, the predominant symptoms are bleeding irregularities or bulk-related symptoms. Symptoms often depend on fibroid location in the uterine cavity and size. Submucosal fibroids are a major cause of abnormal uterine bleeding, particularly heavy and/or prolonged bleeding, and should be considered in any patient presenting with menstrual changes.[12] Intermenstrual or postpartum bleeding are less likely with fibroids and should prompt investigation for another endometrial pathologic condition. Bulk symptoms related to fibroids can include symptoms of abdomino-pelvic pain and bloating. Depending on location and size, leiomyomas can result in bowel and bladder issues.

Data does not suggest that fibroids are a cause of infertility.[13] Most patients with fibroids do not have any complications during pregnancy other than pain[14] and overall, women with leiomyomas are at low risk for obstetric complications compared with women without leiomyomas.[15,16]

Table 1 International federation of gynecology and obstetrics fibroid classification system		
SM-Submucosal[a]	0	Pedunculated Intracavity
	1	<50% intramural
	2	>50% intramural
	3	Contacts endometrium; 100% intramural
O-Other	4	Intramural
	5	Subserous >50% intramural
	6	Subserous <50% intramural
	7	Subserous pedunculated
	8	Other (eg, cervical)

[a] Hybrid classification: Two numbers are listed together by hyphen. By convention, first number refers to relationship with endometrium and second to relationship to serosal surface.

Diagnostic considerations/imaging/differential diagnosis

Workup for possible leiomyomas should be considered in patients presenting with abnormal uterine bleeding and chronic abdomino-pelvic pain. Leiomyomas should also be in the differential in patients presenting with nonspecific bloating, dyspareunia, and bowel or bladder dysfunction. In addition to a detailed history, a physical examination should include a focused abdominal and pelvic examination including a bimanual. On bimanual examination, consideration showed be given to the size, contour, and mobility of the uterus. A mobile uterus with irregular contours is suggestive of a leiomyomatous uterus.

The diagnostic imaging of choice for fibroids is transvaginal ultrasound because it is inexpensive, safe, and readily available. Sensitivity and specificity of transvaginal ultrasound (TVUS) for detecting fibroids are 99% and 91%, respectively.[17] Fibroids on ultrasound usually are hypoechoic, well-circumscribed round masses. Additional diagnostics may include saline infused sonography for infertility workup and hysteroscopy if a hysteroscopic resection is planned. MRI can distinguish leiomyomas from adenomyosis if needed. Beyond this, MRI is usually reserved for complex surgical planning or if a malignant disease is suspected.

Fibroids are diagnosed clinically or based on TVUS with or without the previous symptoms. Histologic diagnosis is not necessary. Differential diagnoses for uterine lesions in both the presence and absence of symptoms include pathologic condition originating from the myometrium or endometrium. Myometrial lesions in the differential include adenomyosis, leiomyosarcoma, and metastatic disease. Endometrial lesions include polyps, which tend to be much smaller than fibroids, and malignancy (carcinosarcoma and endometrial stromal sarcoma). Finally, blood in the uterine cavity, for instance after a dilation and curettage, may also appear similarly to fibroids on ultrasound.

Unfortunately, both clinically and radiographically, it is hard to distinguish leiomyomas from a malignant lesion such as sarcoma. However, although fibroids are very common, uterine sarcoma is very rare (3 to 7/100,000 in the United States population[18]). Given this, tissue sampling and/or hysterectomy should not be performed for the purpose of excluding malignant disease. Risk factors for uterine sarcoma include advancing age, postmenopausal status, and Black race.[19] A malignancy workup should be considered in women presenting with new fibroid symptoms in the postmenopausal phase. MRI can be useful in the diagnosis of a uterine sarcoma.[20] Any concern for workup of malignancy should be perused in conjunction with gynecologist specialized in this care.

Management

Treatment of fibroids is only considered in symptomatic patients. Otherwise, education should be provided to patients. Fibroids can regress over time, especially in the postpartum period,[21] likely due to the waning of gonadal hormones. As such, expectant management is reasonable for asymptomatic patients and those with mild symptoms. In asymptomatic patients, serial imaging is not usually performed and would only be considered for changes in clinical status. Patients that do present with bleeding or painful, bulky symptoms have both medical and surgical options for treatment. Therapies should be chosen based on the patient's desire to maintain fertility using shared decision-making approaches.

For patients who are not actively trying to conceive, the mainstay in treatment is alleviation of symptoms. With menorrhagia, the initial management includes the use of combined estrogen-progestin contraceptive (oral pills, transdermal patch, or vaginal ring), levonorgestrel-releasing intrauterine devices, and progestin-only pills.

Contraceptive decisions should consider patient preferences and contraindications. If fibroids are submucosal, hysteroscopic myomectomy is also considered a first-line approach.[22] Second-line options for both heavy bleeding and bulk or pain symptoms include gonadotropin-releasing hormone (GnRH) agonists and antagonists and uterine artery embolization (UAE). GnRH medications are also often used as a bridge to surgery for fibroid size reduction but also include hypogonadism side effects. Other lesser used treatment options for bleeding include endometrial ablation. Last-line management for patients who do not desire fertility but have persistent fibroid-related symptoms includes hysterectomy and myomectomy. Hysterectomy involves removal of the uterine corpus (definitive therapy), including the fibroids, whereas myomectomy removes only the fibroids and leaves the uterus in situ. Approach depends on location and size of fibroid. Such treatment decisions would be made in conjunction with gynecology and patient's preferences for ongoing fertility. In general, the most minimally invasive procedure is preferred and standard surgical complications should be considered.[9] Both minimally invasive myomectomy and hysterectomy are associated with improved QOL measures[23] in the short-term and long-term with hysterectomy having significantly greater improvement when stratified by surgical approach. QOL outcomes were similar for patients for abdominal myomectomy and abdominal hysterectomy.

For patients desiring ongoing fertility, if conception is not immediately desired, medical options can be considered. However, for patients desiring to conceive, most medical options preclude pregnancy. In this case, the first-line treatment is hysteroscopic myomectomy. If fibroids are not amendable to this approach, options include open abdominal or laparoscopic myomectomy. UAE can also be considered; however, there are limited available data on reproductive outcomes.[23]

Summary or future considerations

Leiomyomas are the most common benign uterine tumor and can present asymptomatically or with heavy bleeding and bulk symptoms affecting women's QOL. Inequalities exist in the management of fibroids with Black women disproportionately affected by symptoms, QOL, and approaches to treatment. Treatment of fibroids depends on symptoms and includes both medical and surgical modalities. Discussing patient preferences and using shared decision-making is cornerstone to determining appropriate treatment.

ENDOMETRIOSIS
Epidemiology/Risk Factors/Pathophysiology

Endometriosis is a complex disease characterized by ectopic endometrial tissue outside the uterus.[24] It is commonly associated with chronic pelvic pain and infertility.[24] The lack of valid and reliable noninvasive diagnostic tests makes calculating the true incidence of endometriosis challenging[25]; however, studies have shown that it affects 6% to 10% of women of reproductive age, 50% to 60% of patients with chronic pelvic pain, and 50% of women with infertility.[26]

Risk factors for endometriosis include early menarche as well as heavy and prolonged menses.[27] These 2 factors prolong the exposure to endogenous estrogen, which stimulates ectopic and eutopic endometrial tissue.[27] Other factors include menstrual outflow obstruction, short menstrual cycles, and low birth weight.[27]

There are numerous hypotheses regarding the pathogenesis of endometriosis. The most widely recognized theory is implantation via retrograde menstruation.[27] During retrograde menstruation, early endometrial tissues spread to other pelvic regions with eventual invasion of the peritoneum, subsequently leading to ectopic endometrial tissue outside the uterus.[27] This triggers an inflammatory response that is responsible for the manifestations of the disease. This inflammatory response activates pain fibers, resulting in dyspareunia, cyclic menstrual pain, and chronic pelvic pain. The ectopic endometrial tissue responds to hormonal stimulation; therefore, women tend to be more symptomatic during the time of their menses.[28] The most common sites of extrapelvic implants include the gastrointestinal tract, lungs, diaphragm, and abdomen.[27]

Clinical presentation/symptoms

The clinical presentation of endometriosis varies widely in women. Patients may be asymptomatic while others present with menstrual pain, chronic pelvic pain, low back pain, dyspareunia, dyschezia, and dysuria.[27] The menstrual pain is typically dull or sharp and can be either constant or intermittent throughout a cycle. The pain is often aggravated by physical activity or deep vaginal penetration.[27] Infertility has been commonly associated with endometriosis; however, the pathophysiology of infertility in endometriosis is not well understood.[29] Some studies have suggested the toxic effects of the chronic inflammatory state on gametes and embryos, in addition to the formation of scarring tissue and adhesions that distort the pelvic anatomy and impair sperm motility.[26] Additionally, patients with endometriosis reported significantly higher rates of depression, anxiety, and emotional sensitivity compared with the general population.[30] On physical examination, most patients will have normal findings. However, some may have findings suggestive of endometriosis including deep infiltrating nodules palpated in the posterior vaginal fornix, a fixed retroverted uterus, and fixed adnexal masses representing ovarian endometriomas.[31]

Diagnostic Considerations/Imaging/Differential Diagnosis

A diagnosis of endometriosis can be made through history and physical examination as described above; however, the gold standard in diagnosis of endometriosis is biopsy and direct histological visualization of the suspected lesions via laparoscopy.[32]

Noninvasive diagnostic modalities include imaging with either a TVUS or MRI. Both imaging methods can be used to detect endometriomas[33] but TVUS is preferred over pelvic MRI given its lower cost.[26] Pelvic MRI may be considered superior to TVUS when assessing the depth and extent of endometriomas involving the bowel, bladder, and ureters.[27] Unfortunately, neither modality is able to detect overall pelvic endometriosis well enough to replace laparoscopy as the gold standard diagnostic tool.[34]

Several other conditions may present with similar findings. The differential includes chronic pelvic pain, pelvic inflammatory disease, and primary dysmenorrhea, as well as other nongynecological conditions such as irritable bowel syndrome, interstitial cystitis, and myofascial pelvic pain.[29] Often endometriosis can co-occur with these conditions.

Management

The goal of management in patients with endometriosis is symptomatic relief and prevention of disease progression and complications.[7] Approaches to treatment should be individualized and may be focused on symptomatic relief of pelvic pain, and complications of endometriosis such as infertility. Treatment of endometriosis may include medical therapy, surgical therapy, or both.

Medical therapy

Medical therapy can be initiated once a presumptive diagnosis of endometriosis is made. The main goal of medical therapy is to relieve pain associated with endometriosis through multiple mechanisms including decreasing inflammation, suppressing ovulation, and reducing menstrual cycles.

Nonsteroidal anti-inflammatory drugs (NSAIDs) are considered first-line therapy in the treatment of dysmenorrhea.[35] There are no studies that have shown a certain NSAID to be superior over another in the treatment of endometriosis.[36] If patients do not attain adequate symptomatic relief within 3 months of initiating NSAID therapy, they should be started on second-line agents such as hormonal therapy.[37]

First-line hormonal therapy includes combined oral contraception pills and should be considered in patients without contraindications to hormonal therapy. Studies have supported the effect of combined contraceptive pills to reduce pain associated with endometriosis compared with placebo.[38] Combined oral contraceptives can be given cyclically or continuously depending on the severity of the symptoms.[39,40] In women with severe dysmenorrhea who have not responded adequately to cyclic combined contraceptives, switching to continuous therapy with either oral progestins or combined oral contraceptives can provide significant pain relief.[41]

Second-line hormonal therapy includes gonadotrophin releasing hormone analogs (GnRHa) such as leuprolide and goserelin.[6] These agents work by downregulating the signaling of the hypothalamic-pituitary axis, suppressing ovulation, and reducing estrogen levels resulting in a hypoestrogenic state.[37] Side effects of this hypoestrogenic state are similar to menopause, including hot flashes, vaginal dryness, and bone loss. Low doses add back estrogen and progestin can be used to reduce side effects. Additionally, the FDA does not recommend women remain on these agents for more than 6 months given the hypoestrogenic state.[37]

Medical treatment of infertility associated with endometriosis includes agents that will stimulate follicle growth and restore normal ovulation. Agents that have been widely used are clomiphene citrate as well as aromatase inhibitors. Agents that suppress ovulation such as GnRHa and combined contraceptives should not be used in women who wish to conceive as they can delay pregnancy.[32]

Surgical therapy

Surgical modalities used to treat pain associated with endometriosis include the excision of endometrial implants and the disruption of nerve pathways through ablation of uterosacral nerves or hysterectomy.[24] Surgical excision has shown to provide 50% to 80% of symptomatic relief; however, there continues to be recurrence of endometriosis in patients after surgery in about 10% to 50% of patients.[25,28]

Surgery can also be used to treat infertility. The goal is to remove endometrial tissue to restore normal pelvic anatomy that may allow spontaneous conception. This can be achieved through laparoscopic techniques to remove endometrial cysts or through ablation of ectopic tissue.[42] Other lines of treatment in infertility include intrauterine insemination and in vitro fertilization.[43] Women who do not achieve pregnancy after surgery should be referred to reproductive specialists who can assist in the above-mentioned modalities.

SUMMARY

Endometriosis is a complex disorder that typically manifests with chronic pain and infertility. The absence of noninvasive reliable diagnostic tests leads to delay in early diagnosis of endometriosis. Clinical suspicion of endometriosis should prompt the initiation of medical therapy with the goal to provide symptomatic relief and to prevent disease progression. Women should be referred to a gynecologist if they do not attain adequate symptomatic relief with the first-line medical therapy. Women should be referred to reproductive specialist if they are aged older than 35 years with chronic pain and fail to conceive after 6 months.

Table 2
Ovarian cyst types, ultrasound findings, and pathophysiology

Ovarian Cyst Type	Ultrasound Findings and Pathophysiology
Functional-follicular	• Simple cyst <3 cm in diameter • Secondary to the development of an oocyte
Corpus luteum	• Thick-walled cyst <3 cm in diameter
Simple cyst	• Thin-walled cyst without internal elements • Secondary to a follicular/corpus luteum that failed to involute
Hemorrhagic	• Cyst with internal reticular pattern • Secondary to bleeding into a follicular or corpus luteum
Endometrioma	• Cyst with internal homogenous echos • Results of endometrial tissue inside an ovarian cyst
Dermoid—Mature teratoma	• Complex cyst • Derived from all 3-germ cell layers can contain different tissue types • Most common germ cell tumor

OVARIAN CYSTS
Epidemiology/Risk Factors/Pathophysiology

Ovarian cysts are common clinical findings in both premenopausal and postmenopausal women with both high incidence and prevalence.[44,45] Premenopausal women will develop a new functional cyst monthly and among postmenopausal women up to 17% will have an ovarian cyst on TVUS. There are several different types of ovarian cysts as described in **Table 2**.[28,46]

Given the how common ovarian cysts are, the clinical question is when do ovarian cysts require further follow-up, which is determined by a combination of menopausal status, imaging findings, patient symptoms, and potential concern for malignancy. Ovarian cancer is more common in older women with a median age at diagnosis of 63 years.[47] Unfortunately, it remains a deadly disease with a 5-year survival rate of 49% because most cases are still diagnosed with late-stage disease.[48] Therefore, although most ovarian cysts are benign, it is important to fully evaluate women presenting with a new cyst.

Clinical presentation/symptoms

Most cysts will be discovered incidentally either on imaging or physical examination and less commonly will present symptomatically in a patient. Patients who do present with symptoms may experience pain or pressure sensations. Pain can result either from the physical size of the cyst or from rupture of cyst contents, for example, blood from a hemorrhagic cyst, which results in local inflammation. However, given how common cysts are, it is important to do a complete evaluation of a woman presenting with pelvic pain because the ovarian cyst may be an incidental finding rather than the true cause of her pain.

Less commonly, ovarian cysts can present more urgently and even require emergent surgical intervention. For example, a woman could present with symptoms of ovarian torsion with severe unilateral abdominal/pelvic pain[49] or with symptoms of acute blood loss from uncontrolled bleeding secondary to a hemorrhagic cyst. These would require emergent consultation with gynecology and surgical intervention. Finally, if a woman presents with any systemic symptoms such as abdominal bloating, ascites, or early satiety, there should be a higher index of suspicion for an ovarian malignancy.[50]

Diagnostic Considerations/Imaging/Differential Diagnosis

The differential diagnosis for ovarian cysts includes both benign pathologic conditions, such as functional cysts, endometriomas, mature teratomas, hemorrhagic cysts, and cystadenomas, along with malignant findings including epithelial carcinoma, germ cell tumor, sex-cord, or stromal tumors. Additionally, nonovarian pathologic conditions such as paratubal cysts and hydrosalpinx may be found either on palpation of the adnexa or on imaging.[50]

In evaluating a woman presenting with an ovarian cyst, it is important to start with a good review of personal and family history to assess for any risk for a hereditary cancer syndrome such as BRCA1/2, which would increase the concern for malignancy.[50] Assuming there are no concerning findings on history, most ovarian pathologic conditions can be evaluated with the use of TVUS, even if they had previous imaging with computed tomography or MRI because TVUS is the preferred modality. In general, simple cysts up to 10 cm in size are considered benign, whereas cysts with irregularity, septations, solid components, or vascularity are concerning for malignancy.[50] In 2019, the American College of Radiology published consensus guidelines for the reporting of ovarian-adnexal ultrasound findings (O-RADS score) based on the risk for malignancy **(Table 3)**.[46] If TVUS is unable to fully visualize the cysts, MRI may be helpful as the next line imaging modality.

With regard to laboratory evaluation, CA-125 is the most commonly study tumor marker in ovarian cancer; however, it is only specific to epithelial carcinoma and only elevated 50% of the time in stage 1 disease. Additionally, in premenopausal women CA-125 can be elevated secondary to benign causes such as endometriosis, pelvic inflammatory disease, and pregnancy making it less useful in premenopausal women. In postmenopausal women, it is reasonable to order a CA-125 as part of the workup for ovarian pathologic conditions given its increased sensitive in this population. In postmenopausal women, a level of greater than 35 U/mL should prompt referral to a gynecologist oncologist regardless of ultrasound findings. Additionally, premenopausal and postmenopausal patients with concerning ultrasound findings should be referred to a gynecologist oncologist regardless of CA-125 level.[50]

Management

Because most ovarian cysts are benign, they can often be followed with repeat imaging in primary care without surgical intervention. Simple cysts, hemorrhagic cysts, dermoid, and endometriomas can be managed expectantly. Although there are limited data with regards to interval follow-up, the American College of Radiologists recommend repeat TVUS in 8 to 12 weeks for simple and hemorrhagic cysts greater than 5 cm but less than 10 cm. For a simple cyst, if there is diagnostic certainty, no further surveillance is needed.[51] If a hemorrhagic cyst persists or enlarges at follow-up, consider referral to gynecology. For dermoids and endometriomas less than 10 cm, they recommend an optional follow-up in 8 to 12 weeks.[46] Annual surveillance can be considered if the cyst is not surgically removed. Repeat imaging would also be warranted if the diagnosis is uncertain.[50] Given that CA-125 is recommended as part of the workup in postmenopausal women, it would be reasonable to repeat the laboratory at the same time as any follow-up imaging.[50]

Oral contraceptive pills are no longer recommended for the management or suppression of future ovarian cysts based on a 2014 systematic review.[52] Surgical referral would be appropriate for any woman who is symptomatic; however, premenopausal patients should be counselled regarding ovarian reserve and impact of surgery on future fertility.

Table 3
American college of radiology O-RADS for transvaginal ultrasound categories based on 2019 reporting guidelines

O-RADS	Malignancy Risk	Example Findings
0	N/A	Incomplete evaluation
1	N/A	Normal ovary Follicle development Corpus luteum
2	<1%	Simple cyst <10 cm in size Benign lesions—dermoid, hemorrhagic cyst, endometriomas
3	<10%	Larger unilocular cysts ≥10 cm Larger typical benign lesions ≥10 cm Multilocular cysts <10 cm
4	10–<50%	Multilocular cysts ≥10 cm Unilocular cysts with solid components (0–3 papillary projections) Solid cysts
5	≥50%	Unilocular cysts with ≥4 papillary projections Multilocular cysts with solid components Ascites and/or peritoneal nodules

If there is concern for potential malignancy based either on personal or family history, ultrasound findings, or laboratory evaluation, the woman should be referred to a gynecologic oncologist for further workup and management. The data demonstrate that women with ovarian cancer have better survival and are more likely to achieve cytoreduction when their initial surgery is performed by a specially trained a gynecologic oncologist rather than a general gynecologist or general surgeon.[50]

SUMMARY

Ovarian cysts are common pathologic conditions in both premenopausal and postmenopausal women and, generally, are found incidentally. Simple cysts up to 10 cm in size are universally benign and do not require surgical referral. If there is concern for ovarian malignancy based on history, imaging, or laboratory evaluation, the patient should be referred to a gynecologic oncologist.

CLINICS CARE POINTS

- Fibroids do not require a histological diagnosis but rather than be diagnosed based on clinical exam or transvaginal ultrasound.

- Only symtompatic fibroids require management.

- Endometriosis is a clinical diagnosis and the goal of treatment is to control the cyclical pain associated with endometriosis. First line options including NSAID therapy and oral contraceptive pills.

- Simple ovarian cysts up to 10 cm in diameter can be considered benign and do not require additional evaluation.

- If there is a concern for ovarian malignancy a patient should be referred to gynecological oncology for management.

DISCLOSURE

None of the authors has any disclosures.

REFERENCES

1. Baird DD, Dunson DB, Hill MC, et al. High cumulative incidence of uterine leiomyoma in black and white women: ultrasound evidence. Am J Obstet Gynecol 2003;188(1):100–7.
2. Munro MG, Critchley HOD, Fraser IS. The two FIGO systems for normal and abnormal uterine bleeding symptoms and classification of causes of abnormal uterine bleeding in the reproductive years: 2018 revisions. Int J Gynaecol Obstet 2018;143(3):393–408.
3. Ishikawa H, Ishi K, Serna VA, et al. Progesterone is essential for maintenance and growth of uterine leiomyoma. Endocrinology 2010;151(6):2433–42.
4. Parazzini F, La Vecchia C, Negri E, et al. Epidemiologic characteristics of women with uterine fibroids: a case-control study. Obstet Gynecol 1988;72(6):853–7.
5. Wise LA, Palmer JR, Harlow BL, et al. Reproductive factors, hormonal contraception, and risk of uterine leiomyomata in African-American women: a prospective study. Am J Epidemiol 2004;159(2):113–23.
6. Terry KL, De Vivo I, Hankinson SE, et al. Anthropometric characteristics and risk of uterine leiomyoma. Epidemiology 2007;18(6):758–63.
7. Mehine M, Kaasinen E, Mäkinen N, et al. Characterization of uterine leiomyomas by whole-genome sequencing. N Engl J Med 2013;369(1):43–53.
8. Marshall LM, Spiegelman D, Barbieri RL, et al. Variation in the incidence of uterine leiomyoma among premenopausal women by age and race. Obstet Gynecol 1997;90(6):967–73.
9. ACOG Practice Bulletin No. 228: Management of Symptomatic Uterine Leiomyomas: Correction. Obstet Gynecol 2021;138(4):683.
10. Alexander AL, Strohl AE, Rieder S, et al. Examining Disparities in Route of Surgery and Postoperative Complications in Black Race and Hysterectomy. Obstet Gynecol 2019;133(1):6–12.
11. Laughlin SK, Baird DD, Savitz DA, et al. Prevalence of uterine leiomyomas in the first trimester of pregnancy: an ultrasound-screening study. Obstet Gynecol 2009;113(3):630–5.
12. Practice bulletin no. 128: diagnosis of abnormal uterine bleeding in reproductive-aged women. Obstet Gynecol 2012;120(1):197–206.
13. Sundermann AC, Velez Edwards DR, Bray MJ, et al. Leiomyomas in Pregnancy and Spontaneous Abortion: A Systematic Review and Meta-analysis. Obstet Gynecol 2017;130(5):1065–72.
14. Lam SJ, Best S, Kumar S. The impact of fibroid characteristics on pregnancy outcome. Am J Obstet Gynecol 2014;211(4). 395.e391-395.
15. Stout MJ, Odibo AO, Graseck AS, et al. Leiomyomas at routine second-trimester ultrasound examination and adverse obstetric outcomes. Obstet Gynecol 2010; 116(5):1056–63.
16. Segars JH, Parrott EC, Nagel JD, et al. Proceedings from the Third National Institutes of Health International Congress on Advances in Uterine Leiomyoma Research: comprehensive review, conference summary and future recommendations. Hum Reprod Update 2014;20(3):309–33.
17. Dueholm M, Lundorf E, Hansen ES, et al. Accuracy of magnetic resonance imaging and transvaginal ultrasonography in the diagnosis, mapping, and measurement of uterine myomas. Am J Obstet Gynecol 2002;186(3):409–15.

18. Brooks SE, Zhan M, Cote T, et al. Surveillance, epidemiology, and end results analysis of 2677 cases of uterine sarcoma 1989-1999. Gynecol Oncol 2004; 93(1):204–8.

19. Hosh M, Antar S, Nazzal A, et al. Uterine Sarcoma: Analysis of 13,089 Cases Based on Surveillance, Epidemiology, and End Results Database. Int J Gynecol Cancer 2016;26(6):1098–104.

20. Santos P, Cunha TM. Uterine sarcomas: clinical presentation and MRI features. Diagn Interv Radiol 2015;21(1):4–9.

21. Laughlin SK, Hartmann KE, Baird DD. Postpartum factors and natural fibroid regression. Am J Obstet Gynecol 2011;204(6). 496.e491-496.

22. Laughlin-Tommaso SK, Lu D, Thomas L, et al. Short-term quality of life after myomectomy for uterine fibroids from the COMPARE-UF Fibroid Registry. Am J Obstet Gynecol 2020;222(4). 345.e341-345.e322.

23. Hartmann KE, Fonnesbeck C, Surawicz T, et al. AHRQ comparative effectiveness reviews. In: Management of uterine fibroids. Rockville (MD): Agency for Healthcare Research and Quality (US); 2017. p. 49–50.

24. Parasar P, Ozcan P, Terry KL. Endometriosis: Epidemiology, Diagnosis and Clinical Management. Curr Obstet Gynecol Rep 2017;6(1):34–41.

25. Buck Louis GM, Hediger ML, Peterson CM, et al. Incidence of endometriosis by study population and diagnostic method: the ENDO study. Fertil Steril 2011;96(2): 360–5.

26. Giudice LC. Clinical practice. Endometriosis. N Engl J Med 2010;362(25): 2389–98.

27. Alimi Y, Iwanaga J, Loukas M, et al. The Clinical Anatomy of Endometriosis: A Review. Cureus 2018;10(9):e3361.

28. Farkas AHTS, Gonzaga AMR. Fibriods, endometriosis, and ovarian cyts. In: Tilstra SAKD, Mitchell JL, Dolan BM, et al, editors. Sex- and gender-based women's health: a practical guide for primary care. Cham, Switzerland: Springer International; 2020. p. 145.

29. Macer ML, Taylor HS. Endometriosis and infertility: a review of the pathogenesis and treatment of endometriosis-associated infertility. Obstet Gynecol Clin North Am 2012;39(4):535–49.

30. Laganà AS, Condemi I, Retto G, et al. Analysis of psychopathological comorbidity behind the common symptoms and signs of endometriosis. Eur J Obstet Gynecol Reprod Biol 2015;194:30–3.

31. Kuznetsov L, Dworzynski K, Davies M, et al. Diagnosis and management of endometriosis: summary of NICE guidance. BMJ 2017;358:j3935.

32. Tanbo T, Fedorcsak P. Endometriosis-associated infertility: aspects of pathophysiological mechanisms and treatment options. Acta Obstet Gynecol Scand 2017; 96(6):659–67.

33. Brosens I, Puttemans P, Campo R, et al. Diagnosis of endometriosis: pelvic endoscopy and imaging techniques. Best Pract Res Clin Obstet Gynaecol 2004;18(2):285–303.

34. Nisenblat V, Bossuyt PM, Farquhar C, et al. Imaging modalities for the non-invasive diagnosis of endometriosis. Cochrane Database Syst Rev 2016;26(2): CD009591. https://doi.org/10.1002/14651858.CD009591.

35. ACOG Committee Opinion No. 760: Dysmenorrhea and Endometriosis in the Adolescent. Obstet Gynecol 2018;132(6):e249–58.

36. Brown J, Crawford TJ, Allen C, et al. Nonsteroidal anti-inflammatory drugs for pain in women with endometriosis. Cochrane Database Syst Rev 2017;1(1): Cd004753.

37. Kalaitzopoulos DR, Samartzis N, Kolovos GN, et al. Treatment of endometriosis: a review with comparison of 8 guidelines. BMC Womens Health 2021;21(1):397.
38. Harada T, Momoeda M, Taketani Y, et al. Low-dose oral contraceptive pill for dysmenorrhea associated with endometriosis: a placebo-controlled, double-blind, randomized trial. Fertil Steril 2008;90(5):1583–8.
39. Dmitrovic R, Kunselman AR, Legro RS. Continuous compared with cyclic oral contraceptives for the treatment of primary dysmenorrhea: a randomized controlled trial. Obstet Gynecol 2012;119(6):1143–50.
40. Zorbas KA, Economopoulos KP, Vlahos NF. Continuous versus cyclic oral contraceptives for the treatment of endometriosis: a systematic review. Arch Gynecol Obstet 2015;292(1):37–43.
41. Vercellini P, Frontino G, De Giorgi O, et al. Continuous use of an oral contraceptive for endometriosis-associated recurrent dysmenorrhea that does not respond to a cyclic pill regimen. Fertil Steril 2003;80(3):560–3.
42. Casper RF. Introduction: A focus on the medical management of endometriosis. Fertil Steril 2017;107(3):521–2.
43. Kennedy S, Bergqvist A, Chapron C, et al. ESHRE guideline for the diagnosis and treatment of endometriosis. Hum Reprod 2005;20(10):2698–704.
44. Pavlik EJ, Ueland FR, Miller RW, et al. Frequency and disposition of ovarian abnormalities followed with serial transvaginal ultrasonography. Obstet Gynecol 2013;122(2 Pt 1):210–7.
45. Greenlee RT, Kessel B, Williams CR, et al. Prevalence, incidence, and natural history of simple ovarian cysts among women >55 years old in a large cancer screening trial. Am J Obstet Gynecol 2010;202(4):373.e1-9.
46. Andreotti RF, Timmerman D, Strachowski LM, et al. O-RADS US Risk Stratification and Management System: A Consensus Guideline from the ACR Ovarian-Adnexal Reporting and Data System Committee. Radiology 2020;294(1):168–85.
47. American Cancer Society. Ovarian Cancer Risk Factors. 2022. Available at: https://www.cancer.org/cancer/ovarian-cancer/causes-risks-prevention/risk-factors.html#references. Accessed July 21, 2022.
48. American Cancer Society. Survival Rates for Ovarian Cancer. 2022. Available at: https://www.cancer.org/cancer/ovarian-cancer/detection-diagnosis-staging/survival-rates.html. Accessed July 21, 2022.
49. Bridwell RE, Koyfman A, Long B. High risk and low prevalence diseases: Ovarian torsion. Am J Emerg Med 2022;56:145–50.
50. Practice Bulletin No. 174: Evaluation and Management of Adnexal Masses. Obstet Gynecol 2016;128(5):e210–26.
51. ACOG Practice Bulletin. Management of adnexal masses. Obstet Gynecol 2007;110(1):201–14.
52. Grimes DA, Jones LB, Lopez LM, et al. Oral contraceptives for functional ovarian cysts. Cochrane Database Syst Rev 2014;4:Cd006134.

Ovarian, Uterine, and Vulvovaginal Cancers
Screening, Treatment Overview, and Prognosis

Deborah Gomez Kwolek, MD[a,b,*],
Stefanie Gerstberger, MD, PhD[a,c], Sarah Tait, MD[a],
Jeanna M. Qiu, AB[a,b]

KEYWORDS

- Ovarian cancer • Uterine cancer • Vulvar cancer • Vaginal cancer

KEY POINTS

- Ovarian, uterine, and vulvovaginal cancers are not part of routine screening protocols, but the primary-care clinician plays a key role in detection through a focused history, review of systems, and evaluation of concerning symptoms.
- Obesity, estrogen excess, smoking, nulliparity, genetics, diethylstilbestrol, and human papillomavirus are important risk factors for gynecologic malignancies, and patients should be counseled appropriately.
- Postmenopausal bleeding must be evaluated as possible uterine cancer.
- Treatment of gynecologic malignancies is managed by gynecologic oncologists, and often involves a combination of surgery, chemotherapy, and possible radiation treatments.
- Gynecologic cancer survivors need special care including attention to mental, physical, and sexual health care issues.

INTRODUCTION

Gynecologic cancers, uterine, ovarian, and vulvovaginal, affect approximately 96,000 women and result in approximately 29,000 deaths in the United States annually. In 2022, it is estimated that 65,950 US women will be diagnosed with uterine cancer, and all but 12,580 will be cured. For ovarian cancer, 19,880 will be diagnosed, and 12,810 will not survive. Vulvar and vaginal cancers comprise 1% to 2% of cancers and affect approximately 11,000 per year with a combined mortality of 3000 per

[a] Department of Medicine, Massachusetts General Hospital, 55 Fruit Street, Boston, MA 02114, USA; [b] Harvard Medical School, 25 Shattuck Street, Boston, MA 02115, USA; [c] Memorial Sloan Kettering Cancer Center, 1275 York Avenue, New York, NY 10065, USA
* Corresponding author. Department of Medicine, Massachusetts General Hospital, Women's Health and Sex and Gender Medicine Program, 50 Staniford Street, #522, Boston, MA 02114.
E-mail address: dkwolek@mgh.harvard.edu

Med Clin N Am 107 (2023) 329–355
https://doi.org/10.1016/j.mcna.2022.10.016
0025-7125/23/© 2022 Elsevier Inc. All rights reserved.

year.[1–4] There is no current recommended routine screening of asymptomatic women for these malignancies, and thus the diagnosis is usually discovered after patients become symptomatic; in the case of ovarian cancer, this leads to a poor prognosis.[1]

Despite the lack of screening recommendations, primary-care physicians (PCPs) and other primary-care clinicians have an important role in the prevention, detection, and survivorship care of patients with gynecologic malignancies. PCPs should pay close attention to risk factors and early symptoms and educate patients accordingly (**Table 1**).

Gynecologic, gastrointestinal, and urinary symptoms require evaluation, and gynecologic malignancies should be excluded. Past medical history should include the obstetrical and gynecologic history with attention paid to nulliparity, current and past bleeding issues, the use of oral contraceptives and hormonal therapies, a history of diethylstilbestrol (DES) exposure (usually before 1971), prior gynecologic biopsies and surgeries including the pathological findings, and any history of other cancers. The review of systems should screen for symptoms of pain, bleeding, discharge, bloating, urinary issues, dysparunia, and vulvar abnormalities. A sexual history is appropriate for all patients, and especially for cancer survivors.

The family and personal history of malignancies may give clues to a genetic propensity for malignancy, and this history should be updated at preventive visits every 1 to 3 years. Patients with a strong cancer history, or those with a first-degree relative with

Table 1 Overview of gynecologic malignancies			
	Ovarian Cancer	**Uterine Cancer**	**Vulvovaginal Cancer**
Risk factors	Nulliparity; uninterrupted ovulation; genetics	Obesity; unopposed estrogen; SERM[a] use; genetics	HPV[b]; immunosuppression; Lichen Planus; DES exposure[c];
Protective factors	Oral contraceptive use Parity Breastfeeding	Ideal weight Progesterone	HPV vaccination Smoking cessation
Symptoms and early detection	Evaluation of abdominal bloating; pelvic pain; bowel or urinary complaints; abnormal cells on pap test (rare)	Evaluation of heavy premenopausal vaginal bleeding; postmenopausal bleeding; glandular, atypical endometrial, or abnormal squamous cells on pap	Vulvar pruritis, masses or lesions; vaginal bleeding or discharge
Major genetic syndromes	BRCA[d] 1 and 2; Lynch syndrome; offer genetic screening when appropriate based on family history	Lynch syndrome; Cowden syndrome; Offer genetic screening when appropriate based on family history	

[a] SERM, selective estrogen receptor modulator.
[b] HPV, human papillomavirus.
[c] DES, diethylstilbestrol
[d] BRCA, breast cancer gene;[1–4]

ovarian cancer, should be referred for genetic counseling. Prophylactic surgery should be considered in some patients with genetic syndromes with a high probability of future malignancy.

The review and reconciliation of medications should watch for unopposed estrogen and selective estrogen receptor modulator (SERM) use. The general physical examination should pay attention to the body mass index (BMI), hirtutism and stigmata of polycystic ovary syndrome (PCOS), and periodic inspection of the vulva. The pelvic examination is becoming less frequently performed, and cannot be relied upon for screening, except for inspection of the vulva, which may detect lesions requiring further evaluation.[1]

The treatment of gynecologic malignancies is managed by the gynecologic oncologist and may include surgery, radiation, and/or chemotherapy. Younger women may seek fertility-preserving treatments if future childbearing is a concern. Survivorship care technically begins when the patient is diagnosed with cancer. Survivors may have sequelae such as a surgical menopause, a negative self-esteem/body image, fear of sexual relations, incontinence, pain or difficulty with intercourse, anxiety, depression, posttraumatic stress disorder (PTSD), or neuropathies.

The role of the PCP in the prevention, early detection, and survivorship care cannot be overstated. The skill of the PCP in gaining trust, providing patient education, and overcoming barriers to access of care will help lessen morbidity and mortality. With the current social determinants of health realities, health inequities, and at-risk populations, the role of the PCP in advocacy and policy change takes on increased importance.

OVARIAN CANCER
Introduction

Ovarian cancer is the leading cause of death from gynecological malignancies and the second most common gynecological malignancy after uterine cancer.[2,3] The average age at diagnosis is 63 years old, with a 1.1% lifetime risk of developing ovarian cancer in women of average risk.[3] Ninety-five percent of malignant ovarian tumors are of epithelial cell origin, with the most common subtype being high-grade serous carcinoma.[5] The remainder are either germ cell tumors, which are more common in young women and girls, or sex cord-stromal tumors.[5]

Genetic predisposition, such as breast cancer gene (BRCA) mutations, Lynch syndrome, or Ashkenazi Jewish heritage; inflammation; and uninterrupted ovulation increase the risk of ovarian cancer. BRCA1 mutation carriers have a 44% lifetime risk of ovarian cancer and BRCA2 mutation carriers have a 17% lifetime risk.[6] Patients with the genetic predisposition for ovarian cancer should be referred to specialty care providers to consider prophylactic bilateral salpingo-oophorectomy and patients with a strong family history of breast and ovarian cancer should be referred for genetic counseling. Factors that contribute to chronic inflammation, such as endometriosis, cigarette smoking, and PCOS, also increase the risk of ovarian cancer.[7,8] Factors that decrease ovulation over the lifetime, such as the history of pregnancy, history of breast feeding, and combined oral contraceptive use, reduce the risk of ovarian cancer through ovarian rest, reducing the frequency of ovarian cell division and therefore, the risk of DNA damage.[9,10] Use of combined oral contraceptives for more than 10 years results in a decreased relative risk of ovarian cancer by 50%, an intervention estimated to have saved hundreds of thousands of lives from ovarian cancer.[11,12]

The clinical symptoms of ovarian cancer are often nonspecific and easily missed. The most common symptoms include bloating, fullness, and abdominal pressure (71%); abdominal or lower back pain (52%); lack of energy (43%); and urinary symptoms (33%).[13,14] Notably, symptoms of increased abdominal size, bloating, and pelvic pain are seen in 43% of patients with ovarian cancer, but only 8% of patients without cancer, suggesting that this may be an early specific symptom.[14] An ovarian cancer symptom index indicates that further investigation is warranted for patients if any of the following symptoms are present for less than one year and occur more than 12 days per month: pelvic or abdominal pain, urinary urgency or frequency, increased abdominal size or bloating, and difficulty eating or early satiety.[15]

Screening and Diagnosis

There is currently no recommended screening method for ovarian cancer. Challenges in establishing an effective screening method for ovarian cancer include the need for invasive follow-up and the difficulty in identifying early-stage malignancies due to a lack of symptoms and signs. Suspected ovarian cancer cannot be biopsied because of the risk of seeding the peritoneum; as a result, any positive screening test would warrant an oophorectomy for further investigation.[16] In addition, the low prevalence of ovarian cancer results in many false positives when screening is attempted, exposing people to unnecessary surgeries and morbidity. The Prostate, Lung, Colon, Ovarian (PLCO) Cancer Screening Trial reported that of 3285 subjects, 5% of each screening round had false-positive results from CA-125 or transvaginal ultrasound (TVUS). Of these, 1080 underwent surgical follow-ups, of whom 163 subjects (15%) had at least one serious complication.[7] Screening methods may also be inadequate because some aggressive types of ovarian cancer are not restricted to the ovary even in early stages.[17]

Thus far, randomized controlled trials using CA-125 levels and TVUS as screening methods have shown no significant effect on mortality among asymptomatic, postmenopausal women. Abnormal CA-125 level has a positive predictive value (PPV) for invasive ovarian cancer of 3.7%, whereas abnormal TVUS has a PPV of 1.0%; if both tests are abnormal, the PPV is 23.5%.[16] The Shizuoka Cohort Study of Ovarian Cancer Screening showed that by using annual CA-125 levels, there was a nonsignificant increase in the identification of ovarian cancer.[18] The PLCO Cancer Screening Trial tested annual screening with simultaneous CA-125 levels and TVUS and found no statistically significant reduction in mortality from ovarian cancer.[19]

The UK Collaborative Trial of Ovarian Screening, the largest trial to date, tested multimodal screening, annual TVUS, and no screening.[20] The multimodal approach stratified participants based on a risk of ovarian cancer algorithm into three groups for future screening: normal (annual screening), intermediate (repeat CA-125 in 3 months), and (repeat CA-125 and TVUS in 6 weeks). The annual TVUS group also stratified participants into normal (annual screening), unsatisfactory (repeat in 3 months), and abnormal (repeat in 6 weeks). The results found a nonsignificant decrease in mortality among the multimodal (15%) and annual TVUS (11%) screening groups. In the multimodal screening group, findings suggested that 641 patients would need to be screened to prevent 1 death from ovarian cancer. Regarding other screening methods, pelvic examinations do not have sufficient sensitivity or specificity to be reliable methods of screening for ovarian cancer.[21–23] New screening tests are being developed that look for tumor cells in endocervical brushings.[24]

The most recent guidelines from the United States Prevention Services Task Force do not recommend screening for ovarian cancer among asymptomatic women (class D) as the risks of harm from screening outweigh the benefits at this time.[25] However, patients with known genetic predisposition who have not had salpingo-oophorectomy may elect to have screening with TVUS and/or CA-125, though this is of uncertain benefit.[26]

Treatment

Treatment of most ovarian cancer involves a combination of surgery and chemotherapy. Decision of treatment is initially determined based on imaging findings or diagnostic laparoscopy to estimate tumor burden.[27] Surgical and pathological staging occurs during surgery, which typically includes hysterectomy, unilateral or bilateral salpingo-oophorectomy, pelvic and paraaortic lymph node dissection, cytology of pelvic washings and the surface of the diaphragm, and omentectomy (**Table 2** and **Fig. 1**).[28] When metastases are present, cytoreduction is performed to reduce the cancer burden to less than 1 cm of residual disease, which may include bowel or liver resection.[28]

Most chemotherapy regimens use platinum-based drugs, such as carboplatin or cisplatin, and paclitaxel.[29,30] Intraperitoneal chemotherapy has shown a long-term survival benefit compared with intravenous chemotherapy, in part due to increased drug concentration in the abdominopelvic cavity.[31] However, intraperitoneal chemotherapy is also associated with more complications compared with intravenous, such as higher toxicities, worse quality of life during treatment (though it was comparable one year after treatment), and catheter complications.[32,33] For early-stage ovarian cancer, observation after surgery is recommended for stage 1A or 1B; however, adjuvant chemotherapy is recommended for patients with stage IC or stage II disease, clear cell, or high-grade histology.[34,35] For advanced ovarian cancer, neoadjuvant chemotherapy followed by interval debulking surgery is considered, as it may decrease perioperative morbidity and increase the likelihood of sufficient resection (<1 cm) during cytoreductive surgery; however, studies thus far have only shown that neoadjuvant therapy is noninferior compared with debulking surgery and adjuvant chemotherapy.[36,37]

Since 2016, the FDA has approved targeted therapies, including poly-ADP ribose polymerase (PARP) inhibitors (Olaparib, niraparib, rucaparib, veliparib) and angiogenesis inhibitors (bevacizumab) for maintenance therapy of ovarian cancer based on multiple trials showing an increase in progression-free survival.[38] Maintenance therapy is currently used after surgery and adjuvant therapy in the initial diagnosis of stage III or IV disease or after recurrence more than 6 months after prior platinum-based chemotherapy.[38] As many ovarian cancers are homologous-repair deficient with mutations in genes like *BRCA*, PARP inhibitors cause single- and double-strand breaks in DNA that cause cell death because the cells cannot perform homologous recombination.[39] Common side effects include gastrointestinal and hematologic toxicities, such as anemia, and rarely myelodysplastic syndrome or acute myeloid leukemia.[40] Bevacizumab is an anti-vascular endothelial growth factor (*VEGF*) monoclonal antibody that inhibits angiogenesis, which causes slowing of tumor growth and may enhance the effects of chemotherapy (**Fig. 3**).[41] It is currently approved for use in combination with chemotherapy and as maintenance monotherapy.[38] Notable side effects include hypertension, which can be medically managed, wound healing complications, and bowel perforation, after which the drug must be discontinued.[42]

Prognosis and Surveillance

Overall, the prognosis remains poor for ovarian cancer. Early-stage, localized ovarian cancer has a 5-year relative survival of 93%; however, only 5% of cases are caught at that stage. Most ovarian cancers are diagnosed when they have metastasized, with a 5-year relative survival of 30.8%.[3] Young age, good performance status, and decreased residual tumor volume are positive prognostic indicators.[43,44] Clear-cell or mucinous histology is associated with worse progression-free survival and overall survival compared with serous histology.[43] Maximal cytoreductive surgery is one of

Table 2
Ovarian cancer staging, 5-year survival, and treatment

FIGO Stage	Stage Description	5-year Survival	Treatment
IA IB IC1,2,3	The cancer is only in the ovary (or ovaries) or fallopian tube(s). IA—confined to one ovary, no surface involvement, no rupture upon removal IB—both ovaries, no surface involvement, no rupture upon removal IC1—confined to one or both ovaries, surgical spill IC2—confined to one or both ovaries, capsule rupture before surgery, surface involvement IC3—malignant cells in pelvic wash	78% to 93%	If completely resected, observation. If high-risk features, treated with three to six cycles of platinum-based chemotherapy.
IIA IIB	The cancer is in one or both ovaries or fallopian tubes and has spread to other organs within the pelvis (such as the uterus, bladder, sigmoid colon, or rectum) IIA—extension or implant into the uterus or fallopian tubes IIB—extension or implant into other pelvic organs	61% to 82%	If completely resected, adjuvant chemotherapy, typically paclitaxel plus carboplatin for six cycles
IIIA IIIB IIIC	No longer confined to the pelvis; has spread into the abdomen IIIA1—cancer spread to pelvic and or para-aortic lymph nodes IIIA2—microscopic tumor involvement in upper abdominal tissues or organs IIIB—macroscopic tumor < 2 cm in size involving upper abdominal tissues or organs IIIC—Macroscopic tumor > 2 cm in size involving upper abdominal tissues or organs	28% to 63%	Surgical cytoreduction, intravenous or intra-peritoneal adjuvant platinum-based chemotherapy, consideration of maintenance therapy with poly ADP-ribose polymerase inhibitors (PARPi) or bevacizumab.
IVA IVB	Cancer has spread to the inside of the spleen or liver, or outside the abdomen IVA—malignant pleural effusion IVB—parenchymal liver or spleen metastasis, distant metastasis	19%	Platinum-based chemotherapy before or after surgical cytoreduction, consideration of maintenance therapy with PARPi or bevacizumab.

From [Prifti, C.A., Kwolek, D., Growdon, W.B., Palamara, K. (2020). Gynecologic Malignancies. In: Tilstra, S.A., Kwolek, D., Mitchell, J.L., Dolan, B.M., Carson, M.P. (eds) Sex- and Gender-Based Women's Health. Springer, Cham. https://doi.org/10.1007/978-3-030-50695-7_15. 15.9']; with permission

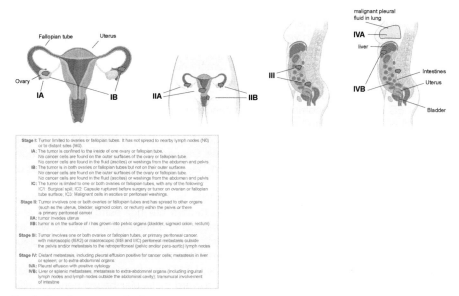

Fig. 1. Ovarian cancer staging.

the strongest prognostic factors in patients with advanced ovarian cancer; a 10% increase in cytoreduction is associated with a 5.9% increase in median survival time.[45]

Recurrence of ovarian cancer is common. Recurrence occurs in 25% of patients with early-stage disease and more than 80% of patients with advanced disease.[46] Unfortunately, treatment after recurrence is rarely curative with a median survival of 2 years after recurrence.[47] Factors associated with 5-year survival after recurrence include secondary debulking surgery, a favorable response to second-line chemotherapy, and $\geq$ 3 treatment regimens after recurrence.[47] For surveillance of recurrence, the National Comprehensive Cancer Network (NCCN) guidelines indicate follow-up with the gynecological oncologist every few months for the first 5 years, after which surveillance care may transition to the PCP for annual visits.[26] As 26% to 50% of recurrences occur within the pelvis, a pelvic examination is indicated at each surveillance visit.[46] CA-125 levels are measured if they were elevated during active disease. Radiographic imaging with CT or PET-CT is often performed, although both have wide-ranging sensitivity and specificity.[46] If the cervix was removed during surgery, pap smears are no longer required.

Survivorship management after ovarian cancer treatment involves managing both the psychological effects and the side effects of treatment. Patients may experience neuropathy from platinum-based chemotherapy; gastrointestinal symptoms from surgery; sudden and severe menopausal symptoms from the removal of ovaries; depression, anxiety or PTSD; and sexual dysfunction.[1,48]

UTERINE CANCER
Introduction

Uterine cancer is the 4th most common cancer in women, after lung, breast, and colorectal cancers, and the most common gynecological malignancy in the United States.[49] Uterine cancers are broadly divided into two classes—endometrial cancer (EC), which comprises 97% of uterine malignancies, and uterine sarcomas, which represent 3% of cases.[50,51]

Endometrial cancer

EC is a malignancy of the inner lining of the uterus and most commonly presents with abnormal uterine bleeding in women aged 55 to 64 years, with a mean age of 63 at diagnosis.[2,49,52] Endometroid carcinomas typically present at an early stage and tend to have a favorable prognosis. These tumors are further subdivided into Type I and Type II based on histology, and differ in their incidence, clinical course, and responsiveness to hormones (**Table 3**).

Type I EC is the most common uterine cancer, comprising 80% to 85% of EC.[53] These tumors are associated with estrogen excess and are well to moderately differentiated tumors of endometroid histology (grade 1 or 2). They respond to progestins and tend to have an overall favorable prognosis. Despite this, the incidence and mortality of EC is rising in the United States, which may be associated with rising rates of obesity.[54]

Type II EC, which comprises the remaining 15% to 20% of all EC, is more aggressive with a less favorable prognosis. These tumors are not estrogen-driven and include higher grade, poorly differentiated (grade 3) endometroid tumors, as well as tumors of non-endometroid histology including papillary serous carcinomas, clear cell, mucinous, carcinosarcomas, and undifferentiated carcinomas.

Although historically the division into type I and II EC has been useful for risk stratification, more recently there has been a shift toward molecular-based genomic risk stratification. Commonly found mutations in EC are phosphate and tensin homologue (PTEN) loss, KRAS, p53, genes in the DNA mismatch repair pathway mutated in Lynch syndrome, and BRCA1. The Cancer Genome Atlas (TCGA) has identified four molecular subtypes of EC that naturally cluster into different profiling patterns with distinct survival differences.[55] These subtypes are divided into POLE mutated (excellent prognosis, endometroid), MSI hypermutated (intermediate prognosis, high MSI/deficient MMR, mutations in MLH1, MSH2, PMS2, MSH6—Lynch syndrome), copy number low (intermediate-to-good prognosis, common mutations in PTEN, PIK3CA, CTNNB1, and ARID1A), and copy number high (poor prognosis, p53 mutation, serous-like).[53,55]

Table 3
Classification of uterine cancers

	Endometrial Type I	Endometrial Type II	Sarcoma
Percentage of uterine cancers	80%	10% to 15%	5%
Major risk factors	Estrogen excess	BRCA 1 and 2 for serous carcinoma	Genetics and history of radiation
Cancer subtypes	Endometrial adenocarcinoma (grade 1 or 2)	Poorly differentiated endometrial adenocarcinoma (grade 3), clear cell and uterine serous carcinomas, and carcinosarcomas	Leiomyosarcomas and endometrial stromal sarcoma, adenosarcomas, rhabdomyosarcoma, and malignant epithelioid tumors
Prognosis	Good	Poor	Poor

From [Prifti, C.A., Kwolek, D., Growdon, W.B., Palamara, K. (2020). Gynecologic Malignancies. In: Tilstra, S.A., Kwolek, D., Mitchell, J.L., Dolan, B.M., Carson, M.P. (eds) Sex- and Gender-Based Women's Health. Springer, Cham. https://doi.org/10.1007/978-3-030-50695-7_15. Table 15.2¹]; with permission. Data from Trope CG, Abeler VM, Kristensen GB. Diagnosis and treatment of sarcoma of the uterus. A review. Acta oncologica. 2012;51(6):694-705. Felix AS, Weissfeld JL, Stone RA, Bowser R, Chivukula M, Edwards RP. Factors associated with Type I and Type II endometrial cancer. Cancer causes & control. 2010;21(11):1851-1856.

Uterine sarcoma

Uterine sarcomas arise from the myometrium or connective tissue elements of the endometrium. They are rare and account for 3% of uterine cancers.[51] The most common subtypes are leiomyosarcoma, endometrial stromal sarcoma, and undifferentiated uterine sarcoma. Leiomyosarcoma makes up 70% of all uterine sarcomas and 1% of all uterine cancers. Their presentation is similar to EC with a mean age at diagnosis of 60 years and patients often present with complaints of abnormal uterine bleeding or abdominal fullness.

Risk factors. Type I EC arises from prolonged excessive estrogenic stimulation of the endometrial lining of the uterus without adequate opposition by progestin. This leads to endometrial hyperplasia, which can progress into atypical endometrial hyperplasia, the precursor lesion that can ultimately transform endometrioid cancer.

Patients often have a thickened endometrial stripe on pelvic ultrasound. Risk factors for excess estrogen include obesity, anovulation, estrogen-producing tumors such as granulosa cell tumors or thecomas, hormone replacement therapy with unopposed estrogen, tamoxifen use, nulliparity, early menarche or late menopause, and PCOS. Obesity increases estrogen exposure through peripheral conversion of androstenedione to estrone in adipocytes, which in turn stimulates endometrial proliferation.[56] Women with BMI above 30 have a two- to sevenfold increased risk of EC. In wealthy countries an increase in EC has been noticed with increased body weight; one study showed that 75% of women diagnosed with EC before age 25 were obese.[57–59] Anovulation leads to continuous unopposed estrogen exposure as without ovulation the corpus luteum (which produces progesterone) is not formed. Estrogen replacement therapy without progesterone has an eightfold increased risk of EC. Oral contraceptive pills are associated with decreased EC risk.[58]

Tamoxifen is an SERM commonly used as a treatment in hormone receptor-positive breast cancer. In breast tissue tamoxifen is an estrogen antagonist; however, its effect on the endometrium is to act as an agonist. Women on tamoxifen therapy for breast cancer treatment or prevention have a two- to threefold risk in EC and should be routinely asked about symptoms of abnormal uterine bleeding.[60] Despite this increased risk, routine TVUS or endometrial biopsy (EMB) are not recommended in asymptomatic patients on tamoxifen therapy due to a low specificity and low PPV for detecting malignancy.[61–63]

Other, nonhormonal risk factors for EC include age, diabetes, and genetic predisposition. For both type I and type II EC, age is a significant risk factor with 90% of cases occurring in women aged 50 years and older.[64] Only 20% of diagnosed women are premenopausal: among women with predisposing genetic cancer syndromes, there is a higher incidence of EC in premenopausal women as compared with in sporadic cases.[65] Diabetes is thought to be associated with higher EC rates through increased inflammation, co-morbid obesity, and metabolic syndrome.[66]

Several genetic syndromes have been associated with EC, including Lynch syndrome (also known as hereditary non-polyposis colorectal cancer [HNPCC]), Cowden syndrome (autosomal PTEN harmatoma syndrome), and BRCA1/BRCA2 mutations. Patients with Lynch syndrome have an increased risk for colon, ovarian cancer, gliomas, and other GI cancers, and a lifetime risk of 40% to 60% for developing EC.[67–69] Lynch patients require intensive screening for a variety of cancers, starting in their 20s, including yearly EMB starting by age 35.[65,70] Lynch patients are followed by gynecology for annual screening, and prophylactic hysterectomy with bilateral salpingo-oophorectomy should be considered after the completion of childbearing.[65]

Given the rare occurrence of uterine sarcomas, identifying risk factors has been more challenging; however, obesity, pelvic radiation, and long-term tamoxifen use have been associated with increased risk for leiomyosarcomas.[61,71–73] Hereditary leiomyomatosis and renal cell carcinoma syndrome (LHRCC) and hereditary childhood retinoblastoma are genetic syndromes associated with an increased risk of developing leiomyosarcoma.

Racial disparities have been observed for the more aggressive Type II EC as well as for uterine sarcomas. Black women are more commonly diagnosed with the more aggressive type II EC for reasons that are not well understood and leiomyosarcoma is twice as common in Black women than in White women.[74,75]

Smoking, progestin-only contraceptives such as intrauterine devices (IUDs), and combined oral contraceptives have been associated with a decreased risk of developing EC.[76–79]

Screening and Diagnosis

Routine screening is not recommended for uterine cancers in the asymptomatic patient with the exception of patients with genetic syndromes. Routine pap smears for the detection of cervical cancer may incidentally detect uterine cancer if abnormal cells are present such as atypical glandular cells or atypical endometrial cells. Approximately 90% of patients with endometrial carcinoma present with uterine bleeding. Postmenopausal bleeding is the classical presentation, followed by women over 45 with abnormal uterine bleeding.

In postmenopausal women, a TVUS usually excludes endometrial malignancy if the endometrial stripe is < 4 mm.[80] A thicker stripe or persistent bleeding for > 3 to 6 months with prior negative workup requires EMB. In premenopausal women, the thickness of the endometrial stripe is nondiagnostic, therefore for women age 45 and above or with risk factors, evaluation with EMB should be performed after excluding pregnancy. Diagnosis is usually made by EMB; however, office EMB has a false negative rate of 10%. In a patient with a negative EMB, close follow-up is warranted. If there is a high suspicion of malignancy, or if bleeding continues or recurs, an EMB should be repeated, possibly followed by a fractional dilation and curettage (D&C). Further workup may include additional endometrial and endocervical sampling, and/or colposcopy, or TVUS. Hysteroscopy can be helpful in evaluating specific lesions in the endometrium such as a polyp when a patient has persistent or recurrent undiagnosed bleeding.

There is no validated blood screening test for EC. In patients with extrauterine disease, CA-125 marker can be useful in monitoring clinical response; however, in young patients, CA-125 levels can be falsely elevated due to peritoneal inflammation, infection, or radiation injury, and levels can be falsely low in patients with isolated vaginal metastases.[81–83]

EC is classified by the International Federation of Gynecology and Obstetrics (FIGO) grading and staging system (**Table 4** and **Fig. 2**). Grading is based on histology and divided into grade 1 (well differentiated), grade 2 (moderately differentiated), and grade 3 (poorly differentiated). Grades 1 and 2 are classified as type I EC, whereas Grade 3 categorizes as type II EC. Before initiating treatment, uterine cancers must also be staged. Uterine cancers are not staged by imaging, but by surgery. Before surgery a complete physical examination, pelvic examination, as well as computed tomography (CT) chest/abdomen/pelvis are performed to determine the extent of tumor involvement and distant metastasis.

Standard surgical staging is done with total hysterectomy with bilateral salpingo-oophorectomy (TH/BSO), washings, and an examination of the entire abdominal

Table 4
Tumor-node-metastasis and International Federation of Gynecology and Obstetrics surgical staging for endometrial carcinoma

TNM	FIGO Stage	Primary Tumor
TX		Primary tumors cannot be assessed
T0		No evidence of a primary tumor
T1, N0, and M0	I	Tumor confined to corpus uteri
T1a, N0, and M0	IA	Tumor confined to endometrium or invading <50% of myometrium
T1b, N0, and M0	IB	Tumor invading $\geq$50% of myometrium
T2, N0, and M0	II	Uterine cervical extension
T3, N0, and M0	III	Tumor extends outside the uterus
T3a, N0, and M0	IIIA	Tumor involves serosa and/or adnexa (direct extension or metastasis)
T3b, N0, and M0	IIIB	Vaginal involves vagina or parametria (direct extension or metastasis)
T1-3, N1-N2, and M0	IIIC1-IIC2	Tumor with pelvic or paraaortic lymph node metastasis
T4, any N, and any M0	IVA	Tumor invades bladder and/or bowel mucosa
T4, any N, and M1	IVB	Distant metastasis

Data from Lewin SN. Revised FIGO staging system for endometrial cancer. *Clinical obstetrics and gynecology.* 2011;54(2):215-218.

cavity. Lymph node dissection identifies patients requiring adjuvant treatment with radiation therapy and/or systemic therapy. The NCCN guidelines recommend lymphadenectomy for selected EC patients and paraaortic lymphadenectomy for high-risk patients. Lymphadenectomy in uterine sarcomas is currently not indicated by NCCN guidelines as there is generally a low incidence of lymph node involvement in early disease.[51,84] Sentinel lymph node (SLN) biopsy can be considered as an alternative to full lymphadenectomy in uterine-confined disease.[51] SLN biopsy was found in

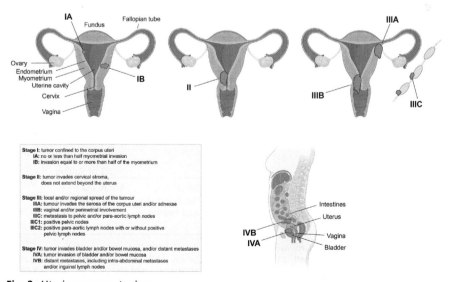

Fig. 2. Uterine cancer staging.

these patients to result in accurate prediction of pelvic lymph node metastasis with less than 5% false negative rate, a sensitivity of 97%, and a negative predictive value of 99.6%.[85,86] Staging is classified according to the 2010 FIGO/TNM classification system based on the level of invasion of the tumor into normal tissue (Please see **Fig. 2**).

Treatment

Early-stage EC is considered low risk and surgery is done with curative intent. Most women undergo simple hysterectomy ± BSO. Women with high-risk EC or uterine sarcomas have a poor prognosis following hysterectomy alone and a more extensive hysterectomy is recommended ± debulking surgery. Radical hysterectomy includes total hysterectomy with BSO plus removal of the parametrium and the upper one-third of the vagina. The various types of hysterectomies that can be performed range from Type I–Type V (**Table 5**). A type I hysterectomy is simple, and type III is radical. Types IV and V include greater excision of the vagina, and partial exenteration with the removal of ureter/bladder or rectum segments, respectively. In EC, the use of laparoscopy has been shown to have equivalent oncologic outcomes with decreased surgical morbidity when compared with open surgery.[87]

An increasing number of women in their reproductive age are diagnosed with EC and may want to preserve their fertility. Counseling women undergoing gonadotoxic therapies should include fertility preservation and future reproduction. Fertility-sparing options can be considered for low grade 1 EC with disease limited to the endometrium by MRI or TVUS, and absence of suspicious or metastatic disease on imaging; however, it is currently not recommended as standard of care. For these patients, continuous progestin-based therapy is considered (Megestrol, Medroxyprogesterone, Progestin IUD) with response assessed by endometrial evaluation every 3 to 6 months by D&C or EMB. TH/BSO is encouraged after childbearing is complete or the progression of disease is detected on endometrial sampling. Response rate to oral progestin ranges between 48% and 76%, whereas recurrence rates are reported between 35% and 40% and TH/BSO is recommended after childbearing is complete.[88,89]

Debulking surgeries for metastatic stage IV disease are controversial and considered only for recurrent pelvic/intraabdominal disease for highly selected patients.

Table 5
Types of hysterectomy

Type of Hysterectomy	Supracervical	Simple	Radical
Description	Removal of the uterine body; cervix left in place	Uterus, cervix, fallopian tubes, and ovaries removed	Total hysterectomy and BSO, plus removal of parametrium (connective tissue surrounding the uterus) and upper 1/3 of vagina
Sample indications	Benign conditions	Endometrial cancer, early-stage cervical cancer, and ovarian cancer	Stage IA2—IIA cervical cancer

From [Prifti, C.A., Kwolek, D., Growdon, W.B., Palamara, K. (2020). Gynecologic Malignancies. In: Tilstra, S.A., Kwolek, D., Mitchell, J.L., Dolan, B.M., Carson, M.P. (eds) Sex- and Gender-Based Women's Health. Springer, Cham. https://doi.org/10.1007/978-3-030-50695-7_15. Table 15.5[1]]; with permission.

For nonsurgical candidates and higher stage diagnoses, standard of care includes adjuvant external beam radiation therapy (EBRT) or brachytherapy, as well as consideration of systemic therapy, endocrine-, immuno- or targeted therapies.

Systemic therapy for EC centers usually around platin-based regimens such as carboplatin/paclitaxel or cisplatin-based combination therapies. Preferred regimens for uterine sarcomas are Doxorubicin or docetaxel/gemcitabine. Patients on such regimens will need a cardiac echocardiogram before starting therapy due to the cardiac toxicities of these therapies. Targeted therapies include Trastuzumab (targeting the human epidermal growth factor receptor [HER] receptor) for human epidermal growth factor receptor 2 (HER2) positive serous carcinoma, bevacizumab (an anti-VEGF binding antibody that inhibits angiogenesis) in combination with platin-based regimens, tyrosine kinase inhibitors (eg, Lenvatinib), and mTOR inhibitors (temsirolimus, everolimus) as a single agent or in combination with aromatase inhibitors (**Table 6**).[90,91]

Endocrine therapies include progestational agents (medroxyprogesterone and megrestol), tamoxifen, aromatase inhibitors (eg, letrozole), and fulvestrant (an estrogen receptor antagonist). These are generally used for patients with low-grade, hormone-receptor-positive disseminated metastases.[51] Recent advances in immunotherapies have been made and anti-PDL1/PDL-1 immune checkpoint inhibitors such as pembrolizumab, nivolumab, avelumab, and dostarlimab are now approved for second-line therapy in recurrent or metastatic disease, their application being most commonly for tumors with high mutational burden and defects in DNA mismatch repair (see **Fig. 3**).[92–96]

Prognosis and Surveillance

The overall prognosis for EC Type I is usually good, with only 4% of female-cancer-related deaths attributable to uterine cancer.[49] The majority of patients are diagnosed at an early stage (67%), with 5-year survival rates of 80% to 90% for Stage I disease, 80% for Stage II, 50% to 70% for Stage III, and approximately 20% for Stage IV disease.[53] Prognosis of EC Type II and uterine sarcomas is generally poor. These tumors are characterized by more aggressive behavior and extrauterine involvement is common as well as the risk of recurrence and distant metastases is higher. They are more common in older patients. The 5-year survival rate for Leiomyosarcoma stage I disease is only 55% and falls to 21.7% for stage IV disease.[97]

The greatest recurrence in EC patients is within the first 2 years of treatment. The most common site for the recurrence of Stage I disease is the vagina. Thus, following therapy, patients should be seen every 3 to 4 months for 2 years for a gynecological examination. Most vaginal recurrences are treated with radiation therapy. Surveillance imaging is only recommended if patients show signs or symptoms of recurrence. In these cases, whole-body PET/CT imaging is the recommended choice of imaging.[98]

Large health disparities have been found in historically marginalized groups. Incidence of invasive uterine cancers at diagnosis is higher in Black compared with White women and mortality among Black women is nearly twice as high compared with any other racial or ethnic group.[99] The absolute 5-year survival rates starkly differ between Black and White women by 21%, with 63% and 84%, respectively.[100] For years, a higher mortality has been reported among Black women compared with White women with uterine cancer at every stage, grade, histologic subtype, and for every age group. The disparity in mortality persisted despite controlling for sociodemographic factors, comorbid conditions, and histopathologic variables. Factors underlying these differences are noted in the inequities of health care. Black and Hispanic women are diagnosed more frequently at a later advanced stage.[101,102] Studies found they were less

Table 6
Overview of mechanisms of actions of drugs used for endometrial cancer

Category:	Mechanism of Action:
Hormone therapy:	
Progestational agents: medroxyprogesterone acetate and megestrol acetate	Decrease estrogen levels and gonadotropin levels and oppose estrogen-driven proliferation.
Tamoxifen	Selective estrogen receptor modulator
Fulvestrant	Binds to estrogen receptor monomers inhibiting receptor dimerization, activation, and translocation to the nucleus, leading to accelerated degradation of the estrogen receptor.
Aromatase inhibitors (eg, letrozole)	Inhibit the aromatase enzyme, which catalyzes the conversion of androgens to estrogens, thereby reducing estrogen levels.
Targeted therapy:	
Temsirolimus and everolimus	mTOR inhibitor, inhibits downstream signaling for protein synthesis and inhibits cell growth.
Trastuzumab	Antibody targeting Her2 receptor. Inhibits Her2 receptor homodimerization, preventing Her2-mediated signaling. Also facilitate antibody-dependent cellular cytotoxicity, leading to cell death of cells that express HER2 (see **Fig. 3**)
Bevacizumab	The antibody that binds to circulating VEGF, inhibits VEGF binding to VEGF receptors, thereby inhibiting VEGF-mediated endothelial cell proliferation and angiogenesis (see **Fig. 3**)
Systemic chemotherapy (commonly given as a two-drug regimen):	
Platin-based chemotherapy: cisplatin and carboplatin	Crosslink with DNA, thereby activating apoptosis.
Anthracycline: doxorubicin and liposomal doxorubicin (doxil)	Inhibit topoisomerase 2, interfering with DNA replication.
Taxols: paclitaxel and docetaxel	Bind to microtubules and inhibit cell cycle.
Immunotherapy:	
Nivolumab, dorstalimab, and avelumab	Anti-PD1 antibody: binds PD1 receptor on T cells, thereby inhibiting the interaction of PD1 with PDL-1 on tumor cells, which allows T cells to remain active against cancer cells (see **Fig. 3**)

likely to receive surgery for treatment,[103–105] and if they did receive surgery, they less likely received minimally invasive laparoscopic procedures.[106] Furthermore, even though Black and Hispanic women more frequently have positive lymph nodes, fewer of them received lymph node sampling or sentinel lymph biopsies, and they were less likely to receive chemotherapy and overall guideline-concordant care.[104,107–109] Socioeconomic status and level of education were also found to be associated with worse outcomes.[110]

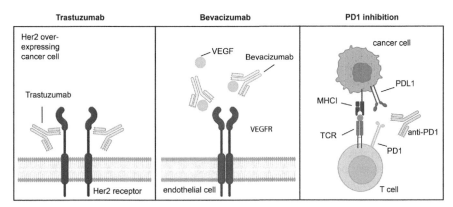

Fig. 3. Mechanisms of actions of trastuzumab, bevacizumab, and immunotherapy PD1 inhibition.

Survivorship care in patients with uterine cancer is similar to that of patients with ovarian cancer, and attention to menopausal symptoms, bowel and bladder issues, surgical adhesions, depression, anxiety, and sexual issues is warrented.[1]

VULVOVAGINAL CANCERS
Introduction

Although vulvovaginal cancers are the least common of all gynecologic malignancies, they nonetheless impact a significant number of patients.[111] In 2022, 6,330 women are expected to be diagnosed with vulvar cancer, and 8,870 women are expected to be diagnosed with vaginal or other genital cancers.[49] Vulvovaginal cancers typically present as asymptomatic lesions but may also present with vulvar or vaginal complaints including pruritus, irritation, pain, bleeding, or discharge. The vast majority of vulvar cancers are diagnosed at an early stage, whereas the stage at diagnosis for vaginal cancers is more variable.[112,113] Most vulvovaginal malignancies are squamous cell in origin and related to human papillomavirus (HPV) or chronic inflammatory processes such as lichen sclerosis.[114–117] Other notable risk factors for vulvovaginal cancers include age, tobacco use, and immunodeficiency. DES exposure in utero increases the risk of clear cell adenocarcinoma, a rare type of vaginal cancer.[118]

To reduce the risk of vulvovaginal cancers, routine HPV vaccination is recommended for all persons aged 11 to 12 years and up to age 26.[119] Smoking cessation should be encouraged for all patients, especially for patients found to have premalignant or malignant vulvovaginal lesions. Lastly, routine HIV testing is recommended to detect states of immunodeficiency that may predispose patients to HPV-related carcinogenesis.

Screening and Diagnosis

Screening tests are not recommended for vulvar or vaginal cancer. Instead, detection is mediated primarily through the thorough evaluation of all vulvovaginal complaints and by the routine physical examination. The review of systems at annual visits should include questions pertaining to vulvovaginal complaints. A pelvic examination should be performed as indicated for cervical cancer screening or evaluation of gynecologic complaints and should include a thorough inspection of the vulva and vagina with palpation of the vaginal walls. The most common site of vaginal tumors is in the posterior upper one-third of the vagina and may be missed on routine speculum examinations.[120] A significant portion of vaginal cancers are found incidentally during pap testing.[121]

All suspicions lesions, including lesions for which a definitive diagnosis is unclear, lesions with a presumed diagnosis that do not respond to initial therapy, and lesions with atypical appearance, should undergo biopsy. A colposcope can be useful to better evaluate vulvovaginal lesions that are incompletely visualized or in women with persistent symptoms without evidence of a lesion on gross inspection. Application of acetic acid turns HPV-infected areas white and can be used to help visualize lesions, although this is non-specific. Further evaluation of documented or suspected lesions is typically performed by a gynecologist, as most primary-care offices do not have the equipment for a complete evaluation.[119]

Treatment

Vulvar cancer

Vulvar malignancies range from vulvar intraepithelial neoplasia (VIN), a premalignant condition, to invasive disease. VIN falls into three categories: vulvar low-grade squamous intraepithelial lesion (LSIL), vulvar high-grade squamous intraepithelial lesion (HSIL), and differentiated VIN. Treatment of VIN depends on its categorization.[122] Vulvar LSIL is typically benign and self-limited and, as such, treatment centers on close surveillance. Vulvar HSIL is considered a true premalignant lesion and is typically treated with excision, laser ablation, or topical therapy with imiquimod.[119] Differentiated VIN is more likely to be associated with invasive vulvar malignancy than HSIL. If histopathology shows differentiated VIN, or if there is a concern for occult invasion, treatment should involve wide local excision to definitively rule out invasive disease. Women with a complete response to therapy at 6 and 12 months can be monitored with an annual visual inspection.[119]

Treatment of invasive vulvar cancer similarly depends upon staging (**Table 7**).[122] Early-stage disease (T1 and smaller T2) can be treated with partial or total vulvectomy with or without inguinofemoral lymph node evaluation depending on the size and extent of the disease. If margins are positive at the time of initial resection, patients may require adjuvant treatment with EBRT ± concurrent chemotherapy. For locally advanced diseases (larger T2 and T3), primary treatment involves EBRT and concurrent chemotherapy (to the tumor ± inguinofemoral lymph nodes depending on nodal involvement). If there is evidence of residual disease following initial treatment, the residual disease is resected. Initial treatment of metastatic disease involves EBRT and/or systemic therapy. Importantly, evidence has shown that the treatment modality pursued varies significantly based on factors such as patient race/ethnicity, age, and insurance status.[123,124]

Vaginal cancer

Similar to vulvar disease, vaginal cancers also range from non-invasive, premalignant disease (vaginal intraepithelial neoplasia or VaIN) to invasive disease. Given the rarity of vaginal cancers, there are no randomized controlled trials supporting treatment guidelines. Treatment approaches are instead adopted from those used in cervical and anal cancers.

VaIN falls into two categories: vaginal LSIL and vaginal HSIL. Treatment of VaIN depends upon its categorization. Vaginal LSIL is monitored with close surveillance, including an annual physical examination and HPV/cytology co-testing for 2 years following the diagnosis. There are multiple treatment options for Vaginal HSIL that

Table 7
Vulvar cancer staging

International Federation of Gynecology and Obstetrics (FIGO) Stage	Stage Grouping	Description
IA	T1a	Tumor ≤2 cm confined to the vulva and/or perineum with stromal invasion ≤1 mm
	N0	No involved lymph nodes
	M0	No distant metastasis
IB	T1b	Tumor >2 cm confined to the vulva and/or perineum with stromal invasion >1 mm
	N0	No involved lymph nodes
	M0	No distant metastasis
II	T2	Tumor of any size with extension to adjacent perineal structures
	N0	No involved lymph nodes
	M0	No distant metastasis
IIIA	T1 to T2	
	N1a or N1b	One or two lymph node metastases <5 mm OR one lymph node metastasis ≥5 mm
	M0	No distant metastasis
IIIB	T1 to T2	
	N2a or N2b	≥3 lymph node metastases <5 mm OR ≥2 lymph node metastasis ≥5 mm
	M0	No distant metastasis
IIIC	T1 to T2	
	N2c	Lymph nodes with extranodal extension
	M0	No distant metastasis
IVA	T3	Tumor of any size with extension to any of the following: proximal two-thirds of urethra, proximal two-thirds of vagina, bladder, or rectum
	N3	Fixed or ulcerated regional lymph node metastasis
	M0	No distant metastasis
IVB	Any T	
	Any N	
	M1	Distant metastasis (including pelvic lymph node metastasis)

Data from Beller U, Quinn MA, Benedet JL, et al. Carcinoma of the vulva. FIGO 26th Annual Report on the Results of Treatment in Gynecological Cancer. *Int J Gynaecol Obstet.* 2006;95 Suppl 1:S7-27. doi: 10.1016/S0020-7292(06)60028-3

are all variably supported by the evidence, including surgical excision, laser ablation, ultrasonic surgical aspiration, and topical therapy with imiquimod.

Initial treatment of invasive vaginal cancer depends upon the stage (**Table 8**). For stage I disease, primary treatment typically involves surgical excision; however, tumors > 2 cm and/or tumors in anatomically challenging locations, including the mid to lower vagina, are often treated with upfront radiation given the challenges associated with surgical resection.[125] For more advanced diseases (stages II–IV), patients are typically treated with either chemotherapy or radiation.[126]

Table 8		
Vaginal cancer staging		
International Federation of Gynecology and Obstetrics Stage	**Stage Grouping**	**Description**
IA	T1a	Tumor ≤2 cm confined to the vagina
	N0	No involved lymph nodes
	M0	No distant metastasis
IB	T1b	Tumor >2 cm confined to the vagina
	N0	No involved lymph nodes
	M0	No distant metastasis
IIA	T2a	Tumor ≤2 cm invading paravaginal tissues
	N0	No involved lymph nodes
	M0	No distant metastasis
IIB	T2b	Tumor >2 cm invading paravaginal tissues but not pelvic wall
	N0	No involved lymph nodes
	M0	No distant metastasis
III	T3	Tumor extending to the pelvic sidewall and/or causing kidney dysfunction
	N1	Pelvic or inguinal lymph node metastasis
	M0	No distant metastasis
IVA	T4	Tumor invading the bladder, rectum, and/or extending beyond the pelvis
	Any N	
	M0	No distant metastasis
IVB	Any T	
	Any N	
	M1	Distant metastasis

Data from Hacker NF, Eifel PJ, van der Velden J. Cancer of the vagina. *Int J Gynaecol Obstet.* 2012;119 Suppl 2:S97-99. doi: 10.1016/S0020-7292(12)60022-8

Prognosis and Surveillance

Vulvar cancer

Average survival following vulvar cancer diagnosis for women in the United States is 72.1% at 5 years; however, this depends in large part on stage at the time of diagnosis. Lymph node involvement is considered the most important prognostic factor.[127] Localized disease (stages I and II) has an average 5-year survival rate of 86%, locally advanced disease (stages III and IVa) has an average 5-year survival of 53%, and advanced disease (stage IVb) has an average 5-year survival rate of 19%.[128] For noninvasive vulvar cancer (VIN), recurrence rates range from 9% to 50% following treatment.[119]

Vaginal cancer

Average survival following vaginal cancer diagnosis similarly varies based upon the stage at diagnosis. Localized disease has an average 5-year survival rate of 66%, the regional disease has a 5-year survival of 54%, and advanced disease has a 5-year survival of 24%.[129] For VaIN, less than 10% of lesions progress to invasive disease.[121] Vaginal cancers associated with high-risk HPV have the highest rates of relapse and disease progression.[121,130]

Surveillance

Routine imaging for surveillance in women with a prior history of vulvovaginal cancer is not recommended. Instead, a thorough history and physical examinations are recommended every 3 to 6 months for 2 years after diagnosis, every 6 o 12 months for 3 to 5 years after diagnosis, and annually thereafter to elicit signs and symptoms of disease recurrence. The Society of Gynecologic Oncology currently recommends that women with a prior history of vulvovaginal cancer undergo annual pap testing/cytology after completion of treatment, though the evidence behind this recommendation is mixed.[122,131] For vulvar cancers specifically, most recurrence is noted within the first 1 to 2 years following treatment, though recurrence has also been reported in patients more than 5 years out from initial diagnosis.[132] Patients should be educated on symptoms suggestive of recurrence as well as lifestyle modifications to reduce the risk of recurrence, including smoking cessation.

Survivorship care for patients with vulvar or vaginal cancers can be challenging. In addition to the issues mentioned for uterine and ovarian cancer survivors, these patients often have surgery that shortens the vagina or causes disfigurement of the vulva and introitis. In addition, radiation therapy increases the chances of proctitis, rectal bleeding, incontinence, and urgency. Vaginal penetration during intercourse may be painful, difficult, or impossible. Patient education and referral back for expert gynecologic care, pelvic floor physical therapy, and sexual therapy with the patient and partner can mitigate the effect of these complications and lead to increased patient satisfaction and enhanced quality of life.[1]

SUMMARY

Gynecologic malignancies: ovarian, uterine, and vulvovaginal cancers, affect nearly 96,000 women per year in the United States, and result in approximately 30,000 deaths annually. Routine cancer screening protocols as part of primary care do not detect these malignancies. PCPs play an essential role by recognizing risk factors for gynecologic malignancies: obesity, unopposed estrogen, smoking, DES exposure, HPV, and genetic factors, and in counseling patients appropriately. The annual examination with history and review of systems should include screening and evaluation of worrisome symptoms such as vaginal bleeding, abdominal fullness, and vulvar lesions to aid in early detection and improved prognoses. Treatment of gynecologic cancers is managed by gynecologic oncologists, and often involves a combination of surgery, chemotherapy, and possible radiation treatments. Survivor care is managed by the primary-care clinician. Expert attention to the mental, physical and sexual health of patients will ensure the best outcomes and quality of life for each individual.

CLINICS CARE POINTS

- Gynecologic malignancies are not part of routine screening protocols, but the primary-care clinician can pay a key role in detection through a focused history and review of systems and the evaluation of concerning symptoms.

- Obesity, estrogen excess, smoking, nulliparity, genetics, diethylstilbestrol, and human papillomavirus are important risk factors for gynecologic malignancies, and patients should be counseled appropriately.

- Postmenopausal bleeding must be evaluated as possible uterine cancer.

- Treatment of gynecologic malignancies is managed by gynecologic oncologists, and often involves a combination of surgery, chemotherapy, and possible radiation treatments.

- Gynecologic Cancer survivors need special care including attention to mental, physical, and sexual health care issues.

DISCLOSURES

Drs D. Gomez Kwolek, S. Gerstberger and S. Tait, and J.M. Qiu have no relevant financial disclosures or conflicts of interest.

ACKNOWLEDGMENTS

The authors would like to acknowledge the previous work of Drs Christine Prifti, Deborah Kwolek, Whitfield Board Growdon, and Kerri Palamara which influenced this article. Gynecologic Malignancies: Prifti, C.A., Kwolek, D., Growdon, W.B., Palamara, K. (2020). Gynecologic Malignancies. In: Tilstra, S.A., Kwolek, D., Mitchell, J.L., Dolan, B.M., Carson, M.P. (eds) Sex- and Gender-Based Women's Health. Springer, Cham. https://doi.org/10.1007/978-3-030-50695-7_15.[1]

REFERENCES

1. Prifti C, Kwolek D, Growdon W, et al. Gynecologic malignancies. In: Tilstra SA, Kwolek D, Mitchell JL, et al, editors. Sex- and gender-based women's health. Cham, Switzerland: Springer International Publishing; 2020. p. 231–55.
2. Program NCIS. Cancer Stat Facts: Uterine Cancer. 2018. https://seer.cancer.gov/statfacts/html/corp.html. Accessed October 16, 2022.
3. Program NCIS. Cancer Stat Facts: Ovarian Cancer. 2018. https://seer.cancer.gov/statfacts/html/ovary.html. Accessed October 16, 2022.
4. Society AC. Special Section: Rare Cancers in Adults. 2017. https://www.cancer.org/content/dam/cancer-org/research/cancer-facts-and-statistics/annual-cancer-facts-and-figures/2017/cancer-facts-and-figures-2017-special-section-rare-cancers-in-adults.pdf. Accessed October 16, 2022.
5. Desai A, Xu J, Aysola K, et al. Epithelial ovarian cancer: An overview. World J Transl Med 2014;3(1):1–8.
6. Kuchenbaecker KB, Hopper JL, Barnes DR, et al. Risks of Breast, Ovarian, and Contralateral Breast Cancer for BRCA1 and BRCA2 Mutation Carriers. JAMA 2017;317(23):2402–16.
7. Maccio A, Madeddu C. Inflammation and ovarian cancer. Cytokine 2012;58(2):133–47.
8. Savant SS, Sriramkumar S, O'Hagan HM. The Role of Inflammation and Inflammatory Mediators in the Development, Progression, Metastasis, and Chemoresistance of Epithelial Ovarian Cancer. Cancers 2018;10(8):251.
9. King SM, Hilliard TS, Wu LY, et al. The impact of ovulation on fallopian tube epithelial cells: evaluating three hypotheses connecting ovulation and serous ovarian cancer. Endocr Relat Cancer 2011;18(5):627–42.
10. Fathalla MF. Incessant ovulation—a factor in ovarian neoplasia. Lancet 1971;298(7716):163.
11. Havrilesky LJ, Moorman PG, Lowery WJ, et al. Oral contraceptive pills as primary prevention for ovarian cancer: a systematic review and meta-analysis. Obstet Gynecol 2013;122(1):139–47.
12. Beral V, Doll R, Hermon C, et al. Ovarian cancer and oral contraceptives: collaborative reanalysis of data from 45 epidemiological studies including 23,257 women with ovarian cancer and 87,303 controls. Lancet 2008;371(9609):303–14.
13. Olson S. Symptoms of ovarian cancer. Obstet Gynecol 2001;98(2):212–7.

14. Goff BA, Mandel LS, Melancon CH, et al. Frequency of symptoms of ovarian cancer in women presenting to primary care clinics. JAMA 2004;291(22): 2705–12.

15. Goff BA, Mandel LS, Drescher CW, et al. Development of an ovarian cancer symptom index: possibilities for earlier detection. Cancer 2007;109(2):221–7.

16. Buys SS, Partridge E, Greene MH, et al. Ovarian cancer screening in the Prostate, Lung, Colorectal and Ovarian (PLCO) cancer screening trial: findings from the initial screen of a randomized trial. Am J Obstet Gynecol 2005;193(5): 1630–9.

17. Kurman RJ, Visvanathan K, Roden R, et al. Early detection and treatment of ovarian cancer: shifting from early stage to minimal volume of disease based on a new model of carcinogenesis. Am J Obstet Gynecol 2008;198(4):351–6.

18. Kobayashi H, Yamada Y, Sado T, et al. A randomized study of screening for ovarian cancer: a multicenter study in Japan. Int J Gynecol Cancer 2008; 18(3):414–20.

19. Buys SS, Partridge E, Black A, et al. Effect of screening on ovarian cancer mortality: the Prostate, Lung, Colorectal and Ovarian (PLCO) Cancer Screening Randomized Controlled Trial. JAMA 2011;305(22):2295–303.

20. Jacobs IJ, Menon U, Ryan A, et al. Ovarian cancer screening and mortality in the UK Collaborative Trial of Ovarian Cancer Screening (UKCTOCS): a randomised controlled trial. Lancet 2016;387(10022):945–56.

21. Padilla LA, Radosevich DM, Milad MP. Accuracy of the pelvic examination in detecting adnexal masses. Obstet Gynecol 2000;96(4):593–8.

22. Padilla LA, Radosevich DM, Milad MP. Limitations of the pelvic examination for evaluation of the female pelvic organs. Int J Gynaecol Obstet 2005;88(1):84–8.

23. Guirguis-Blake JM, Henderson JT, Perdue LA. Periodic Screening Pelvic Examination: Evidence Report and Systematic Review for the US Preventive Services Task Force. JAMA 2017;317(9):954–66.

24. Wang Y, Li L, Douville C, et al. Evaluation of liquid from the Papanicolaou test and other liquid biopsies for the detection of endometrial and ovarian cancers. Sci Transl Med 2018;10(433):eaap8793.

25. US Preventive Services Task Force, Grossman DC, Curry SJ, et al. Screening for Ovarian Cancer: US Preventive Services Task Force Recommendation Statement. JAMA 2018;319(6):588–94.

26. Daly MB, Pal T, Berry MP, et al. Genetic/Familial High-Risk Assessment: Breast, Ovarian, and Pancreatic, Version 2.2021, NCCN Clinical Practice Guidelines in Oncology. J Natl Compr Canc Netw 2021;19(1):77–102.

27. Arora T, Mullangi S, Lekkala MR. Ovarian cancer. In: StatPearls. StatPearls Publishing; 2022. Available at: http://www.ncbi.nlm.nih.gov/books/NBK567760/. Accessed May 12, 2022.

28. Hacker NF, Rao A. Surgery for advanced epithelial ovarian cancer. Best Pract Res Clin Obstet Gynaecol 2017;41:71–87.

29. McGuire WP, Hoskins WJ, Brady MF, et al. Cyclophosphamide and cisplatin compared with paclitaxel and cisplatin in patients with stage III and stage IV ovarian cancer. N Engl J Med 1996;334(1):1–6.

30. Ozols RF, Bundy BN, Greer BE, et al. Phase III trial of carboplatin and paclitaxel compared with cisplatin and paclitaxel in patients with optimally resected stage III ovarian cancer: a Gynecologic Oncology Group study. J Clin Oncol Off J Am Soc Clin Oncol 2003;21(17):3194–200.

31. Tewari D, Java JJ, Salani R, et al. Long-term survival advantage and prognostic factors associated with intraperitoneal chemotherapy treatment in advanced

ovarian cancer: a gynecologic oncology group study. J Clin Oncol 2015;33(13): 1460–6.

32. Monk BJ, Chan JK. Is intraperitoneal chemotherapy still an acceptable option in primary adjuvant chemotherapy for advanced ovarian cancer? Ann Oncol Off J Eur Soc Med Oncol 2017;28(suppl_8):viii40–5.

33. Wenzel LB, Huang HQ, Armstrong DK, et al, Gynecologic Oncology Group. Health-related quality of life during and after intraperitoneal versus intravenous chemotherapy for optimally debulked ovarian cancer: a Gynecologic Oncology Group Study. J Clin Oncol 2007;25(4):437–43.

34. Young RC, Walton LA, Ellenberg SS, et al. Adjuvant therapy in stage I and stage II epithelial ovarian cancer. Results of two prospective randomized trials. N Engl J Med 1990;322(15):1021–7.

35. Winter-Roach BA, Kitchener HC, Dickinson HO. Adjuvant (post-surgery) chemotherapy for early stage epithelial ovarian cancer. Cochrane Database Syst Rev 2009;3:CD004706.

36. Vergote I, Trope CG, Amant F, et al. Neoadjuvant chemotherapy or primary surgery in stage IIIC or IV ovarian cancer. N Engl J Med 2010;363(10):943–53.

37. Morrison J, Haldar K, Kehoe S, et al. Chemotherapy versus surgery for initial treatment in advanced ovarian epithelial cancer. Cochrane Database Syst Rev 2012;8:CD005343.

38. Walsh CS. Latest clinical evidence of maintenance therapy in ovarian cancer. Curr Opin Obstet Gynecol 2020;32(1):15–21.

39. Liu JF, Konstantinopoulos PA, Matulonis UA. PARP inhibitors in ovarian cancer: current status and future promise. Gynecol Oncol 2014;133(2):362–9.

40. LaFargue CJ, Dal Molin GZ, Sood AK, et al. Exploring and comparing adverse events between PARP inhibitors. Lancet Oncol 2019;20(1):e15–28.

41. Garcia A, Singh H. Bevacizumab and ovarian cancer. Ther Adv Med Oncol 2013;5(2):133–41.

42. Randall LM, Monk BJ. Bevacizumab toxicities and their management in ovarian cancer. Gynecol Oncol 2010;117(3):497–504.

43. Winter WE, Maxwell GL, Tian C, et al. Prognostic factors for stage III epithelial ovarian cancer: a gynecologic oncology group study. J Clin Oncol 2007; 25(24):3621–7.

44. Klar M, Hasenburg A, Hasanov M, et al. Prognostic factors in young ovarian cancer patients: an analysis of four prospective phase III intergroup trials of the AGO Study Group, GINECO and NSGO. Eur J Cancer Oxf Engl 1990 2016;66:114–24.

45. Bristow RE, Tomacruz RS, Armstrong DK, et al. Survival effect of maximal cytoreductive surgery for advanced ovarian carcinoma during the platinum era: a meta-analysis. J Clin Oncol 2002;20(5):1248–59.

46. Salani R, Backes FJ, Fung Kee Fung M, et al. Posttreatment surveillance and diagnosis of recurrence in women with gynecologic malignancies: society of Gynecologic Oncologists recommendations. Am J Obstet Gynecol 2011; 204(6):466–78.

47. Soyama H, Takano M, Miyamoto M, et al. Factors favouring long-term survival following recurrence in ovarian cancer. Mol Clin Oncol 2017;7(1):42–6.

48. Stavraka C, Ford A, Ghaem-Maghami S, et al. A study of symptoms described by ovarian cancer survivors. Gynecol Oncol 2012;125(1):59–64.

49. Siegel RL, Miller KD, Fuchs HE, et al. Cancer statistics, 2022. CA Cancer J Clin 2022;72(1):7–33.

50. Trope CG, Abeler VM, Kristensen GB. Diagnosis and treatment of sarcoma of the uterus. A review. Acta Oncol 2012;51(6):694–705.
51. Network NCC. NCCN clinical practice guidelines in oncology: uterine Neoplasms, version 1.2022. NCCN; 2022. Available at: https://www.nccn.org/professionals/physician_gls/pdf/uterine.pdf. Accessed October 16, 2022.
52. National Cancer Institute. Surveillance, epidemiology, and end results program. cancer stat facts: uterine cancer. Available at: https://seer.cancer.gov/statfacts/html/corp.html. Accessed December 12, 2020.
53. Chelmow D, Brooks R, Cavens A, et al. Executive summary of the uterine cancer evidence review conference. Obstet Gynecol 2022;139(4):626–43.
54. Sorosky JI. Endometrial Cancer Obstet Gynecol 2012;120(2 Pt 1):383–97.
55. Cancer Genome Atlas Research Network, Kandoth C, Schultz N, et al. Integrated genomic characterization of endometrial carcinoma. Nature 2013;497(7447):67–73.
56. Renehan AG, Zwahlen M, Egger M. Adiposity and cancer risk: new mechanistic insights from epidemiology. Nat Rev Cancer 2015;15(8):484–98.
57. Smith RA, Eschenbach AC, Wender R, et al. American Cancer Society guidelines for the early detection of cancer: update of early detection guidelines for prostate, colorectal, and endometrial cancers. Also: update 2001–testing for early lung cancer detection. CA Cancer J Clin 2001;51(1):38–75.
58. Setiawan VW, Yang HP, Pike MC, et al. Type I and II endometrial cancers: have they different risk factors? J Clin Oncol Off J Am Soc Clin Oncol 2013;31(20):2607–18.
59. Rosen MW, Tasset J, Kobernik EK, et al. Risk Factors for Endometrial Cancer or Hyperplasia in Adolescents and Women 25 Years Old or Younger. J Pediatr Adolesc Gynecol 2019;32(5):546–9.
60. Braithwaite RS, Chlebowski RT, Lau J, et al. Meta-analysis of vascular and neoplastic events associated with tamoxifen. J Gen Intern Med 2003;18(11):937–47.
61. Committee Opinion No. 601: Tamoxifen and uterine cancer. Obstet Gynecol 2014;123(6):1394–7.
62. Fung MF, Reid A, Faught W, et al. Prospective longitudinal study of ultrasound screening for endometrial abnormalities in women with breast cancer receiving tamoxifen. Gynecol Oncol 2003;91(1):154–9.
63. Bertelli G, Venturini M, Del Mastro L, et al. Tamoxifen and the endometrium: findings of pelvic ultrasound examination and endometrial biopsy in asymptomatic breast cancer patients. Breast Cancer Res Treat 1998;47(1):41–6.
64. Braun MM, Overbeek-Wager EA, Grumbo RJ. Diagnosis and Management of Endometrial Cancer. Am Fam Physician 2016;93(6):468–74.
65. Meyer LA, Broaddus RR, Lu KH. Endometrial cancer and Lynch syndrome: clinical and pathologic considerations. Cancer Control J Moffitt Cancer Cent 2009;16(1):14–22.
66. Luo J, Beresford S, Chen C, et al. Association between diabetes, diabetes treatment and risk of developing endometrial cancer. Br J Cancer 2014;111(7):1432–9.
67. Smith RA, Cokkinides V, Brawley OW. Cancer screening in the United States, 2012: a review of current American Cancer Society guidelines and current issues in cancer screening. CA Cancer J Clin 2012;62(2):129–42.
68. Crispens MA. Endometrial and ovarian cancer in lynch syndrome. Clin Colon Rectal Surg 2012;25(2):97–102.

69. Kwon JS, Scott JL, Gilks CB, et al. Testing women with endometrial cancer to detect Lynch syndrome. J Clin Oncol 2011;29(16):2247–52.

70. Manchanda R, Saridogan E, Abdelraheim A, et al. Annual outpatient hysteroscopy and endometrial sampling (OHES) in HNPCC/Lynch syndrome (LS). Arch Gynecol Obstet 2012;286(6):1555–62.

71. Felix AS, Cook LS, Gaudet MM, et al. The etiology of uterine sarcomas: a pooled analysis of the epidemiology of endometrial cancer consortium. Br J Cancer 2013;108(3):727–34.

72. Lavie O, Barnett-Griness O, Narod SA, et al. The risk of developing uterine sarcoma after tamoxifen use. Int J Gynecol Cancer 2008;18(2):352–6.

73. Mark RJ, Poen J, Tran LM, et al. Postirradiation sarcoma of the gynecologic tract. A report of 13 cases and a discussion of the risk of radiation-induced gynecologic malignancies. Am J Clin Oncol 1996;19(1):59–64.

74. Ricci S, Stone RL, Fader AN. Uterine leiomyosarcoma: Epidemiology, contemporary treatment strategies and the impact of uterine morcellation. Gynecol Oncol 2017;145(1):208–16.

75. Cote ML, Ruterbusch JJ, Olson SH, et al. The Growing Burden of Endometrial Cancer: A Major Racial Disparity Affecting Black Women. Cancer Epidemiol Biomark Prev Publ Am Assoc Cancer Res Cosponsored Am Soc Prev Oncol 2015; 24(9):1407–15.

76. Zhou B, Yang L, Sun Q, et al. Cigarette smoking and the risk of endometrial cancer: a meta-analysis. Am J Med 2008;121(6):501–8.e3.

77. Jareid M, Thalabard JC, Aarflot M, et al. Levonorgestrel-releasing intrauterine system use is associated with a decreased risk of ovarian and endometrial cancer, without increased risk of breast cancer. Results from the NOWAC Study. Gynecol Oncol 2018;149(1):127–32.

78. Iversen L, Fielding S, Ø Lidegaard, et al. Contemporary hormonal contraception and risk of endometrial cancer in women younger than age 50: A retrospective cohort study of Danish women. Contraception 2020;102(3):152–8.

79. Michels KA, Pfeiffer RM, Brinton LA, et al. Modification of the associations between duration of oral contraceptive use and ovarian, endometrial, breast, and colorectal cancers. JAMA Oncol 2018;4(4):516–21.

80. Karlsson B, Granberg S, Wikland M, et al. Transvaginal ultrasonography of the endometrium in women with postmenopausal bleeding–a Nordic multicenter study. Am J Obstet Gynecol 1995;172(5):1488–94.

81. Price FV, Chambers SK, Carcangiu ML, et al. CA 125 may not reflect disease status in patients with uterine serous carcinoma. Cancer 1998;82(9):1720–5.

82. Patsner B, Orr JW, Mann WJ. Use of serum CA 125 measurement in posttreatment surveillance of early-stage endometrial carcinoma. Am J Obstet Gynecol 1990;162(2):427–9.

83. Rose PG, Sommers RM, Reale FR, et al. Serial serum CA 125 measurements for evaluation of recurrence in patients with endometrial carcinoma. Obstet Gynecol 1994;84(1):12–6.

84. Giuntoli RL, Metzinger DS, DiMarco CS, et al. Retrospective review of 208 patients with leiomyosarcoma of the uterus: prognostic indicators, surgical management, and adjuvant therapy. Gynecol Oncol 2003;89(3):460–9.

85. Rossi EC, Kowalski LD, Scalici J, et al. A comparison of sentinel lymph node biopsy to lymphadenectomy for endometrial cancer staging (FIRES trial): a multicentre, prospective, cohort study. Lancet Oncol 2017;18(3):384–92.

86. Holloway RW, Abu-Rustum NR, Backes FJ, et al. Sentinel lymph node mapping and staging in endometrial cancer: A Society of Gynecologic Oncology

literature review with consensus recommendations. Gynecol Oncol 2017;146(2): 405–15.

87. Walker JL, Piedmonte MR, Spirtos NM, et al. Recurrence and survival after random assignment to laparoscopy versus laparotomy for comprehensive surgical staging of uterine cancer: Gynecologic Oncology Group LAP2 Study. J Clin Oncol 2012;30(7):695–700.

88. Gunderson CC, Fader AN, Carson KA, et al. Oncologic and reproductive outcomes with progestin therapy in women with endometrial hyperplasia and grade 1 adenocarcinoma: a systematic review. Gynecol Oncol 2012;125(2):477–82.

89. Gallos ID, Yap J, Rajkhowa M, et al. Regression, relapse, and live birth rates with fertility-sparing therapy for endometrial cancer and atypical complex endometrial hyperplasia: a systematic review and metaanalysis. Am J Obstet Gynecol 2012;207(4):266.e1-12.

90. Slomovitz BM, Jiang Y, Yates MS, et al. Phase II study of everolimus and letrozole in patients with recurrent endometrial carcinoma. J Clin Oncol 2015;33(8): 930–6.

91. Oza AM, Elit L, Tsao MS, et al. Phase II study of temsirolimus in women with recurrent or metastatic endometrial cancer: a trial of the NCIC Clinical Trials Group. J Clin Oncol 2011;29(24):3278–85.

92. Oaknin A, Tinker AV, Gilbert L, et al. Clinical activity and safety of the anti-programmed death 1 monoclonal antibody dostarlimab for patients with recurrent or advanced mismatch repair-deficient endometrial cancer: a nonrandomized phase 1 clinical trial. JAMA Oncol 2020;6(11):1766–72.

93. Azad NS, Gray RJ, Overman MJ, et al. Nivolumab is effective in mismatch repair-deficient noncolorectal cancers: results from arm Z1D-A subprotocol of the NCI-MATCH (EAY131) study. J Clin Oncol 2020;38(3):214–22.

94. Marabelle A, Le DT, Ascierto PA, et al. Efficacy of Pembrolizumab in Patients With Noncolorectal High Microsatellite Instability/Mismatch Repair-Deficient Cancer: Results From the Phase II KEYNOTE-158 Study. J Clin Oncol 2020; 38(1):1–10.

95. Marabelle A, Fakih M, Lopez J, et al. Association of tumour mutational burden with outcomes in patients with advanced solid tumours treated with pembrolizumab: prospective biomarker analysis of the multicohort, open-label, phase 2 KEYNOTE-158 study. Lancet Oncol 2020;21(10):1353–65.

96. Makker V, Rasco D, Vogelzang NJ, et al. Lenvatinib plus pembrolizumab in patients with advanced endometrial cancer: an interim analysis of a multicentre, open-label, single-arm, phase 2 trial. Lancet Oncol 2019;20(5):711–8.

97. Zivanovic O, Jacks LM, Iasonos A, et al. A nomogram to predict postresection 5-year overall survival for patients with uterine leiomyosarcoma. Cancer 2012; 118(3):660–9.

98. Atri M, Zhang Z, Dehdashti F, et al. Utility of PET/CT to evaluate retroperitoneal lymph node metastasis in high-risk endometrial cancer: results of ACRIN 6671/ GOG 0233 trial. Radiology 2017;283(2):450–9.

99. Henley SJ, Miller JW, Dowling NF, et al. Uterine Cancer Incidence and Mortality - United States, 1999-2016. MMWR Morb Mortal Wkly Rep 2018;67(48):1333–8.

100. American Cancer Society. Cancer facts & figures. 2021. Available at: https:// www.cancer.org/content/dam/can-cer-org/research/cancer-facts-and-statistics/ annual-cancer-facts-and-figures/2021/cancer-facts-and-figures-2021.pdf. Accessed July 1, 2021.

101. Madison T, Schottenfeld D, James SA, et al. Endometrial cancer: socioeconomic status and racial/ethnic differences in stage at diagnosis, treatment, and survival. Am J Public Health 2004;94(12):2104–11.
102. Long B, Liu FW, Bristow RE. Disparities in uterine cancer epidemiology, treatment, and survival among African Americans in the United States. Gynecol Oncol 2013;130(3):652–9.
103. Bregar AJ, Alejandro Rauh-Hain J, Spencer R, et al. Disparities in receipt of care for high-grade endometrial cancer: A National Cancer Data Base analysis. Gynecol Oncol 2017;145(1):114–21.
104. Rauh-Hain JA, Buskwofie A, Clemmer J, et al. Racial disparities in treatment of high-grade endometrial cancer in the Medicare population. Obstet Gynecol 2015;125(4):843–51.
105. Randall TC, Armstrong K. Differences in treatment and outcome between African-American and white women with endometrial cancer. J Clin Oncol Off J Am Soc Clin Oncol 2003;21(22):4200–6.
106. Fleury AC, Ibeanu OA, Bristow RE. Racial disparities in surgical care for uterine cancer. Gynecol Oncol 2011;121(3):571–6.
107. Kaspers M, Llamocca E, Quick A, et al. Black and Hispanic women are less likely than white women to receive guideline-concordant endometrial cancer treatment. Am J Obstet Gynecol 2020;223(3):398.e1–18.
108. Huang AB, Huang Y, Hur C, et al. Impact of quality of care on racial disparities in survival for endometrial cancer. Am J Obstet Gynecol 2020;223(3):396.e1–13.
109. Rodriguez VE, LeBrón AMW, Chang J, et al. Racial-ethnic and socioeconomic disparities in guideline-adherent treatment for endometrial cancer. Obstet Gynecol 2021;138(1):21–31.
110. Whetstone S, Burke W, Sheth SS, et al. Health disparities in uterine cancer: report from the uterine cancer evidence review conference. Obstet Gynecol 2022;139(4):645–59.
111. Yagi A, Ueda Y, Kakuda M, et al. Descriptive epidemiological study of vaginal cancer using data from the Osaka Japan population-based cancer registry: Long-term analysis from a clinical viewpoint. Medicine (Baltimore) 2017;96(32).
112. Stroup AM, Harlan LC, Trimble EL. Demographic, clinical, and treatment trends among women diagnosed with vulvar cancer in the United States. Gynecol Oncol 2008;108(3):577–83.
113. Yang J, Delara R, Magrina J, et al. Management and outcomes of primary vaginal Cancer. Gynecol Oncol 2020;159(2):456–63.
114. Saraiya M, Watson M, Wu X, et al. Incidence of in situ and invasive vulvar cancer in the US, 1998-2003. Cancer 2008;113(10 Suppl):2865–72.
115. Wu X, Matanoski G, Chen VW, et al. Descriptive epidemiology of vaginal cancer incidence and survival by race, ethnicity, and age in the United States. Cancer 2008;113(10 Suppl):2873–82.
116. HP N, Bulten J, Hollema H, et al. Differentiated vulvar intraepithelial neoplasia is often found in lesions, previously diagnosed as lichen sclerosus, which have progressed to vulvar squamous cell carcinoma. Mod Pathol 2011;24(2):297–305.
117. Faber MT, Sand FL, Albieri V, et al. Prevalence and type distribution of human papillomavirus in squamous cell carcinoma and intraepithelial neoplasia of the vulva. Int J Cancer 2017;141(6):1161–9.
118. Pitkin RM, Herbst AL, Kurman RJ, et al. Vaginal and cervical abnormalities after exposure to stilbestrol in utero. Obstet Gynecol 2003;102(2):222. Obstet Gynecol 1972;40:287-298.

119. Committee Opinion No.675: Management of Vulvar Intraepithelial Neoplasia published correction appears in Obstet Gynecol. 2017. Obstet Gynecol. 2016;128(4):e178–e182.

120. Gadducci A, Fabrini MG, Lanfredini N, et al. Squamous cell carcinoma of the vagina: natural history, treatment modalities and prognostic factors. Crit Rev Oncol Hematol 2015;93(3):211–24.

121. Jentschke M, Hoffmeister V, Soergel P, et al. Clinical presentation, treatment and outcome of vaginal intraepithelial neoplasia. Arch Gynecol Obstet 2016;293(2): 415–9.

122. National Comprehensive Cancer Network. Vulvar Cancer (Version 1.2022). Available at: https://www.nccn.org/professionals/physician_gls/pdf/vulvar.pdf. Accessed May 22, 2022.

123. Tergas AI, Tseng JH, Bristow RE. Impact of race and ethnicity on treatment and survival of women with vulvar cancer in the United States. Gynecol Oncol 2013; 129(1):154–8.

124. Chase DM, Lin CC, Craig CD, et al. Disparities in Vulvar Cancer Reported by the National Cancer Database: Influence of Sociodemographic Factors. Obstet Gynecol 2015;126(4):792–802.

125. Hacker NF, Eifel PJ, van der Velden J. Cancer of the vagina. Int J Gynaecol Obstet Off Organ Int Fed Gynaecol Obstet 2012;119(Suppl 2):S97–9.

126. Di Donato V, Bellati F, Fischetti M, et al. Vaginal cancer. Crit Rev Oncol Hematol 2012;81(3):286–95.

127. Maggino T, Landoni F, Sartori E, et al. Patterns of recurrence in patients with squamous cell carcinoma of the vulva. A multicenter CTF Study. Cancer 2000; 89(1):116–22, 2-4.

128. National Cancer Institute. SEER cancer statistics factsheets: vulvar cancer. 2018. Available at: https://seer.cancer.gov/statfacts/html/vulva.html. Accessed May 22, 2022.

129. National Cancer Institute. Surveillance, Epidemiology, and End Results (SEER) Program Populations (1969-2020). Available at: www.seer.cancer.gov/popdata. Accessed May 22, 2022.

130. Frega A, French D, Piazze J, et al. Prediction of persistent vaginal intraepithelial neoplasia in previously hysterectomized women by high-risk HPV DNA detection. Cancer Lett 2007;249(2):235–41.

131. Salani R, Khanna N, Frimer M, et al. An update on post-treatment surveillance and diagnosis of recurrence in women with gynecologic malignancies: Society of Gynecologic Oncology (SGO) recommendations. Gynecol Oncol 2017; 146(1):3–10.

132. Gonzalez Bosquet J, Magrina JF, Gaffey TA, et al. Long-term survival and disease recurrence in patients with primary squamous cell carcinoma of the vulva. Gynecol Oncol 2005;97(3):828–33.

Genitourinary Syndrome of Menopause

Shanice Cox, MS, BS[a,1], Ryan Nasseri, MD[b,1], Rachel S. Rubin, MD[c,2],
Yahir Santiago-Lastra, MD[b,1],*

KEYWORDS

- Atrophic vaginitis • Genitourinary syndrome of menopause • Menopause
- Vulvovaginal atrophy • Women's sexual health • Urinary urgency

KEY POINTS

- Genitourinary syndrome of menopause (GSM) is a chronic, progressive disease with pervasive and bothersome genitourinary symptoms that can worsen with age or arise years after the onset of menopause.
- Diagnosis of GSM is made with a thorough history and examination, ruling out alternative diagnoses and identifying hallmark physical examination findings.
- Several non-pharmacologic and pharmacologic treatments are available but vaginal hormones are the most effective in reducing symptomatology and preventing recurrent urinary tract infections.
- Vaginal estradiol is safe for women with a history of hormonally sensitive gynecologic cancers.

INTRODUCTION

Urogenital health is essential to maintaining the quality of life after menopause. Genitourinary syndrome of menopause (GSM), first recognized in 2014, is characterized by a variety of unpleasant genital, sexual, and urinary symptoms that may occur alone or concurrently and are unrelated to other medical disorders.[1] GSM is a chronic, progressive disorder—early diagnosis and appropriate management can positively impact urogenital health and quality of life. Despite the significance of early detection and therapy, the illness is often underdiagnosed and undertreated. In this review, we emphasize how to identify GSM in postmenopausal, hypoestrogenic, and hypoandrogenic women and review evidence-based treatments with an in-depth summary of pharmaceuticals and adjuvant therapies.

[a] Texas Christian University School of Medicine; [b] UC San Diego Health; [c] Georgetown University
[1] Present address: 9400 Campus Point Drive, MC 7897, La Jolla, CA 92037, USA
[2] Present address: 6171 Executive Blvd, Rockville, MD 20852, USA
* Corresponding author.
E-mail address: ysantiagolastra@health.ucsd.edu

Med Clin N Am 107 (2023) 357–369
https://doi.org/10.1016/j.mcna.2022.10.017
0025-7125/23/© 2023 Elsevier Inc. All rights reserved.

medical.theclinics.com

Clinical Presentation

GSM (previously described as vulvovaginal atrophy or atrophic vaginitis) can include genital symptoms of dryness, burning, and irritation; sexual symptoms of loss in lubrication, discomfort or pain, decreased libido, difficulty with arousal and orgasm; and urinary symptoms of frequency, urgency, dysuria, and recurrent urinary tract infections (UTIs). Risk factors for GSM include menopause, premature ovarian failure, surgically-induced menopause (eg, bilateral oophorectomy), postpartum loss of placental estrogen, elevated prolactin secondary to lactation, absence of vaginal childbirth, decreased frequency and abstinence of sexual intercourse, history of radiation or chemotherapy, concomitant autoimmune disorders, smoking, alcohol abuse and lack of exercise (**Box 1**).[2] GSM can also occur in hormone-depleted states, due to systemic, pharmacologic, and iatrogenic states (**Box 2**).[3] As estrogen and androgens decline, blood flow to the vagina and vulva also decreases, resulting in impaired vaginal lubrication, vaginal burning, dryness, irritation, and increased pH which can affect sexual function and cause dyspareunia.[4]

GSM symptoms are present in nearly 50% of postmenopausal women and 15% of premenopausal women, as the symptoms associated with GSM can occur during any reproductive stage.[5] Relative low estrogen states (see **Box 2**) can occur in premenopausal women, altering circulating hormonal levels and microbiota. Fewer than 10% of women with GSM symptoms use prescribed therapy; this disparity between prevalence and treatment can be attributed to a lack of patient and provider education and a failure to recognize symptoms. Clinicians should understand the functional

---

Box 1
Signs and symptoms of GSM

Urinary
  Frequency
  Urgency
  Post-void pain
  Dysuria
  Nocturia
  Hematuria
  Bacteriuria
  Recurrent urinary tract infections
  Prominence of urethral meatus

Genital
  Dryness
  Imitation/Burning/Itching of vagina and /or vulva
  Leukorrhea
  Erythema
  Tissue fragility/fissures/petechiae
  Decreased vaginal moisture/elasticity
  Labial shrinkage/labial fusion
  Loss of vaginal rugae
  Clitoral hood retraction
  Vaginal stenosis and shortening

Sexual
  Decreased lubrication with sexual activity
  Dyspareunia
  Post-coital bleeding
  Decreased arousal/orgasm/desire
  Hypertonic pelvic floor
  Pelvic pain

Box 2
Causes of relative estrogen deficiency in premenopausal women

Systemic
Post-partum estrogen deficiency
Prolactinemia during breastfeeding
Hypoestrogenic states (e.g.autoimmune disorders thyroid conditions,pituitary tumrs)

Pharmacological
Oral contraceptive use
Medroxyprogesterone
Danazol
Aromatase inhibitors
Selective estrogen receptor modulators (SERMs)
  Tamoxifen
Gonadotropin-releasing hormone agonist analogs
  Leuprolide
  Nafarelin
Gender affirming hormone therapy

Iatrogenic
Bilateral oophorectomy (i.e surgical menopause)
Post-radiation ovarian failure
Chemotherapy

---

urogenital and vulvar architecture as well as the symptoms and efficacy of GSM therapies to close this knowledge gap (Fig. 1A).

Pathophysiology

Symptoms of GSM arise from a decline in circulating estrogens and androgens and a decrease in the number of estrogen and androgen receptors in the genitourinary tract.[3] The microarchitecture of the genitourinary tract is supported by androgens like testosterone that are converted intracellularly to estrogens. Dehydroepiandrosterone (DHEA) is the only source of intracellular androgens and estrogens in postmenopausal women, as sex hormone synthesis declines significantly after menopause.[4] In addition, DHEA production drops by up to 60% with age, contributing to an overall deficit in bioavailable estrogen.[6]

This age-related decline is of significant impact to the genitourinary system, as estrogen plays a crucial role in the vaginal microbiota. In response to estrogen stimulation, the vaginal epithelial cells produce glycogen. This is converted to lactic acid by lactobacilli, maintaining the vaginal pH within the range of 3.5 to 4.5.[7] This acidic environment and the presence of lactobacilli inhibit the proliferation of pathogenic organisms that may cause UTIs.[8,9] Additionally, the presence of lactobacilli has an inverse relationship with vaginal dryness.[10] Similar to the vulvar and vaginal epithelium, the urethra and bladder have estrogen receptors that play an important role in maintaining healthy, mature urothelium. Clinical evidence suggests estrogen influences the etiology of UTIs. In particular, postmenopausal women frequently experience recurrent UTIs, which is characterized by at least three acute UTI episodes each year. In addition to bacterial factors that promote persistence in the urine bladder, low estrogen levels create structural and chemical alterations in the urogenital tract that promote UTI. Increased residual urine volume and alterations in vaginal microbiota are known risk factors. Local estrogen supplementation can at least partially correct these alterations. The treatment restores a vaginal microflora dominated by lactobacilli and enhances epithelial differentiation and integrity in the urogenital tract. This estrogenic action on the epithelium is characterized by an increase in antimicrobial peptide

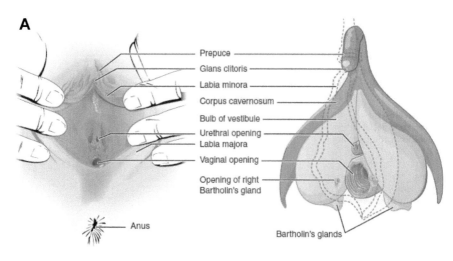

Vulva: External anterior view

Vulva: Internal anterolateral view

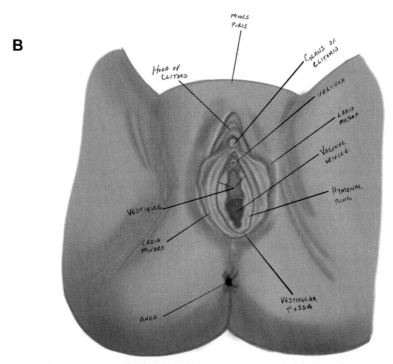

Fig. 1. (*A*) Internal and external vulvar Anatomy. (*B*) External vulvar anatomy. (*From* J. Gordon Betts, Kelly A. Young, James A. Wise, Eddie Johnson, Brandon Poe, Dean H. Kruse, Oksana Korol, Jody E. Johnson, Mark Womble, Peter DeSaix, OpenStax, Anatomy and Physiology, Apr 25, 2013, © Jan 27, 2022 OpenStax. Access for free at https://openstax.org/books/anatomy-and-physiology/pages/1-introduction. Licensed under a Creative Commons Attribution License CC BY 4.0.)

production and a tightening of intercellular connections, preventing bacteria from accessing cells where they can hide and subsequently trigger a new infection.[8]

Consequently, a decline in estrogen reduces glycogen and lactic acid, resulting in a higher pH (>5) and weakened resistance to colonization by Enterobacteriaceae.[9] It leads to a reduction in the collagen content of the bladder trigone, a thinning of the urethral mucosa, a decrease in pelvic floor muscle tone, and a reduction in the sensitivity of alpha-adrenergic receptors at the bladder neck and urethral sphincter.[11,12] Thus, tissues experience a loss of elasticity and flexibility, as well as a decrease in blood supply, resulting in urinary pain and sexual dysfunction.

DISCUSSION
Effective Diagnosis of Genitourinary Syndrome of Menopause

The diagnosis of GSM is primarily clinical, based on history and physical examination.

History. Owing to the sensitive nature of the topic, physicians should explain it openly while making patients feel safe and at ease. This is best accomplished with the patient dressed. A thorough history should then be taken, including a comprehensive description of the patient's symptoms. In addition, a detailed sexual history, including sexual activities and behavior such as decreased arousal, desire, and orgasm, and whether over-the-counter or at-home regimens alleviated symptoms, as well as a gynecologic history. Particularly in premenopausal women, a specific examination of systems focusing on genitourinary symptoms and comorbidities may exclude other probable organic causes (see **Box 2**). **Box 1** outlines the primary GSM signs and symptoms that may be discovered during the history and physical examination and should be used to direct the physical examination.[2]

Physical examination. A comprehensive examination should include an external visual evaluation as depicted in Fig. 1B, musculoskeletal and sensory evaluations, and a bimanual evaluation if the patient can tolerate it. During the physical examination, the following must be assessed:

- Symmetry and size of genital tissues
- Evidence of vaginal atrophy, stenosis, or dermatologic changes to the vulvar vestibule
- Areas of induced pain, especially in the vulvar vestibule and pelvic floor muscles
- Visible lesions such as urethral caruncles, sub-urethral masses, excoriations secondary to itching or scars from prior surgeries
- Presence of pelvic organ prolapse
- Pelvic floor muscle tone and voluntary control
- Presence and character of vaginal discharge
- Presence or absence of vaginal rugae

GSM may also be diagnosed by other objective findings, such as an elevated vaginal pH > 5, a decrease in superficial cells, or an elevated proportion of parabasal cells on the vaginal maturation index. A blood test does not confirm or disprove the diagnosis of GSM, as no set level of sex steroids has been established below which most women will develop GSM-related symptoms.

Other supportive tools used to quantify the severity and patient response to treatment are the Vaginal Health Index (VHI) and Vulvar Health Index. They provide a standardized measure of reported physical examination findings that evaluate five domains: vaginal elasticity, vaginal secretions, pH, epithelial mucous membrane, vaginal hydration allows the clinician to assess severity on a numerical scale and track changes over time. Total score ranges from 5 to 25, with lower scores corresponding to greater severity of GSM (**Table 1**).

Therapeutic Options

The principal purpose of treatment is to relieve symptoms, restore vaginal pH, and prevent the recurrence of UTIs. Women with vulvovaginal discomfort caused by sexual activity may benefit from a multimodal therapeutic approach. Low-dose vaginal hormone therapy is the foundation of treatment and can be administered in the form of vaginal creams, intravaginal tablets, or intravaginal rings. **Table 2** outlines the various formulations and associated administration route and their considerations. The goal of vaginal hormone therapy is to preserve tissue integrity, elasticity, and flexibility. As indicated in **Tables 2** and **3**, other available treatments include nonhormonal vaginal lubricants for use before sex, long-acting vaginal moisturizers for symptom control, laser therapy, and pelvic floor physical therapy. Although all of these methods can provide significant symptom relief, vaginal estrogen therapy is the gold standard treatment.

Estrogen: Owing to the direct action of estrogen on urogenital cells, systematic reviews of vaginal estrogen therapy in patients with GSM have revealed significant improvements in symptoms of vaginal dryness, dyspareunia, and urogenital symptoms, as well as anatomic improvements in vaginal tissues, increased lactobacillus and decreased vaginal pH.[13–15] Data from clinical trials indicate that local estrogen therapy reduces recurrent UTIs and improves lower urinary tract symptoms. Studies of the effectiveness of vaginal estrogen supplementation have shown both objective and subjective measures of success, including improvements in approximately 90% of women who apply the medication for a 90-day period. A 2006 Cochrane review comparing 19 efficacy trials reported that all products tested alleviated symptoms with similar effectiveness. These results are superior to those obtained by oral estrogen supplementation. Additionally, several trials have shown a reduction in the incidence of recurrent UTIs. The major benefit of vaginal estrogen in UTI prevention is restoring the urobiome to its protective state by lowering the vaginal pH and reducing dysbiosis by restoring adequate levels of *Lactobacilli* and other protective vaginal flora. Vaginal estrogen can also improve lower urinary tract symptoms by directly impacting vaginal innervation.[16] Vaginal innervation is highly sensitive to estrogen, and postmenopausal women have greater vaginal innervation density, which helps explain the more profound dysesthesia symptoms like vaginal itching, urinary urgency, burning, dryness and discomfort. Administration of localized topical estrogen reduces innervation more dramatically than systemic hormone replacement therapy, which explains why topical treatment is preferred to systemic hormone therapy in the treatment of these symptoms.[17]

Vaginal estrogen therapy has minimal systemic absorption that may result in headache, breast tenderness, nausea, vomiting, upset stomach, bloating and weight changes. Aside from the early but minimal systemic absorption, vaginal estrogen supplementation can also result in rare and often transient side effects such as vulvovaginal pruritus, genital candidiasis, leukorrhea, vaginitis, vaginal discomfort, vaginal pain, asymptomatic bacterial vaginosis, vaginal hemorrhage, and UTIs.[18] Systematic reviews and long-term observational studies have not shown an association between vaginal estrogen therapy and the likelihood of developing endometrial cancer or an increase in endometrial thickness. A 2019 meta-analysis found no correlation between vaginal estrogen use and the risk of developing breast cancer.[19] Contraindications for low-dose vaginal estrogen are few but include unexplained postmenopausal vaginal hemorrhage and caution in the presence of active hormone-sensitive gynecologic

Table 1
Vaginal health index[36]

Parameters	1	2	3
pH	>6.5	5–6.5	<5
Moisture/consistency	No moisture	Minimal moisture/ superficial layer of scanty mucous	Normal moisture/ flocculent fluid
Rugosity	None	Minimal	Good
Elasticity	Poor	Fair	Excellent
Length of vagina	<4 cm	4 to 6 cm	>6 cm
Epithelial integrity	Petechiae present	Petechiae after scraping	Normal, not friable
Vascularity	Minimal	Fair	Good

malignancies.[20] This concern is often escalated in breast cancer survivors who often suffer from GSM. These symptoms may be alleviated by vaginal estrogen therapy. However, there are concerns of risks of recurrence of breast cancer and death following treatment. In particular, GSM symptoms represent a major barrier to compliance with aromatase inhibitor (AI) therapy in breast cancer survivors. Recent data suggest that vaginal estrogen supplementation was not associated with increased risk of recurrence or mortality in early breast cancer survivors.[21] Additionally, there is emerging data that supports the use of prasterone (vaginal DHEA) to treat GSM symptoms in breast cancer survivors treated with aromatase inhibitors. This data suggests that vaginal estrogen favorably improves symptoms of GSM over plain moisturizer alone, without adversely increasing circulating estrogen levels or affecting recurrence risk or mortality. However, the label warnings persist against use in breast cancer survivors. Enough data exists for the North American Menopause Society (NAMS) to recommend low-dose vaginal estrogen treatment if there is no improvement when using non-hormonal treatments. NAMS recommends the lowest effective dose (0.005% vaginal estriol gel). In patients receiving aromatase inhibitors, the use of low-dose vaginal estrogen has been discouraged by the American Cancer Society, due to fear of vaginal estrogen's potential interference with adjuvant treatments. Taking into account these factors, and the current accrual of more long-term data, breast cancer survivors should confer with their physicians and oncologists before using local estrogen therapies. When deemed safe, these women should use the lowest effective dose of the vaginal estrogen, as recommended by the American College of Obstetricians and Gynecologists, the American Cancer Society, and the NAMS.[22]

Vaginal DHEA: Prasterone is a plant-derived version of endogenous DHEA which is an inactive steroid converted into biologically active estrogens and androgens.[6] A recent retrospective cohort study found that vaginal prasterone reduced UTI recurrence in women over 12 months; however, further randomized controlled trials are needed.[23] Additionally, improvements were noted in vaginal pH, vaginal maturation index, tissue structure, urinary urgency, and incontinence. There are no studies directly comparing vaginal DHEA to vaginal estrogen in efficacy or hormone levels, and for this reason, there can be no current recommendation of prasterone versus estrogen in the treatment of GSM in breast cancer survivors. However, there is increasingly robust data that prasterone improves GSM symptoms and is a suitable alternative to vaginal estrogen, as we await comparative effectiveness data.[6,24]

SERM: Ospemifene is a third-generation selective estrogen receptor modulator (SERM) that can exert variable effects on estrogen receptors and significantly improve the structure and pH levels of the vagina. It reduces dyspareunia, overactive bladder

Table 2
Summary of available vaginal hormone therapy preparations

Brand Name	Preparation	Dosing	Administration	Consideration
Estring	Estradiol vaginal ring	2 mg estradiol reservoir	Releases 7.5 µg per day for 90 d	<2% risk of vaginal ulcers[7]
Vagifem, Yuvafem, Imvexxy	Estradiol vaginal suppository	4, 10 µg estradiol	1 vaginal tablet daily for 2 wk followed by 1 tablet twice weekly	
Estrace	Estradiol vaginal cream	0.1 mg estradiol per g cream	2–4 g daily for 1–2 wk followed by 1–2 g daily for 1–2 wk Maintenance: 1 g 1–3 times weekly	No randomized controlled trials in the past 10 y[37]
Premarin	Estradiol vaginal cream	0.625 mg conjugated equine estrogens per g cream	Cyclically: 0.5–2 g daily for 21 d/mo Continuosly: 0.5 g twice weekly	There was a small and transient increase in circulating estradiol seen[7]
Intrarosa[38]	Dehydroepiandrosterone (DHEA) vaginal suppository	6.5 mg prasterone	1 insert daily at bedtime using the applicator	Contraindicated in women with undiagnosed abnormal vaginal/uterine bleeding
Ospemifene	Third generation selective estrogen receptor modulator (SERM)	60 mg tablet	By mouth with food daily	Contraindicated in patients with active arterial thromboembolic disease, abnormal postmenopausal vaginal bleeding, hormonally dependent neoplasias
Laser or radiofrequency device	Fractional microablative carbon dioxide laser or erbium: YAG	Emission wavelength: 1064 nm	Three laser treatment sessions over a specified time period (usually one session every 4 to 6 weeks)	Not FDA approved to treat GUSM, experimental

Table 3
Summary of non-prescriptive vaginal therapy

Treatment	Use	Symptomatic Relief	Considerations
Vaginal Moisturizer (replens, vagisil, feminease, moist again, K-Y liquibeads, hyalo GYN)	Routinely, typically two or 3 days per week, not just during sexual activity	Mild–moderate symptoms; improve coital comfort and increase vaginal moisture, but they do not reverse most atrophic vaginal changes	Some have bacteriocidal properties that disrupt the vaginal microbiome
Lubricant silicone-based (Pjur, ID millennium) Water-based (astroglide, slippery stuff, K-Y jelly) Oil-based (Pjur, ID millennium)[39]	Used as needed, before intercourse	Relieve discomfort during intercourse, reduce friction and trauma to the tissues	Silicone- main ingredient glycol and its metabolite glycerine, degraded into sugar can predispose to candidal growth water- evaporate quickly, require reapplication and may exacerbate symptoms oil- latex breakdown
Pelvic floor muscle training (PMFT)[40]	As needed, for patients with contraindication to hormone therapy and women with high-tone pelvic floor dysfunction	Improved vaginal blood flow parameters, increased pelvic floor muscle strength, and improved vaginal atrophy index	
Vaginal dilators and vibrators	Consistent use	Increase vaginal elasticity, decrease dyspareunia with deep penetration, stimulate blood flow and preserve vaginal function in women with or without sexual partner	Vaginal shortening or stenosis not improved in conjunction with hormone therapy

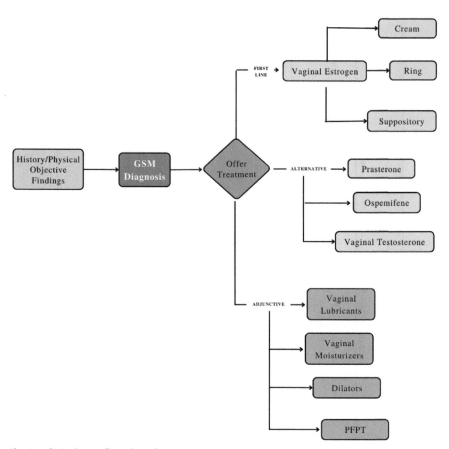

Fig. 2. Clinical care flowchart for GSM management.

symptoms, stress incontinence, and sexual function after 4 weeks of use, and it has a minimal effect on the endometrium.[25–27] Vulvoscopic photographs at 20 weeks identified improvements in anatomic changes due to GSM, including vaginal stenosis and rugae, meatal prominence, and vestibular changes. Ospemifene is a good alternative in women who cannot apply vaginal estrogen in cream or tablet format and who have other anatomic factors that do not permit the application of an estrogen ring[28]

Laser technologies Yttrium Aluminum Garnet (YAG) laser: Laser energy stimulates collagen synthesis, elastin production, vasodilation, and angiogenesis of vaginal tissues, however, limited investigations have found laser technologies to be effective in restoring vaginal architecture and improvement in symptoms related to GSM.[29–32] Unfortunately, this method has not been approved by the FDA, and has only been used in experimental settings.

Vaginal testosterone: The discovery of the androgen receptor and of the essential enzymes involved in androgen synthesis suggests that androgens play a crucial role in the differentiation of the vagina as well as in sustaining trophic and functional effects in postnatal life. Testosterone is necessary for the complex neurovascular processes that control arousal and lubrication (vascular smooth muscle relaxation via the nitric oxide-cyclic GMP-phosphodiesterase type 5 (NO/cGMP/PDE5) pathway, nerve fiber density, and neurotransmission), the integrity of vaginal tissue structure (including non-vascular smooth muscle thickness and contractility, and collagen fiber compactness), and both.[33] In the vagina, nociception, inflammation, and mucus secretion have all been reported to be modulated by testosterone. Small studies have shown some potential benefits with vaginal testosterone use, but intravaginal testosterone is not yet Food Drug Administration (FDA)-approved due to lacking high-quality data. In postmenopausal women with breast cancer on aromatase inhibitors, vaginal testosterone has been shown to improve Vaginal Maturity Index (VMI), dyspareunia, and dryness symptoms without affecting serum estradiol levels.[34,35] Further high-quality studies are needed to evaluate the safety and efficacy of testosterone on GSM symptoms.

SUMMARY AND CLINICAL CARE POINTS

GSM describes a chronic and progressive condition with a variety of genital, sexual, and urinary symptoms that require early recognition and appropriate management guided by patient symptoms and goals to preserve urogenital health. Patients with symptoms of GSM should receive lifelong treatment and regular clinical evaluations for symptom resolution for nonhormonal treatment options and hormonal options when symptom resolution is inadequate or UTIs persist (Fig. 2).

CLINICS CARE POINTS

- Utilize history and physical and objective findings to diagnose GSM.
- Offer treatment for symptomatic patients that include nonhormonal, over-the-counter vaginal moisturizers and lubricants, as well as hormonal treatments like vaginal estrogen.
- Pelvic floor muscle training, vaginal vibrators or dilators can be excellent adjunctive therapy and should be discussed with the patient.
- Low-dose vaginal estrogen can be used in any of its formulations including estradiol cream, suppository, or ring system. Patient preference, ease of application, rate of systemic absorption and cost should guide selection of therapy.
- If patient is seeking alternative therapy in lieu of vaginal estrogen without any contraindications to estrogen, consider the following options: DHEA in for of prasterone, oral ospemifene, and vaginal testosterone.
- If patient has breast cancer and symptoms of GSM, providers may suggest treatment with vaginal estrogen, DHEA, or testosterone.

DISCLOSURE

The authors have nothing to disclose.

REFERENCES

1. Portman DJ, Gass MLS, Vulvovaginal Atrophy Terminology Consensus Conference Panel. Genitourinary syndrome of menopause: new terminology for vulvovaginal atrophy from the International Society for the Study of Women's Sexual Health and the North American Menopause Society. Menopause N Y N 2014;21(10):1063–8.
2. Nappi RE, Cucinella L, Martini E, et al. The role of hormone therapy in urogenital health after menopause. Best Pract Res Clin Endocrinol Metab 2021;35(6): 101595.
3. Gandhi J, Chen A, Dagur G, et al. Genitourinary syndrome of menopause: an overview of clinical manifestations, pathophysiology, etiology, evaluation, and management. Am J Obstet Gynecol 2016;215(6):704–11.

4. Labrie F, Archer DF, Martel C, et al. Combined data of intravaginal prasterone against vulvovaginal atrophy of menopause. Menopause N Y N 2017;24(11): 1246–56.

5. Cagnacci A, Xholli A, Sclauzero M, et al. Vaginal atrophy across the menopausal age: results from the ANGEL study. Climacteric J Int Menopause Soc 2019; 22(1):85–9.

6. Labrie F, Archer DF, Koltun W, et al. Efficacy of intravaginal dehydroepiandrosterone (DHEA) on moderate to severe dyspareunia and vaginal dryness, symptoms of vulvovaginal atrophy, and of the genitourinary syndrome of menopause. Menopause N Y N 2018;25(11):1339–53.

7. Tzur T, Yohai D, Weintraub AY. The role of local estrogen therapy in the management of pelvic floor disorders. Climacteric J Int Menopause Soc 2016;19(2): 162–71.

8. Lüthje P, Hirschberg AL, Brauner A. Estrogenic action on innate defense mechanisms in the urinary tract. Maturitas 2014;77(1):32–6.

9. Caretto M, Giannini A, Russo E, et al. Preventing urinary tract infections after menopause without antibiotics. Maturitas 2017;99:43–6.

10. Brotman RM, Shardell MD, Gajer P, et al. Association between the vaginal microbiota, menopause status, and signs of vulvovaginal atrophy. Menopause N Y N 2014;21(5):450–8.

11. Robinson D, Cardozo LD. The role of estrogens in female lower urinary tract dysfunction. Urology 2003;62(4 Suppl 1):45–51.

12. Goldstein I. Recognizing and treating urogenital atrophy in postmenopausal women. J Womens Health 2010;19(3):425–32.

13. Phillips NA, Bachmann GA. Genitourinary syndrome of menopause: common problem, effective treatments. Cleve Clin J Med 2018;85(5):390–8.

14. Biehl C, Plotsker O, Mirkin S. A systematic review of the efficacy and safety of vaginal estrogen products for the treatment of genitourinary syndrome of menopause. Menopause N Y N 2019;26(4):431–53.

15. Weber MA, Kleijn MH, Langendam M, et al. Local oestrogen for pelvic floor disorders: a systematic review. PLoS One 2015;10(9):e0136265.

16. Raz R, Stamm WE. A controlled trial of intravaginal estriol in postmenopausal women with recurrent urinary tract infections. N Engl J Med 1993;329(11):753–6.

17. Griebling TL, Liao Z, Smith PG. Systemic and topical hormone therapies reduce vaginal innervation density in postmenopausal women. Menopause N Y N 2012; 19(6):630–5.

18. Krause M, Wheeler TL, Snyder TE, et al. Local effects of vaginally administered estrogen therapy: a review. J Pelvic Med Surg 2009;15(3):105–14.

19. Collaborative Group on Hormonal Factors in Breast Cancer. Type and timing of menopausal hormone therapy and breast cancer risk: individual participant meta-analysis of the worldwide epidemiological evidence. Lancet Lond Engl 2019;394(10204):1159–68.

20. Pitkin J, British Menopause Society medical advisory council. BMS - Consensus statement. Post Reprod Health 2018;24(3):133–8.

21. Cold S, Cold F, Jensen MB, et al. Systemic or vaginal hormone therapy after early breast cancer: a danish observational cohort study. J Natl Cancer Inst 2022;20: djac112.

22. Mension E, Alonso I, Cebrecos I, et al. Safety of prasterone in breast cancer survivors treated with aromatase inhibitors: the VIBRA pilot study. Climacteric J Int Menopause Soc 2022;28:1–7.

23. Rubin * R, Moyneur E, Tjoa ML, et al. Mp30-15 prevalence of urinary tract infections in women with genitourinary syndrome of menopause and the impact of vaginal prasterone on urinary tract infections. J Urol 2020;203(Supplement 4): e443–4.

24. Collà Ruvolo C, Gabrielli O, Formisano C, et al. Prasterone in the treatment of mild to moderate urge incontinence: an observational study. Menopause N Y N 2022; 29(8):957–62.

25. Cui Y, Zong H, Yan H, et al. The efficacy and safety of ospemifene in treating dyspareunia associated with postmenopausal vulvar and vaginal atrophy: a systematic review and meta-analysis. J Sex Med 2014;11(2):487–97.

26. McCall JL, DeGregorio MW. Pharmacologic evaluation of ospemifene. Expert Opin Drug Metab Toxicol 2010;6(6):773–9.

27. Schiavi MC, Sciuga V, Giannini A, et al. Overactive bladder syndrome treatment with ospemifene in menopausal patients with vulvovaginal atrophy: improvement of sexuality? Gynecol Endocrinol Off J Int Soc Gynecol Endocrinol 2018;34(8): 666–9.

28. Goldstein SW, Winter AG, Goldstein I. Improvements to the vulva, vestibule, urethral meatus, and vagina in women treated with ospemifene for moderate to severe dyspareunia: a prospective vulvoscopic pilot study. Sex Med 2018;6(2): 154–61.

29. Karcher C, Sadick N. Vaginal rejuvenation using energy-based devices. Int J Womens Dermatol 2016;2(3):85–8.

30. Sipos AG, Kozma B, Poka R, et al. The effect of fractional CO2 laser treatment on the symptoms of pelvic floor dysfunctions: pelvic floor distress inventory-20 questionnaire. Lasers Surg Med 2019;51(10):882–6.

31. Lang P, Dell JR, Rosen L, et al. Fractional CO2 laser of the vagina for genitourinary syndrome of menopause: Is the out-of-pocket cost worth the outcome of treatment? Lasers Surg Med 2017;49(10):882–5.

32. Naumova I, Castelo-Branco C. Current treatment options for postmenopausal vaginal atrophy. Int J Womens Health 2018;10:387–95.

33. Maseroli E, Vignozzi L. Testosterone and vaginal function. Sex Med Rev 2020; 8(3):379–92.

34. Witherby S, Johnson J, Demers L, et al. Topical testosterone for breast cancer patients with vaginal atrophy related to aromatase inhibitors: a phase I/II study. Oncologist 2011;16(4):424–31.

35. Dahir M, Travers-Gustafson D. Breast cancer, aromatase inhibitor therapy, and sexual functioning: a pilot study of the effects of vaginal testosterone therapy. Sex Med 2014;2(1):8–15.

36. Nappi RE, Martini E, Cucinella L, et al. Addressing vulvovaginal atrophy (VVA)/ genitourinary syndrome of menopause (GSM) for healthy aging in women. Front Endocrinol 2019;10:561.

37. Dalley AF. The American Association of Clinical Anatomists (AACA): the other American anatomy association. Anat Rec 1999;257(5):154–6.

38. Eriksen B. A randomized, open, parallel-group study on the preventive effect of an estradiol-releasing vaginal ring (Estring) on recurrent urinary tract infections in postmenopausal women. Am J Obstet Gynecol 1999;180(5):1072–9.

39. Potter N, Panay N. Vaginal lubricants and moisturizers: a review into use, efficacy, and safety. Climacteric J Int Menopause Soc 2021;24(1):19–24.

40. Mercier J, Morin M, Tang A, et al. Pelvic floor muscle training: mechanisms of action for the improvement of genitourinary syndrome of menopause. Climacteric J Int Menopause Soc 2020;23(5):468–73.

Affirming Care for Transgender Patients

Rebecca Green, MD, MS[a],*, Kristen L. Eckstrand, MD, PhD[b], Morgan Faeder, MD, PhD[c], Sarah Tilstra, MD, MS[a], Eloho Ufomata, MD, MS[a]

KEYWORDS

- Transgender • Gender affirmation • Hormone therapy • Transgender health

KEY POINTS

- Transgender individuals encounter a lack of education of clinicians on topics related to the health care of transgender patients.
- Medical gender affirmation is an individualized process.
- Clinicians can serve as facilitators to gender affirmation through medical and surgical approaches, including hormone therapy and gender-affirming surgeries.

INTRODUCTION/HISTORY/DEFINITIONS/BACKGROUND

Gender is distinct from sex. Sex is determined by factors including reproductive organs, chromosomes, and hormones, which lead to individuals being assigned male at birth, assigned female at birth, or assigned as intersex. Gender is a social construct which varies depending on cultural norms and behaviors. Gender identity is a deeply felt internal sense of self, which may correspond (cisgender) or not correspond (transgender) with assigned sex at birth.[1,2] As of 2015, there are an estimated 1.4 million transgender individuals in the United States, and this number has likely increased in the intervening years.[3] In addition, there are individuals who identify as nonbinary. According to the Human Rights Campaign, "non-binary people may identify as being both a man and a woman, somewhere in between, or as falling completely outside of these categories. While many also identify as transgender, not all non-binary people do. Non-binary can also be used as an umbrella term encompassing identities such as agender, bigender, genderqueer, or gender fluid."[1]

[a] Department of Medicine, University of Pittsburgh School of Medicine, UPMC General Internal Medicine Clinic, Montefiore 9S, 200 Lothrop Street, Pittsburgh, PA 15213, USA; [b] Department of Psychiatry, University of Pittsburgh School of Medicine, Loeffler Building #301, 121 Meyran Avenue, Pittsburgh, PA 15213, USA; [c] University of Pittsburgh School of Medicine, UPMC Psychiatry CL, 3600 Forbes Avenue, Suite 306, Pittsburgh, PA 15213, USA
* Corresponding author.
E-mail address: greenre@upmc.edu

Med Clin N Am 107 (2023) 371–384
https://doi.org/10.1016/j.mcna.2022.10.011
0025-7125/23/© 2022 Elsevier Inc. All rights reserved.

Gender dysphoria refers to distress that stems from a gender identity that is incongruent with sex assigned at birth. Importantly, not all transgender individuals experience gender dysphoria.[4] Individuals may choose to affirm their gender in any number of ways including name and pronouns, choice of hairstyle and clothing, gender markers on legal documentation, hormone therapy (HT), vocal therapy, and gender-affirmation surgery.

Transgender individuals face a myriad of health disparities and inequities related to bias, stigma, and discrimination within the medical institution, as well as a lack of education of clinicians on topics related to the health care of transgender patients.[5–7]

Not all providers or clinics may feel "ready" to provide gender-affirming care, but everyone should feel empowered and confident that they can. Many resources exist to facilitate the development of clinical spaces and a competent workforce, with motivation and buy-in from key stakeholders. The "LGBTQ Primary Care Toolkit[8]" is comprehensive online resource cosponsored by the National Institutes of Health (NIH) and the National Institute on Minority Health that can be used to guide clinic-led organizational change and provide recommendations and resources for clinics caring for sexual and gender diverse patients.

FACILITATING MEDICAL GENDER AFFIRMATION

Gender affirmation is a deeply personal process, and medical gender affirmation can look different depending on the individual's personal goals. The standard of care is an individualized approach, wherein a person may choose some aspects of medical or surgical gender affirmation but not others.

Given this individualized approach, obtaining the gender and medical history is a keystone to medical gender affirmation. It sets the stage for the development of trust between the patient and health care provider. This process begins by creating a welcoming clinical environment. In the largest survey of transgender individuals to date, one-quarter of respondents reported experiencing a negative encounter with a health care provider and viewed doctors' offices as unsafe spaces.[9] Some approaches to creating a welcoming environment include

- Educating all staff on sensitive cultural awareness of gender diversity
- Creation of inclusive clinical intake forms
- Appropriately documenting gender identity including name and pronouns in the electronic medical record
- The use of inclusive language by all members of the clinical team
- Signage indicating that the environment aims to be inclusive of all gender identities
- Access to "all gender" bathrooms

In obtaining a medical history, it is important to use open-ended questions, avoid any assumptions about the patient, and mirror the patient's language for self-description if it is respectful and neutral. The goal of the history is to learn about

- The patient's gender identity, chosen name, and pronouns
- Their current and future goals for medical and surgical gender affirmation
- Their experience with gender dysphoria, if any
- Any past or current treatments including HT, surgeries, esthetic procedures and social or legal gender affirmation
- Organs which are present, either surgically removed or created absent, that is, an organ inventory
- The patient's overall medical, family, and social histories

Before performing a physical examination, it is helpful to understand if there are any aspects of the examination which might exacerbate gender dysphoria or create discomfort for the patient. Of note, examination of genitalia should only be conducted when medically necessary, for example, for cervical cancer screening or operative planning.

There are many evidence-based benefits to medical gender affirmation, including improved mental health after gender-affirming surgeries[10]; decreased suicidal ideation with access to HT[11]; and improved psychological functioning, well-being, and overall quality of life with HT.[12,13]

According to the World Professional Association for Transgender Health (WPATH), there are four criteria for initiating HT

1. Persistent, well-documented gender dysphoria
2. Capacity to make an informed decision and consent to treatment
3. Age of majority
4. Concomitant medical or psychiatric conditions are controlled.[4]

Written informed consent is not required before initiating treatment, however, a comprehensive conversation between patient and clinician is necessary in order to ascertain the patient's goals for treatment and discuss expectations, benefits, and risks of HT.

USING A TRAUMA-INFORMED APPROACH

Traumatic events are direct or witnessed unpredictable, unexpected occurrences that threaten an individual's life or self-preservation. Exposure to trauma is a near-ubiquitous experience, with 89% of individuals reporting one or more trauma exposures by the time they reach 18.[14] Transgender and gender diverse individuals are four times more likely to report exposure to violent traumatic events.[15] Within the health care setting, 33% of transgender and gender diverse people report being exposed to negative experiences in the past year, with common experiences including repeated misgendering, critical or discriminatory language, intrusive questions related to genitalia and/or sexual practices, and unwanted components of the physical examination.[16]

Not all individuals who are exposed to trauma report experiencing physiologic or emotional sequelae, and few predictive markers exist to determine whether—and when—trauma exposures will lead to heightened stress responses or negative emotional reactions.[17] Because trauma exposure is ubiquitous and the sequelae of trauma cannot be objectively predicted, it is recommended that all individuals involved in health care adopt a trauma-informed care (TIC) approach.[17] This is particularly true with populations that are more likely to have experienced a higher frequency of trauma exposures, such as transgender and gender diverse individuals.

TIC is "a strengths-based framework that emphasizes physical, psychological, and emotional safety for both providers and survivors, and creates opportunities for survivors to rebuild a sense of control and empowerment"[18] TIC operates on four key assumptions (the 4 Rs)

- *Realize* the widespread impact of trauma on individuals and communities.
- *Recognize* the signs and symptoms of trauma, including heightened arousal, avoidance, intrusion, and negative changes in thoughts and mood.
- *Respond* by applying principles of TIC into policies, procedures, and practices.
- *Resist* re-traumatization by reducing or eliminating exposures that could trigger trauma reactions.[19]

Adherence to six principles is required for a complete TIC approach.

- *Safety* prioritizes physical and psychological safety in the physical environment and interpersonal relationships
- *Trustworthiness and Transparency* focuses on trust through transparent decisions.
- *Peer Support* integrates those with shared experiences to promote healing and mutual self-help.
- *Collaboration and Mutuality* aims to reduce the power differential between patients and providers to support shared decision-making.
- *Empowerment, Voice, and Choice* values the strengths and resilience of individuals.
- *Cultural, Historical, and Gender Issues* acknowledges the importance of services responsive to the needs of diverse patients.

Some simple primary care practices for transgender individuals rooted in TIC include using the correct name, pronouns, and gender; focusing on building a trusting relationship during initial visits; screening for trauma, including in health care, and validating the difficulty of those experiences; determining possible alternatives or modifications to physical examinations when re-traumatization may occur; planning how to perform the sensitive components of the physical examination using shared decision-making; asking for assent to perform the physical examination; narrating the physical examination so patients are aware of what is happening; and debriefing after challenging experiences, including emphasizing the importance of the patient–provider relationship.[20] Because a comprehensive TIC approach requires engagement across all levels of the health care system, the abilities of a single care provider may not be sufficient to meet the health care needs of all individual patients. However, the actions of a single provider may be sufficient to support interpersonal and physical safety for a patient and allow for a trusting and affirming patient–provider relationship.

MEDICAL AND SURGICAL GENDER AFFIRMATION FOR TRANSGENDER WOMEN
Medical Gender Affirmation

Hormone therapy
There are several medications that, as monotherapy or in combination, are used for feminizing treatment. Estrogen preparations of 17-beta-estradiol are available in oral, transdermal, intramuscular, and subcutaneous forms. This is a bioidentical estrogen to that produced by the ovary. All formulations of estrogen can produce the same degree of physical changes, though transdermal estradiol is the least thrombogenic. Antiandrogen therapy with spironolactone and/or a 5-alpha-reductase inhibitor (such as finasteride) can help reduce testosterone levels and activity, thereby decreasing masculine characteristics including body hair and male pattern baldness. The addition of progesterone to feminizing HT regimens is less well studied. Some patients and clinicians report that progesterone enhances breast development and improves mood, however, large-scale studies have not replicated these findings.[21] Dosing guidelines are available via the Endocrine Society guidelines, or the University of California, San Francisco, UCSF Primary Care Guidelines.[21,22]

Feminizing HT yields, to a variable extent, several physical changes. Early changes include a reduction in spontaneous erections, decreased libido, and softening of the skin. Later changes include the redistribution of body fat, decreased muscle mass, breast growth, testicular atrophy, and thinning of facial and body hair. Although these physical changes are first noticeable within the first year of treatment, it may take up to 5 years of HT to see full effects.[4,21]

Feminizing HT carries some potential risks. Clinicians must thoroughly assess the patient's risk factors including age, weight, smoking status, and family history and address modifiable risk factors when present. The primary risk of estrogen is venous thromboembolism. Estrogen also increases the risk of hypertriglyceridemia, and can increase liver enzymes, blood pressure, and cause weight gain.[4] The effect of estrogen on cardiovascular risk is controversial, and existing data across predominantly retrospective cohort studies are mixed, with some studies showing increased risks of myocardial infarction and stroke in transgender women compared with cisgender men and cisgender women, and other studies are showing no difference.[23,24] Risks of spironolactone are hypotension and hyperkalemia. Active hormone-sensitive malignancy and unstable cardiac disease are contraindications to beginning HT.

The goals of titration of feminizing HT are to: suppress testosterone; attain physiologic levels of estrogen consistent with those found in cisgender women; and achieve the outwardly appearance and features desired by the patient. If planning to use spironolactone, clinicians should check the creatinine and potassium before initiating treatment. At 3, 6, and 12 months, estradiol as well as free and total testosterone levels help guide dose titration. If taking spironolactone, check creatinine and potassium at these intervals as well. After 1 year, estradiol, free and total testosterone, as well as creatinine and potassium if warranted, should be monitored annually.[21]

Electrolysis

Although estrogen therapy causes thinning of body and sometimes facial hair, it does not eliminate it completely. Transgender women seeking more permanent hair removal can pursue electrolysis or laser hair removal. In addition to removing unwanted facial and body hair, these procedures can help prepare areas of skin for vaginoplasty surgery. Electrolysis and laser hair removal can be painful; topical anesthetics can help mitigate pain.[21]

Vocal therapy

Feminizing HT does not affect voice pitch. Thus, some transgender women elect to work with a speech–language pathologist with training in transgender health to learn to speak with more feminine tones and speech patterns.[21]

Surgical Gender Affirmation

Breast augmentation

Breast augmentation surgery for transgender women, performed by a plastic surgeon, creates a more feminine chest contour. There are no definitive guidelines as to the timing of surgical breast augmentation with regard to HT. Choice and timing of surgery is an individual decision based on informed conversations between patient and surgeon.[21,25]

Orchiectomy

Transgender women may pursue orchiectomy, with or without vaginoplasty. Performed by a plastic surgeon or urologist, surgically removing the testes drastically reduces the amount of testosterone produced. As such, after orchiectomy, patients typically require much lower doses of estrogen, and no longer need testosterone suppressing medications such as spironolactone.

Vaginoplasty

Creation of a neovagina is within the scope of practice of plastic surgeons and urologists. The most common technique inverts the skin of the penis to form a vaginal canal, uses the scrotal skin to create labia majora, and uses a portion of the glans penis to create a sensate clitoris.[25] A dilation regimen is required postoperatively to ensure the vaginal canal retains its depth and girth.[21]

Facial feminization surgery

To achieve more feminine facial features, plastic surgeons use a variety of techniques including hairline advancement, cheek, lip, and chin augmentation, jaw reduction, and tracheal shaving.[25]

MEDICAL AND SURGICAL GENDER AFFIRMATION FOR TRANSGENDER MEN
Medical Gender Affirmation

Hormone therapy

The mainstay of masculinizing HT is testosterone. Testosterone comes in multiple formulations: topical creams and gels, transdermal patch, and intramuscular or subcutaneous injections. The selection of route of administration should be made through shared decision-making between patient and clinician based on patient tolerability and preference. Dosing guidelines are available in the Endocrine Society guidelines or the UCSF Primary Care Guidelines.[21,22]

Early physical changes seen with testosterone therapy include oily scan and acne. Later changes include growth of facial and body hair, redistribution of body fat, cessation of menses, clitoral enlargement, deeper voice, and increased muscle mass. Male pattern baldness is possible, but unpredictable. It takes 1 to 5 years of HT to see full physical effects.[21]

Testosterone therapy can impact fertility, but to variable extents between individuals. Although physiologic levels of testosterone usually suppress menstruation in transgender men, testosterone alone is not effective contraception. If patients wish to avoid pregnancy and partner with a person capable of producing sperm, contraception is still needed. We recommend shared decision-making with the individual patient to choose the right form of contraception. Hormonal, nonhormonal, short, long acting, or permanent options are all reasonable, however, many patients want to avoid systemic estrogen, as this can induce dysphoria.

There are some risks of testosterone therapy that clinicians must discuss with patients before initiating treatment. Testosterone increases the production of red blood cells and can lead to polycythemia.[21] Elevated liver enzymes, hyperlipidemia, and sleep apnea are possible as well.[4] Weight gain and acne are common side effects early in treatment, however, tend to subside with time.[4] In individuals with preexisting risk factors, testosterone can also increase the risk of type 2 diabetes, hypertension, and destabilize those with underlying psychiatric disorders.[4] The effect of testosterone on cardiovascular risk is controversial. Observational and retrospective cohort studies have shown multiple and often contradictory outcomes. Ultimately, evidence has demonstrated an increased risk of hypertension and hyperlipidemia in transgender men on HT, but no clear association between these risk factors and elevated risk of stroke and myocardial infarction.[23,24]

Goals when titrating testosterone are to attain physiologic levels of testosterone consistent with those of cisgender men and to achieve the outwardly appearance and features desired by the patient. Before initiating treatment, clinicians should check the patient's hemoglobin and hematocrit. At 3, 6, and 12 months, hemoglobin and hematocrit should be checked to monitor for polycythemia. In addition, free and total testosterone should be checked at these intervals to guide dose titration. If polycythemia has not developed after 1 year, hemoglobin and hematocrit should be monitored annually[17](**Table 1**).

Vocal therapy

Unlike estrogen therapy, testosterone treatment in transgender men affects the pitch of the voice, both deepening and lowering it. Some transgender men will still pursue vocal therapy with a speech–language pathologist trained in transgender health to learn to speak in a more masculine manner.[17]

Surgical Gender Affirmation

Chest reconstruction

Performed by a plastic surgeon, subcutaneous mastectomy or chest reconstruction removes breast tissue and reshapes the chest to achieve a more masculine contour. Of note, this procedure is not equivalent to a mastectomy performed for treatment or prevention of breast cancer; residual breast tissue can remain, and development of breast cancer is still possible.[4,17]

Hysterectomy

Some transgender men may choose to undergo hysterectomy, with or without bilateral salpingectomy and oophorectomy. This procedure, performed by a gynecologist, can alleviate dysphoria by removing gender incongruent organs and eliminating menstrual bleeding and associated symptoms.[4,17]

Genital reconstruction

There are multiple surgical options for transgender men that aim to balance achieving male-appearing genitals with sexual function, the ability to void standing, and esthetics. These procedures may be performed by plastic surgeons or urologists. Metoidioplasty uses hormonally enlarged clitoral tissue to create a neophallus.[26] Phalloplasty uses a free flap of skin from the arm or leg to create a neophallus.[17] Scrotoplasty uses the labia majora, with or without testicular implants, to create a scrotum.[26] Some transgender men may choose to undergo vaginectomy, or surgical removal of the vagina, as well.

Facial masculinization

In facial masculinization procedures, plastic surgeons use a variety of techniques including forehead lengthening, cheek augmentation, jaw reshaping and chin contouring, and enhancing the laryngeal prominence to create more masculine facial features.[25]

MEDICAL AND SURGICAL GENDER AFFIRMATION FOR NONBINARY INDIVIDUALS

Nonbinary individuals may decide to pursue various options for medical gender affirmation to best fit their own gender affirmation goals. One commonly used strategy is microdosing of hormones or the use of low-dose hormone therapy. Microdosing can help facilitate the development of physical characteristics, which affirm an individual's gender identity.

Fertility Considerations

Many transgender individuals want biologically related children.[4,27] The effects of gender-affirming therapy on gonadal function and fertility are not well understood. The available data show a variable impact on fertility from HT. As such, both WPATH

Table 1
Medications for Gender Affirmation

Class/Route	Name	Low–High Dose	Notes
Feminizing Hormone Therapy			
Estradiol			
Oral (can be given sublingually)	Estradiol	1–8 mg/d	Can divide to twice daily dosing if more than 4 mg
Parenteral (intramuscular or subcutaneous)	Estradiol cypionate Estradiol valerate	2–10 mg/wk 5–30 mg/2 wk	Can divide dose for once weekly dosing
Topical	Estradiol transdermal	50–400 mcg	Maximum dose of a single patch available is 100 mcg Lowest venous thromboembolism (VTE) risk
Antiandrogens			
Oral	Spironolactone Finasteride Bicalutamide	50–300 mg/d 1–5 mg/d	In divided doses Used as an adjunct, typically for hair loss Has been used in transgender populations, however, no clear dosing schedule; concern is hepatotoxicity
Masculinizing Hormone Therapy			
Testosterone			
Parenteral (intramuscular or subcutaneous)	Testosterone cypionate Testosterone enanthate	50–100 mg/wk 50–100 mg/wk	Can double dose for every 2 week dosing
Topical	Testosterone gel 1.6% Testosterone transdermal patch	50–100 mg/d 2–8 mg/d	

Note: These are typical regimens and typical dosing schedules for transgender individuals, lower doses may be appropriate based on individual patient goals and clinical responses, for example, microdosing.

and the Endocrine Society guidelines recommend that clinicians counsel individuals on fertility preservation before initiating HT.[4,22]

There are multiple options for fertility preservation for transgender individuals. It is important to note that these treatments can be expensive (with limited insurance coverage), time intensive, and may not be available in all settings. Early referral to a fertility specialist is important if reproduction is within the patient's goals. Individuals can undergo sperm cryopreservation, or testicular sperm extraction, oocyte cryopreservation, and/or embryo cryopreservation. In addition, there are many experimental and innovative options coming down the pike.[28]

Sex and gender-specific screenings in transgender patients

The evidence for routine sex-specific screenings for transgender individuals lacks the frequently robust data that exist for screening cisgender patients. As such, many of the recommendations are based on expert opinion or evidence extrapolated from data from cisgender individuals.

Cervical cancer screening

All individuals with a cervix, including transgender men, should be screened routinely for cervical cancer beginning at age 21 per the US Preventive Services Task Force and the American Society of Colposcopy and Cervical Pathology.[29,30]

Cervical cancer screening can be a physically painful and emotionally dysphoric and non-affirming experience for transgender men. However, there are steps physicians can take to make the procedure more tolerable. Using the smallest available speculum, providing the patient agency over inserting the speculum and offering the patient the option to have a support person present can help mitigate distress. For patients who have taken testosterone, prescribing estradiol 1% cream for the patient to apply vaginally for 1 to 2 weeks before the examination can help mediate pain related to testosterone-induced vaginal atrophy.

Prostate cancer screening

Several cohort studies have shown that transgender women have a lower incidence of prostate cancer than cisgender men.[31,32] However, when prostate cancer occurs in transgender women, it is typically associated with worse outcomes.[31] There are no guidelines for prostate cancer screening specific to transgender women. The most recent recommendations according to the US Preventive Services Task Force calls for shared decision-making between patient and clinician on whether to screen with a prostate-specific antigen (PSA) test between the ages of 55 and 69 years.[29]

Screening for osteoporosis

Sex steroids are integral to the development and maintenance of bone density. As such, gender-affirming HT in transgender men and transgender women has been associated with increased bone density, though this has not correlated with reduced fracture risk.[33] There are no definitive, evidence-based guidelines for screening for osteoporosis in transgender individuals. The UCSF guidelines recommends screening transgender men and women with dual-energy x-ray absorptiometry beginning at age 65 years.[17] Screening of transgender men and transgender women ages 50 to 64 years should be based on the assessment of individual risk factors. Patients who have undergone gonadectomy and have had at least 5 years without hormone replacement should also be screened for osteoporosis.[17]

Breast cancer screening

Although population-based statistics of breast cancer incidence in transgender patients are lacking, screening for breast cancer must be considered in both transgender men and transgender women. One of the largest studies of breast cancer incidence in transgender patients is derived from a retrospective cohort study in the Netherlands, which included transgender men and transgender women who received gender-affirming HT which showed a higher incidence of breast cancer in transgender women as compared with cisgender men and a lower incidence of breast cancer in transgender women as compared with cisgender women.[34] Meanwhile, transgender men had a lower incidence of breast cancer than cisgender women, but a higher incidence of breast cancer than cisgender men.[34] In the United States, a retrospective cohort study from the Veterans Health Administration showed similar trends.[35]

Transgender women. Given that estrogen exposure is thought to be the primary driver of malignant changes in breast tissue, recommendations regarding when to begin screening for breast cancer in this patient population are based on years of estrogen exposure. The American College of Radiology's Choosing Wisely campaign advises that digital breast tomosynthesis or mammography may be appropriate in transgender women beginning at age 40 with at least 5 years of estrogen exposure.[36] The University of San Francisco Center for Transgender Excellence recommends biennial mammograms for transgender women beginning at age 50 who have had at least 5 years of estrogen treatment.[17] A more individualized approach may be required for transgender women at higher risk due to family history or BRCA positivity.

Transgender men. According to the American College of Radiology's Appropriate Use Criteria, transgender men who have not undergone chest reconstruction surgery should be screened for breast cancer per the guidelines for cisgender women.[36] Transgender men who have undergone chest reconstruction are still at risk of breast cancer due to the potential presence of residual breast tissue. However, there are no existing guidelines for screening in this patient population. Moreover, mammography in these patients can be technically challenging. If imaging is required to evaluate a concern for breast cancer, MRI or ultrasound may be required.[17,36]

When to Seek Psychiatric Consultation

Although having a gender identity that does not align with sex assigned at birth is no longer considered a psychiatric disorder,[37] there remains discomfort among many medical and surgical practitioners with providing gender-affirming care without prior consultation with behavioral health. According to the current WPATH Standards of Care, prescription of medication for transition is to be done according to an "informed consent" model, whereas surgical procedures require one or two evaluations by a mental health professional, depending on the site of the procedure.[4] Insurance carriers currently require documentation of gender dysphoria to prove medical necessity for surgical procedures.

The question remains, aside from insurance requirements, when is psychiatric consultation in the best interests of the transgender patient? The answer, though seemingly facile, is that a transgender person should be referred to psychiatry for the same reasons as any other patient. Many transgender people have been compelled to see behavioral health providers to access gender-affirming care or have been subjected to conversion therapy. This historical gatekeeping of gender-affirming care, along with a culture that often presents transgender identity alone as being a mental illness, sets up the visit to be an adversarial experience in which the patient is expected to prove their identity, and show that they do not have any psychiatric symptoms which would preclude them from accessing affirming care. Therefore, the referring provider must frame their referral as beneficial to the patient and provide compelling reasoning. They must explicitly state that the referral is not an evaluation necessary to obtain gender-affirming care or based on the assumption that transgender identity is pathologic. It is a referral for evaluation and treatment of symptoms to improve the patient's quality of life.

Even so, providers may have concerns about a psychiatric diagnosis or symptoms affecting the patient's ability to follow up with essential testing or perioperative care. Owing to these concerns, the evaluation in anticipation of gender-affirming surgery has been compared with a pretransplant evaluation. Nevertheless, among transplant patients, a mental health diagnosis is not associated with poor follow-up[38] and is not considered a contraindication to organ transplantation.[33] Thus, the mere presence of a mental health diagnosis alone should not trigger a referral to behavioral health. When providers are concerned about psychosocial factors that may impact a patient's ability to access care, a referral to social work can be invaluable.

Another issue that triggers psychiatric involvement is the concern that psychiatric symptoms may impact the patient's capacity to make informed medical decisions. Importantly, there is no mental health disorder or symptom that a priori precludes capacity to participate in informed consent. In this case, the referral is presented as one of the steps intended to facilitate affirming care, and not to be a roadblock in the process.

In short, a referral to psychiatry should be made following the same reasoning as for any other patient, or when they need an evaluation due to the requirements of their insurance carrier.

SUMMARY

Medical and surgical gender affirmation leads to improved health outcomes and quality of life for transgender individuals who desire it. A safe and welcoming culture, with attention to a trauma-informed approach is necessary given the discrimination that is commonly faced by transgender individuals in health care settings. The standard of care for medical and surgical gender affirmation is an individualized approach, which focuses on the patient's goals as the main driver of care. Last, barriers to care should be minimized.

CLINICS CARE POINTS

- Some transgender or gender diverse individuals can experience gender dysphoria, which refers to the distress that stems from a gender identity that is incongruent with sex assigned at birth.
- Medical and surgical treatments can be used to affirm one's gender, including hormone therapy, surgeries including facial surgeries, chest and genital reconstruction surgeries, and adjunct treatments like hair removal and voice therapy.
- It is important to create and foster a welcoming clinical environment, avoid discrimination and microaggressions, and use a trauma-informed approach.

DISCLOSURE

The authors have no competing commercial or financial conflicts of interest to disclose.

FUNDING SOURCES

Dr K.L. Eckstrand is supported by National Institutes of Health (NIH) grant K23MH128728.

REFERENCES

1. The Human Rights Campaign. Glossary of terms. Available at. https://www.hrc. org/resources/glossary-of-terms.
2. Makadon HJ, Mayer KH, Potter J, et al, editors. Fenway guide to lesbian, gay bisexual, and transgender health. 2nd edition. Philadelphia, PA: American College of Physicians; 2015.
3. Safer JD, Tangpricha V. Care of the transgender patient. Ann Intern Med 2019; 171(1):ITC1–16.
4. World Professional Association for Transgender Health. Standards of care for the health of transsexual, transgender, and gender nonconforming people [7thVersion]. 2012. Available at. https://www.wpath.org/publications/soc.
5. Grant JM, Mottet L, Tanis J, et al. National Transgender Discrimination Survey, [United States], 2008-2009. Inter-university Consortium for Political and Social Research [distributor], 2020-11-19. https://doi.org/10.3886/ICPSR37888.v1.
6. Pregnall AM, Churchwell AL, Ehrenfeld JM. A call for LGBTQ content in graduate medical education program requirements. Acad Med 2021;96(6):828–35.
7. Korpaisarn S, Safer JD. Gaps in transgender medical education among healthcare providers: A major barrier to care for transgender persons. Rev Endocr Metab Disord 2018;19(3):271–5.
8. Willging C, Sturm R, Sklar M, et al. LGBTQ primary care toolkit: a guide for primary care clinics to improve services for sexual and gender minority (SGM) patients. Albuquerque, NM: Pacific Institute for Research and Evaluation; 2021.
9. Grant JM, Lisa A, Justin T, et al. Injustice at every turn: a report of the national transgender discrimination survey. Washington: National Center for Transgender Equality and National Gay and Lesbian Task Force; 2011.
10. Almazan AN, Keuroghlian AS. Association between gender-affirming surgeries and mental health outcomes. JAMA Surg 2021;156(7):611–8.
11. Turban JL, King D, Kobe J, et al. Access to gender-affirming hormones during adolescence and mental health outcomes among transgender adults. PLoS One 2022;17(1):e0261039. Published 2022 Jan 12.
12. Achille C, Taggart T, Eaton NR, et al. Longitudinal impact of gender-affirming endocrine intervention on the mental health and well-being of transgender youths: preliminary results. Int J Pediatr Endocrinol 2020;2020:8.
13. White Hughto JM, Reisner SL. A Systematic Review of the Effects of Hormone Therapy on Psychological Functioning and Quality of Life in Transgender Individuals. Transgend Health 2016;1(1):21–31. https://doi.org/10.1089/trgh.2015.0008.
14. Anda RF, Felitti VJ, Bremner JD, et al. The enduring effects of abuse and related adverse experiences in childhood. A convergence of evidence from neurobiology and epidemiology. Eur Arch Psychiatry Clin Neurosci 2006;256(3):174–86.
15. Flores AR, Meyer IH, Langton L, et al. Gender identity disparities in criminal victimization. Los Angeles, CA: The UCLA Williams Institute of Law; 2021.
16. James SE, Herman JL, Rankin S, et al. The report of the 2015 U.S. Transgender survey. Washington, DC: National Center for Transgender Equality; 2016.
17. McLaughlin KA, Sheridan MA, Humphreys KL, et al. The value of dimensional models of early experience: Thinking clearly about concepts and categories. Perspect Psychol Sci 2021;16(6):1463–72.

18. Hopper EK, Bassuk EL, Olivet J. Shelter from the storm: Trauma-informed care in homelessness services settings. Open Health Serv Policy J 2010;3:80–100.

19. Substance Abuse and Mental Health Service Administration. SAMHSA's concept of trauma and guidance for a trauma-informed approach. Rockville, MD: Substance Abuse and Mental Health Services Administration; 2014.

20. Potter J, Peitzmeier SM, Bernstein I, et al. Cervical cancer screening for patients on the female-to-male spectrum: a narrative review and guide for clinicians. J Gen Intern Med 2015;30(12):1857–64.

21. Deutsch MB, Center of Excellence for Transgender Health. Department of Family and Community Medicine, University of California San Francisco. Guidelines for the primary and gender-affirming care of transgender and gender nonbinary people. 2nd edition. San Francisco: University of California; 2016. Available from: www.transhealth.ucsf.edu/.

22. Hembree WC, Cohen-Kettenis PT, Gooren L, et al. Endocrine treatment of gender-dysphoric/gender-incongruent persons: an endocrine society clinical practice guideline. J Clin Endocrinol Metab 2017;102(11):3869–903 [published correction appears in J Clin Endocrinol Metab. 2018 Feb 1;103(2):699] [published correction appears in J Clin Endocrinol Metab. 2018 Jul 1;103(7): 2758-2759].

23. Aranda G, Halperin I, Gomez-Gil E, et al. Cardiovascular risk associated with gender affirming hormone therapy in transgender population. Front Endocrinol (Lausanne) 2021;12:718200.

24. Connelly PJ, Marie Freel E, Perry C, et al. Gender-Affirming Hormone Therapy, Vascular Health and Cardiovascular Disease in Transgender Adults. Hypertension 2019;74(6):1266–74 [published correction appears in Hypertension. 2020 Apr;75(4):e10].

25. Gender Affirmation Surgeries. American society of plastic surgeons. Available at. https://www.plasticsurgery.org/reconstructive-procedures/gender-affirmation-surgeries. Accessed July 23, 2022.

26. Djordjevic ML, Stojanovic B, Bizic M. Metoidioplasty: techniques and outcomes. Transl Androl Urol 2019;8(3):248–53.

27. Tornello SL, Bos H. Parenting intentions among transgender individuals. LGBT Health 2017;4(2):115–20. https://doi.org/10.1089/lgbt.2016.0153.

28. Cheng PJ, Pastuszak AW, Myers JB, et al. Fertility concerns of the transgender patient. Transl Androl Urol 2019;8(3):209–18. https://doi.org/10.21037/tau.2019. 05.09.

29. U.S. Preventive Services Task Force., & United States. U.S. Preventive services Task Force (USPSTF). Rockville, MD: U.S. Dept. of Health & Human Services, Agency for Healthcare Research and Quality; 2000.

30. Perkins RB, Guido RS, Castle PE, et al. 2019 ASCCP risk-based management consensus guidelines for abnormal cervical cancer screening tests and cancer precursors. J Low Genit Tract Dis 2020;24(2):102–31 [published correction appears in J Low Genit Tract Dis. 2020 Oct;24(4):427].

31. Bertoncelli Tanaka M, Sahota K, Burn J, et al. Prostate cancer in transgender women: what does a urologist need to know? BJU Int 2022;129(1):113–22.

32. Stevenson MO, Tangpricha V. Osteoporosis and bone health in transgender persons. Endocrinol Metab Clin North Am 2019;48(2):421–7.

33. Faeder S, Moschenross D, Rosenberger E, et al. Psychiatric aspects of organ transplantation and donation. Curr Opin Psychiatry 2015;28(5):357–64.

34. de Blok CJM, Wiepjes CM, Nota NM, et al. Breast cancer risk in transgender people receiving hormone treatment: nationwide cohort study in the Netherlands. BMJ 2019;365:l1652.

35. Brown GR, Jones KT. Incidence of breast cancer in a cohort of 5,135 transgender veterans. Breast Cancer Res Treat 2015;149(1):191–8.

36. Expert Panel on Breast Imaging, Brown A, Lourenco AP, et al. ACR Appropriateness Criteria® Transgender Breast Cancer Screening. J Am Coll Radiol 2021; 18(11S):S502–15.

37. American Psychiatric Association. Diagnostic and statistical manual of mental disorders. 5th edition. 2013. https://doi.org/10.1176/appi.books.9780890425596.

38. Evans LD, Stock EM, Zeber JE, et al. Posttransplantation outcomes in veterans with serious mental illness. Transplantation 2015;99(8):e57–65.

Intimate Partner Violence

Jillian Kyle, MD, MS*

KEYWORDS

- Intimate partner violence • Trauma-informed care • Domestic violence
- Physical violence • Sexual violence • Stalking

KEY POINTS

- Intimate partner violence is a common and devastating worldwide public health problem leading to potential long term physical, mental, and financial impacts.
- Knowledge of the numerous IPV risk factors can help providers determine which persons may be in need of extra care, attention, and prevention strategies.
- Providers can serve as an important access point for education, resources, and support for persons experiencing violence.
- Treating all persons in a way that is sensitive to potential trauma can help patients experiencing IPV feel comfortable in the health care setting and potentially seek needed help.

INTRODUCTION

Intimate partner violence (IPV) is a common and potentially devastating problem that affects women across the life span. IPV is defined as physical or sexual violence, stalking behavior, and/or psychological aggression by an intimate partner (**Table 1**). One in 4 women in the United States will experience some form of IPV in their lifetimes.[1] Persons who experience IPV experience higher rates of negative physical and mental health outcomes when compared with those who have never experienced violence.[2,3] Physician awareness of IPV's impact, consequences, treatments, and patient preferences around IPV discussions can lead to improved patient satisfaction and outcomes.

Risk Factors

IPV affects all demographics and can be seen across genders, sexual orientation, age, ethnic identity, and socioeconomic factors. With that in mind, there are certain identifiable risk factors for relationship violence. Although none of these factors individually guarantees harmful relationship outcomes, knowledge of associated risks can be helpful in determining which populations may need extra care, attention, and prevention strategies.

Division of General Internal Medicine, University of Pittsburgh, 5200 Centre Avenue Suite #509, UPMC Shadyside, Pittsburgh, PA 15232, USA
* Corresponding author.
E-mail address: roperj@upmc.edu

Med Clin N Am 107 (2023) 385–395
https://doi.org/10.1016/j.mcna.2022.10.012
0025-7125/23/© 2022 Elsevier Inc. All rights reserved.

Table 1
Intimate partner violence terms

Term	Definition
Intimate partner violence	Physical or sexual violence, stalking behavior, and/or psychological aggression by an intimate partner
Intimate partner	Person with whom an individual has a close personal relationship, which may include many of the following elements (not all are required): emotional connectedness, regular contact including physical contact, couple identity, knowledge of each other's lives
Physical violence	Intentional use of force with potential to cause death, disability, injury, or harm
Sexual violence	Completion or attempt of a sexual act in which the victim has not provided consent or is unable to consent or refuse
Stalking	Repeated and unwanted attention and/or contact that causes fear for one's own or someone else's safety
Psychological aggression	Use of communication, both verbal and nonverbal, to either mentally or emotionally harm another person, or to exert control over another person

From Breiding MJ, Basile KC, Smith SG, Black MC, Mahendra RR. Intimate partner violence surveillance: Uniform definitions and recommended data elements, Version 2.0. Atlanta (GA): National Center for Injury Prevention and Control, Centers for Disease Control and Prevention, 2015.

Individual risk factors are numerous and varied. A 2018 systematic review by Yakubovich and colleagues identified several risk factors at the individual level including nonwhite identities, female education less than high school level, unwanted or unplanned pregnancies, substance use, history of child abuse, adolescent antisocial behaviors, and traditional gender role attitudes.[4] The CDC further identifies young age, a history of depression or suicide attempts, and economic insecurity as additional individual risk factors.[5] It remains clear that membership in marginalized groups significantly increases individual risk. The National Intimate Partner and Sexual Violence Survey (NIPSVS) identified women of multiracial, American Indian/Alaska Native, and non-Hispanic Black as having a greater than 40% lifetime IPV risk as compared with a less than 40% lifetime risk in non-Hispanic Whites, Hispanic, and Asian or Pacific Islander identifying women.[6] There are further discrepancies to note among LGTBQIA patients and relationships. The NIPSVS reports 44% of women who identify as lesbian and 61% of women with bisexual identity have experienced rape, physical violence, or stalking by an intimate partner as compared with 35% of straight-identifying women.[7] Studies of transgender-identifying women have reported up to 6 times higher rates of physical violence than cisgender-identifying women.[8]

Relationship factors include single-parent households, cohabitating relationships, relationship conflict including jealousy or possessiveness, maladaptive dominance and control patterns, and low socioeconomic status.[4,5] Among these many relationship qualities that may increase violence risk relationship dominance and control by one partner over the other is a useful framework for understanding the pathophysiology of many maladaptive relationships. Although previous IPV models viewed violence in the context of a particular conflict or provoking situation, more recent models view violence as part of a greater systematic pattern of fear, intimidation, and isolation, also called "coercive control." In these relationships, efforts are consistently and progressively used to increase the individual's own power and their partner's compliance. A wide variety of means may be used by the violence perpetrator to systematically reduce their partner's autonomy and standing; these measures both include and delve beyond traditional IPV paradigms including physical violence, sexual violence, financial restrictions and dependence, isolation from friends, family, and resources, and emotional trauma. In a study by Dichter and colleagues, women who acknowledged relationships characterized by "coercive control" experienced high rates of all forms of IPV and higher levels of danger than those who experienced more situational violence.[9]

Identifiable community factors include communities with high rates of economic instability, minimal educational opportunities, and low community support for persons experiencing violence and/or unwillingness to intervene.[5] It stands to reason that community cohesiveness and connectedness may provide a potential support network for those experiencing violence to exit relationships and seek care. A strong community may also act as a buffer against isolation, powerlessness, and poor access to jobs and resources that may lead an individual toward seeking control over others.

Impact

IPV results in physical, emotional, and financial negative outcomes for persons who experience violence and their families. Patients experiencing violence may present with symptoms both overt and subtle to multiple health-care settings including primary care, specialty offices, and emergency departments. IPV sequelae are present both during times of violence and long after violence has ended. Providers must be vigilant to signs and symptoms suggestive of violence to appropriately support patients.

Physical health consequences are well documented and include physical injuries; acute illnesses including respiratory, urinary tract, and sexually transmitted illnesses; and chronic and pain-based disorders such as fibromyalgia, menstrual-related and pelvic pain disorders, functional gastrointestinal diseases, and migraine and headache disorders.[10] Studies have variable prevalence of these disorders in patients experiencing IPV in part because stress and trauma may manifest differently in each individual patient. There is no doubt, however, that IPV has both direct and indirect, as well as short-term and long-term, consequences on patient health.

Beyond the physical health of the individual patient, there is significant impact on reproductive, maternal health, and pregnancy outcomes. Reproductive coercion and contraceptive sabotage are well-described control methods among IPV perpetrators.[11] Control and violence do not stop with the introduction of a pregnancy; 1 in 5 teens and 1 in 6 adult pregnant patients report IPV in pregnancy.[12] Rates and severity of violence may in fact increase in pregnancy and the postpartum period with homicide being a leading cause of maternal mortality.[13] IPV is associated with many poor pregnancy outcomes including poor maternal weight gain, low infant birth weight, preterm delivery, stillbirth and fetal demise, uterine rupture, placental abruption, and hemorrhage.[12,13]

Mental health and substance use consequences are also frequently reported among patients experiencing IPV with potentially devastating consequences. Depression, posttraumatic stress disorder (PTSD), anxiety disorders, suicide, and substance use are all common among this population.[14] The risk of these negative mental health effects worsens with increasing IPV severity.[15] Depression is twice as common in women who experience IPV as compared with women who have never experienced IPV.[16] A cross-sectional study in England found that among those who had attempted suicide in the past year, nearly 50% had experienced IPV during their lifetime, with 23% experiencing IPV in the past year. Persons with a suicide attempt within the last year were more than two times more likely to have ever experienced IPV.[17] Prevalence rates for PTSD range from 31% to 84%.[18] Substance use has also been linked to IPV, with women currently experiencing violence being six times more likely to have a substance use disorder diagnosis.[19] It is important to note that the association between mental health, substance use, and IPV is complex. Although IPV most certainly may lead to worsened mental health and substance use as a potential coping mechanism, the relationship is decidedly bidirectional in that worsened substance use and mental health can result in higher risk for IPV as discussed in the "Risk Factors" section.

Financial hardship is both a predictive factor, a violence subtype, and an outcome of IPV for women. It has been well documented that economic insecurity, particularly a partner's job strain, leads to higher rates of physical violence.[20] Economic abuse is also considered a form of IPV. When a partner controls access to financial resources, it limits a woman's ability to achieve parity and to seek refuge and support outside of the relationship. This keeps women from seeking independence due to a lack of resources and the confidence that they can form a self-sufficient life.[21] Financial hardship is also an outcome of IPV. Adams and colleagues found that women with recent IPV experienced reduced job stability and employment, greater hardship in affording housing, food, and bills, and had a more negative outlook on their financial future compared with those with more distant IPV history and those who had never experienced IPV.[22] Beyond the person experiencing IPV, there is also a societal toll in terms of the financial burden of IPV. Medical and mental health services for patients with an IPV history cost an estimated US$10.4 billion yearly.[23]

With the context of IPV in mind, providers can see the patient in front of them less as a chaotic muddle of functional disorders, mental health problems, and social and financial comorbidities but rather as a person with the understandable and far-reaching consequences of prolonged suffering. Understanding the patient's greater story can help providers to better provide appropriate care that is empathetic and patient-centered.

Role of the Provider

Many organizations have traditionally recommended both focused and universal screening policies to identify and then aid patients experiencing violence. The United States Preventative Services Task Force recommends screening for IPV in women of reproductive age and referring to appropriate support services (Grade B Evidence).[24] Additional organizations supporting universal screening policies include the Department of Health and Human Services, the American Medical Association, American Association of Family Physicians, American Academy of Pediatrics, and American College of Obstetrics and Gynecology.[24] When implemented effectively, screening can identify those experiencing IPV, and correlates with high rates of intervention use and relationship departures.[25,26] A variety of screening tools have been used to assist providers with approaching screening in a systematic way (**Table 2**). Although there is wide support for screening, there is little guidance or consensus on the best screening tool, interval, setting, and most appropriate persons for screening, which may leave providers feeling somewhat uncomfortable about how to approach screening in their care setting.

There is some uncertainty regarding the true effectiveness of screening. The World Health Organization (WHO) 2013 practice guideline recommends against routine IPV screening, citing both provider and patient burdens, particularly when resources are limited.[27] The WHO also expresses concern about the possible "check box" nature of asking all patients, which may make the act of asking an emotionless routine rather than a thoughtful and attentive discussion. Although a Cochrane review of screening practices did find that routine screening increased the identification of patients

Table 2
Screening tools

Tool	Acronym	Description	Items
Humiliation, Afraid, Rape, Kick	HARK	4 items assessing IPV in the past year	Within the last year have you been… 1. Humiliated by… 2. Afraid of… 3. Raped or force to have any kind of sexual activity by… 4. Kicked, hit, slapped or otherwise physically hurt by …your partner or ex-partner?
Hurt, Insulted, Threaten, Scream	HITS	4 items assessing IPV frequency	How often does your partner… 1. Physically hurt you? 2. Insult or talk down to you? 3. Threaten you with physical harm? 4. Scream or curse at you?
Extended-Hurt, Insult, Threaten, Scream	E-HITS	5 items including HITS and a sexual violence question	HITS plus… 5. Force you to have sexual activities?
Partner Violence Screen	PVS	3 items that assess IPV in last year and current safety	1. Have you been hit, kicked, punched, or otherwise hurt by someone within the past year? If so, by whom? 2. Do you feel safe in your current relationship? 3. Is there a partner from a previous relationship who is making you feel unsafe now?
Woman Abuse Screening Tool	WAST	8 items	1. In general, how would you describe your relationship? 2. Do you and your partner work out arguments with… 3. Do arguments ever result in you feeling down or bad about yourself? 4. Do arguments ever result in hitting, kicking, or pushing? 5. Do you ever feel frightened by what your partner says or does? 6. Has your partner ever abused you physically? 7. Has your partner ever abused you emotionally? 8. Has your partner ever abused you sexually?

From U.S. Preventative Services Task Force. Screening for Intimate Partner Violence, Elder Abuse, and Abuse of Vulnerable Adults: An Evidence Review for the U.S. Preventive Services Task Force. Available at: https://www.uspreventiveservicestaskforce.org/uspstf/recommendation/intimate-partner-violence-and-abuse-of-elderly-and-vulnerable-adults-screening, accessed October 23, 2018.

experiencing IPV, it did not find that screening improved health outcomes.[25] A 2018 systematic review of 30 studies involving nearly 15,000 patients found no improvements in IPV incidence or quality of life among patients who were screened versus not screened.[28] Although screening does seem to be successful in identifying patients experiencing IPV, it does not ultimately seem to be successful in the measure we care most about: improving lives. One caveat to this is that these studies may not provide enough follow-up time to show the true effectiveness of a physician's intervention because it may take years and many thoughtful conversations to ultimately improve a patient's life trajectory. In addition, although we as providers may see the fundamental goal of our screening and intervention to remove patients from dangerous relationships, the time scale, method, and whether separation is the best choice in the context of their life is a decision for the patient, not the provider. Further study and thoughtful approaches are clearly needed to better understand how screening can most effectively support patients.

Regardless of whether a physician chooses to use routine screening, there is value in offering education, support, and a safe space to discuss violence concerns should the patient choose to disclose. Many earlier studies have shown that women value being asked about violence, desire information on community resources, and appreciate validation and reassurance from their health-care providers.[29] A qualitative study by Chang and colleagues revealed that patients with current or former IPV experience appreciated informational fliers and brochures that can be anonymously reviewed; counseling on safety, relationships, and behavioral health needs; and recognition of an individual's autonomy in deciding best intervention strategies. Women rejected directive or forced interventions including reporting to police, obligatory counseling, or outreach methods that might further endanger them by inadvertently alerting their partner. A physician's best role in the eyes of patients is to be a sounding board, source of support, and connector to resources when and if they are ready to use them.

Moving away from a disclosure-driven screening approach and closer toward women's preferences of education and compassion, there is increasing support for a universal education model. Futures Without Violence, a nonprofit organization working to end violence against women and children, created the *Confidentiality, Universal Education, Empowerment, and Support* (CUES) intervention to assist practitioners with supporting women experiencing violence (**Table 3**).[30] This framework takes a support-first approach instead of approaching violence discussions as a checklist-screening item. To that end, we recommend placing this discussion within the greater context of a patient's social history instead of within a health maintenance section. Providers can initiate a conversation about IPV when discussing a patient's relationship history, any associated stressors, as well as supports. This allows a conversation about the patient's personal life to be given appropriate weight and care.

In the first step, confidentiality, the provider ensures the patient is alone and in a safe space to freely speak. This includes seeing the patient alone in the office (without partners or children present) but also on telemedicine visits where persons may be present but unseen to the provider. It is also essential that patients that require interpreters be provided one and not be expected to hold a discussion about possible violence in front of a family member acting as an interpreter. The provider should assure the patient that their discussion will not be shared, and also discuss confidentiality limits based on their state reporting requirements. Providers should be familiar with their state reporting requirements before holding these discussions (can be located on the Futures without Violence website).

Table 3
Confidentiality, universal education, empowerment, and support framework for IPV discussion

Step	Description	Example Wording
Initiation	Initiate the conversation within the context of the patient's social history, particularly their relationship history. Ask permission before moving forward	"Thank you for telling me about your relationship with *Person X*. Relationship stress is common, and sometimes stress can lead to violence. Is it ok with you if I talk a little further about this?"
Confidentiality	Ensure patients are alone and able to speak freely; Discuss the limits of confidentiality and any reporting requirements	"Before we get started, I want to let you know that I will not share anything we talk about today outside of this office, unless you tell me about X."
Universal Education	Provide information on relationship stress, healthy relationships, availability of resources, and your role as a support person. Let patients know that you talk about this with all your patients to reduce stigma	"While relationship stress and violence are common, they are never deserved. I make sure to talk to all my patients about violence because it can affect health and there is much we can do to help. I want you to know that I am here for you now and in the future if this is something you would like to talk about further." "I'd like to give you a card that I give to all my patients that discusses relationships and our health. One the back of the card there are resources you can contact if you ever need help, and I am also here for you if you need help now or in the future."
Empower & Support	If a patient chooses to share their story, thank them for sharing, validate their experience, provide empathy, and connect to resources	"Thank you so much for sharing your story with me. I am so sorry you are going through this. I want you to know that you do not deserve this. I would be happy to connect you today with some resources if that would be helpful."

Data from Futures without Violence. CUES: Addressing Domestic and Sexual Violence in Health Settings. Futureswithoutviolence.org.

Following a statement of confidentiality, the provider offers universal education. This could involve a statement of the widespread nature of relationship violence, that it is undeserved, and that help is available should the patient need it. Pocket cards are available to aid in this discussion, and include resource information, education on healthy relationships, and the impact of violence on health (can be found on Futures without Violence website). Note that some patients may not be comfortable taking a card if they are worried about negative consequences from their partner—if so, numbers can be placed on phones or in electronic messages depending on the patient's comfort level and preference. Although many patients may thank the provider and choose not to disclose at the time of this discussion, the goal is not for disclosure. Instead, the provider hopes that the patient has heard the words that violence is undeserved and knows that they have a safe place to turn should they decide to seek help or resources.

Although disclosure is not expected in this approach, patients may be comfortable sharing their story with providers who use this empathetic method. If this happens, providers should offer validation, support, gratitude for the patient's willingness to discuss their experience, and warm resource referral. This is the final step in the CUES intervention, support. This may include inviting an in-office social worker to the conversation, providing the domestic violence hotline number, or connecting the patient with a local domestic violence organization skilled at providing counsel to patients. If indicated, providers may provide an opportunity to call or speak to counselors from the office to limit suspicion from partners. Regardless of the patient's decision on whether to pursue resources or not, the provider should support the patient's autonomy. Patients know their personal situations best and will know they have a supportive caregiver within the health-care community should they desire help in the future. Close follow-up should be arranged for the patient with the same provider (if possible) or a colleague for ongoing care and support.

When providers create an environment that is sensitive to trauma, patients benefit from a safe place to seek care. Health-care experiences can be triggering for patients who have experienced IPV. These triggers could be as simple as an off-handed remark, a suggestion to undress for an examination, or a pelvic examination, which could unearth an earlier sexual trauma. We recommend approaching all health-care encounters in a trauma-informed fashion. This offers all patients the necessary sensitivity to ensure they are as comfortable as possible during the visit and can therefore gain as much as possible from the encounter. Ways that providers can approach visits in a trauma-informed way include reviewing patient charts ahead of time to assess for any documentation of an earlier trauma and best avoid potential triggers, acknowledging the importance of support persons in patient comfort, ensuring confidentiality, explaining all elements of the visit and what the patient can expect, normalizing and explaining the nature of all questioning, being mindful of sensitive documentation, and avoiding stigmatizing language.[31] One of the most challenging components of the provider visit may be the physical examination, particularly the pelvic examination. In order to make the patient most comfortable, the provider can review with the patient ahead of time what the examination will include and if there are steps that can be taken to increase comfort, ask permission before touching the patient each time, encourage the patient to adjust or move clothing instead of the provider, describe each component of the examination verbally both before and while it is being performed, use appropriate language (ie, avoiding terms such as "stirrups," "bed," "lie back"), describe any sounds or sensations the patient may experience (ie, demonstrating the clicking sound of a speculum or describing expected temperature of tools), and offer the patient an alternative to an examination when feasible (ie, offer that the patient may complete a self-Pap smear). Staff members such as rooming staff, front desk personnel, and nurses will also benefit from training in trauma informed care to ensure all the health-care team approaches patients in a sensitive manner. By making these small but intentional changes in language and approach, providers can make a significant impact in the patient experience.

SUMMARY

IPV has a tremendous and pervasive effect on the lives of patients with a current or former history of violence. Substantial influences on patient health, mental well-being, finances, and future are common. Discussions of IPV can seem intimidating given the personal and traumatic nature of the topic. Yet with empathy, education, and support, providers can have positive influences on patient lives that do not require extensive training or experience.

CLINICS CARE POINTS

- Confidentiality is essential to IPV discussions with patients; practitioners must be aware and disclose confidentiality limits when discussing violence.
- Educating all patients about violence and its impacts assists patients in recognizing violence and that it is undeserved.
- Support and empathy while recognizing a patient's autonomy is key in caring for patients who experience violence.
- Approaching all patients with "universal precautions" when it comes to potential trauma can help to create a caring environment welcoming to all persons.

DISCLOSURE

The author has nothing to disclose.

FUNDING

Previous completed research in this topic was funded by the Thomas H. Nimick, Jr. Competitive Research Fund and the University of Pittsburgh Division of General Internal Medicine Fellow Award.

REFERENCES

1. Breiding MJ, Basile KC, Smith SG, et al. Intimate partner violence surveillance: Uniform definitions and recommended data elements, Version 2.0. Atlanta (GA): National Center for Injury Prevention and Control, Centers for Disease Control and Prevention; 2015.
2. Chang JC. Intimate partner violence: How you can help female survivors. Cleve Clin J Med 2014;81:439–46.
3. Rees S, Silove D, Chey T, et al. Lifetime prevalence of gender-based violence in women and the relationship with mental disorders and psychosocial function. JAMA 2011;306:513–21.
4. Yakubovich AR, Stockl H, Murray J, et al. Risk and protective factors for intimate partner violence against women: systematic review and meta-analyses of prospective-longitudinal studies. Am J Public Health 2018;108(7):e1–11.

5. National Center for Injury Prevention and Control, Division of Violence Prevention, Centers for Disease Control and Prevention. Intimate Partner Violence: risk and protective factors. 2, 2021.

6. Smith SG, Chen J, Basile KC, et al. The national intimate partner and sexual violence Survey (NISVS): 2010–2012 state report. Atlanta: Centers for Disease Control and Prevention; 2017.

7. Disease Control & Prevention Ctr. NISVS: An Overview Of 2010 findings on victimization by sexual orientation (Jan. 2013). https://www.cdc.gov/violenceprevention/pdf/cdc_nisvs_victimization final-a.pdf.

8. Valentine SE, Peitzmeier SM, King DS, et al. Disparities in exposure to intimate partner violence among transgender/gender nonconforming and sexual minority primary care patients. LGBT Health 2017;4:260–7.

9. Dichter ME, Kristie AT, Crits-Christoph P, et al. Coercive control in intimate partner violence: relationship with women's experience of violence, use of violence, and danger. Psychol Violence 2018;8(5):596–604.

10. Campbell JC. Health consequences of intimate partner violence. Lancet 2002; 359:1331–6.

11. Miller E, Decker MR, McCauley HL, et al. Pregnancy coercion, intimate partner violence and unintended pregnancy. Contraception 2010;81:316–22.

12. Parker B, McFarlane J, Soeken K. Abuse during pregnancy. Obstet Gynecol September 1994;84(3):323–8.

13. Kady El, Dina MD, Gilbert William M, et al. Maternal and neonatal outcomes of assaults during pregnancy. Obstet Gynecol 2005;105(2):357–63.

14. World Health Organization. Global and regional estimates of violence against women: prev.

15. Ferrari G, Agnew-Davies R, Bailey J, et al. Domestic violence and mental health: a cross-sectional survey of women seeking help from domestic violence support services. Glob Health Action 2016;8(9):29890.

16. Satyanarayana VA, Chandra PS, Vaddiparti K. Mental health consequences of violence against women and girls. Curr Opin Psychiatry 2015;28(5):350–6.

17. McManus S, Walby S, Barvosa EC, et al. Intimate partner violence, suicidality, and self-harm: a probability sample survey of the general population in England. Lancet Psychiatry 2022;9(7):574–83.

18. Dutton M, Green B, Kaltman S, et al. Intimate partner violence, PTSD, and adverse health outcomes. J Interpers Violence 2006;21:955–68.

19. Bonomi A, Anderson M, Reid R, et al. Medical and psychosocial diagnoses in women with a history of intimate partner violence. Arch Intern Med 2009;169: 1692.

20. Fox GL, Benson ML, DeMaris AA, et al. Economic distress and intimate violence: testing family stress and resource theories. J Marriae Fam 2004;64(3):793–807.

21. Lin HF, Postmus JL, Hu H, et al. IPV Experiences and financial strain over time: insights from the Blinder-Oaxaca decomposition analysis. J Fam Econ Issues 2022;1–13. https://doi.org/10.1007/s10834-022-09847-y.

22. Adams AE, Tolman RM, Bybee D, et al. The impact of intimate partner violence on low income women's economic well-being: the mediating role of job stability. Violence Against Women 2013;18(12).

23. Liebschutz JM, Rothman EF. Intimate partner violence—What physicians can do. N Engl J Med 2012;267:2071–3.

24. U.S. Preventative Services Task Force. Screening for intimate partner violence, elder abuse, and abuse of vulnerable adults: an evidence review for the U.S. preventive services task force. Available at: https://www.uspreventiveservices

taskforce.org/uspstf/recommendation/intimate-partner-violence-and-abuse-of-elderly-and-vulnerable-adults-screening. Accessed October 23, 2018.

25. O'Doherty L, Hegarty K, Ramsay J, et al. Screening women for intimate partner violence in healthcare settings. Cochrane Database Syst Rev 2015;7:1–84.

26. McCloskey LA, Lichter E, Williams C, et al. Assessing intimate partner violence in health care settings leads to women's receipt of interventions and improved health. Public Health Rep 2006;121:435–44.

27. World Health Organization. Responding to intimate partner violence and sexual violence against women: WHO clinical and policy guideline. WHO; 2013. Available at: https://apps.who.int/iris/bitstream/handle/10665/85240/9789241548595_eng.pdf.

28. Feltner C, Wallace I, Berkman N, et al. Screening for intimate partner violence, elder abuse, and abuse of vulnerable adults: evidence report and systematic review for the US preventative services task force. JAMA 2018;320(16):1688–701.

29. Chang JC, Cluss PA, Ranieri L, et al. Health care interventions for intimate partner violence: what women want. Womens Health Issues 2005;15(1):21–30.

30. Futures without violence. CUES: addressing domestic and sexual violence in health settings. Futureswithoutviolence.org. Accessed October 12, 2022.

31. Ravi A. Providing trauma-informed care. Am Fam Physician 2017;95(1):655–7.